Workbook

INTRODUCTION TO HEALTH OCCUPATIONS

Sixth Edition

Workbook

INTRODUCTION TO HEALTH OCCUPATIONS

Today's Health Care Worker

Sixth Edition

Shirley A. Badasch, M.Ed, RN
Doreen S. Chesebro, B.Ed, LVN

Prentice Hall

Upper Saddle River, New Jersey 07458

Notice: Care has been taken to confirm the accuracy of information presented in this book. The authors, editors, and the publisher, however, cannot accept any responsibility for errors or omissions or for consequences from application of the information in this book and make no warranty, express or implied, with respect to its contents.

The authors and publishers have exerted every effort to ensure that drug selections and dosages set forth in this text are in accord with current recommendations and practice at time of publication. However, in view of ongoing research, changes in government regulations, and the constant flow of information relating to drug therapy and drug reactions, the reader is urged to check the package inserts of all drugs for any change in indications of dosage and for added warnings and precautions. This is particulatly important when the recommended agent is a new and/or infrequently employed drug.

Publisher: *Julie Levin Alexander*
Publisher's Assistant: *Regina Bruno*
Executive Editor: *Maura Connor*
Acquisitions Editor: *Barbara Krawiec*
Editorial Assistant: *Sheba Jalaluddin*
Director of Production and Manufacturing: *Bruce Johnson*
Managing Production Editor: *Patrick Walsh*
Production Liaison: *Mary C. Treacy*
Production Editor: *Emily Bush, Carlisle Publishers Services*
Manufacturing Manager: *Ilene Sanford*
Manufacturing Buyer: *Pat Brown*
Design Director: *Cheryl Asherman*
Senior Design Coordinator: *Maria Guglielmo Walsh*
Senior Marketing Manager: *Nicole Benson*
Marketing Coordinator: *Janet Ryerson*
Product Information Manager: *Rachele Strober*
Compositor: *Carlisle Communications, Ltd.*
Printer/Binder: *Courier Westford*

Pearson Education, LTD.
Pearson Education Australia PTY, Limited
Pearson Education Singapore, Pte. Ltd.
Pearson Education North Asia Ltd.
Pearson Education Canada, Ltd.
Pearson Educación de Mexico, S.A. de C.V.
Pearson Education Japan
Pearson Education Malaysia, Pte. Ltd.
Pearson Education, Upper Saddle River, New Jersey.

Prentice Hall

10 9 8 7
ISBN 0-13-110269-9

Contents

How to Use the Student Workbook

The Student Workbook is designed to help you develop new skills and the knowledge necessary to work in a health care environment. It is an addition to the textbook and guides you in learning to be a health care worker. Completing the worksheets, reports, and assignments reinforces your learning. Showing proficiency in skills gives you confidence when you begin your on site training (on-site training may also be called community classroom or internship).

To use the Student Workbook most effectively:

- Carefully read each objective. Each objective tells you what you are expected to learn and to know.
- Follow the directions. If you are instructed to complete a worksheet before reading, for example, be certain to complete it in the suggested order. Completing it helps you understand the reading material.
- Use your text to help you complete each worksheet assignment. The knowledge that you gain on the worksheet is important for passing the unit or chapter evaluation.
- Your instructor has the key for each worksheet. Check your answers for accuracy. If you have difficulty with answers, return to the text and read the information again. Do not move on until you are certain that you understand all concepts. Each concept builds on another. If you do not learn one concept, the next is more difficult to learn.
- There are also skills that you must show proficiency in. Use the skills check-off sheets, and practice until you can complete the skill. You need these skills when you begin your internship. Some of the skills check-off sheets are included in your workbook. Ask your teacher for additional check-off sheets.
- When you feel confident that you can meet each objective, ask your instructor for the unit or chapter evaluation. The evaluation is a written test and may also include a demonstration of skills.

Successful completion of worksheets, the written evaluation, and demonstration of competency in skills are necessary before you can begin your internship.

Once you complete Chapter 14, select an occupational area from Part Two. To do this:

- Review the worksheets from Chapter 2 to assist you in making a decision about a health care occupation.
- Choose an occupation that matches your abilities, interests, and values.
- Discuss your selection with your instructor.

You may be required to work in the area of your choice on your own. Your instructor will explain exactly what is expected. Follow the same format as in Part One:

- Review your workbook.
- Complete the worksheets in the order assigned. If a worksheet is assigned before reading the text, be certain to complete it first.
- Read the entire chapter.
- Complete all worksheets and skills demonstrations.
- Take the chapter evaluation.

It is very difficult to "play catch-up." Complete the worksheets and check-off sheets when they are assigned.

This Student Workbook and the text can be used in a self-paced program. As you complete each unit or chapter and successfully pass the evaluations, you may proceed to the next unit or chapter.

Your instructor may prefer to have all class members complete the assignments at the same time. In this case, be certain that you follow your instructor's directions.

When you have successfully completed the text and the Student Workbook, you will have gained a basic core of information. This information will be important in the health career you choose. We wish you success in any endeavor you choose to pursue in the health career field.

Survival Skills: Effective Study Habits

You can develop effective study habits and enjoy effective learning. There are some very important skills that help you study. When you learn them and use them, studying and remembering will be easier. These include:

- Planning where you study
- Planning your time
- Knowing your textbook
- Learning to read for key information
- Taking notes
- Preparing for tests and quizzes
- Taking tests and quizzes

PLANNING WHERE YOU STUDY

Choose a place to study that you find quiet and pleasant. Make this area the place you use to study, learn, and remember. Ask yourself:

- Is it quiet here?
- Do I have a desk or table that is large enough?
- Do I have the materials and equipment I need?
- Is my chair comfortable?
- Do I have enough light?
- Is my work space neat?

All of these questions are important. Plan your work area so you can answer **yes** to each question.

PLANNING YOUR TIME

Planning your time gives you a guideline. It keeps you from putting off what you need to do. It also gives you a way to schedule your fun time. Here are important things to remember:

- Study when you are most alert. People are alert at different times. Some are most productive in the morning, some in the evening or late at night.
- Choose when and where to study, and stick to the plan.

- Write exactly what you want to accomplish on your schedule—for example, write, "Learn the normal and abnormal reading of temperature, pulse, respirations, and blood pressure," *not* "do vital signs homework."
- Study 1½ to 2 hours on any one subject. After this amount of time you tire easily and lose concentration. Take a break, and study another subject.
- Plan enough time to learn what you need to know.
- Study as soon after class as possible. Check your notes while they are fresh in your mind. Start the assignments while they are clear in your mind.
- Space your reviews. Review your notes weekly. Review from the beginning to refresh your memory. This helps you remember and improves your scores on tests and quizzes.
- Use "empty" hours during the day to study. Free periods between classes are good study times, and free you later for fun activities.
- Plan study make-up time. Immediately find time to make up study time when you miss a planned time. Adjust your written schedule also.

KNOWING YOUR TEXTBOOK

Your textbook is a guide to learning. Become familiar with your book. It is your friend.

- Think about the title. What is the book about?
- Read the Contents. It tells you what is in the book.
- Read the Preface. This is where the authors tell you about the book.
- Look at the Index. The more words you already know, the easier the text will be for you.
- Look for a glossary. It gives you important definitions of the words in the text.
- Look at a chapter in the book. All the chapters will look alike. Ask yourself:
  - Is there a summary?
  - Are there questions at the end?
- Write in the book if it belongs to you.
  - Define words so you understand them.
  - Write words in your native language if English is your second language.
- Highlight important information.

Use your book. It is your friend.

LEARNING TO READ FOR KEY INFORMATION

Frances P. Robinson, a psychologist at Ohio State University, developed the SQ3R method for reading your assignments. The SQ3R stands for *survey/question/read/recite/review:*

- *Survey* to get the overall idea of what you are studying.
  - Read the unit objectives carefully.
  - Read headings to see what the units and topics are.
  - Look at figures and tables.
  - Read the summaries.
- *Question* to help you remember the information. Ask yourself:
  - What does the work or phrase mean?
  - Think about questions the author asks.
  - Answer each objective.

- *Read* to get key information and answer questions.
  - Read everything, including tables, figures, and illustrations.
  - Think about what the author wants you to know. The objectives tell you what the author wants you to learn.
- *Recite* what you are learning. This helps you find out what you remember and understand. Stop as you read and try to tell yourself what you have read.
  - Recall the main headings.
  - What are the important ideas under each heading?
  - Try to state what you have read without looking at the pages.
  - Check for things you have left out and for errors.
- *Review* what you have read.
  - Go back and review immediately after reading.
  - Look at each heading and ask yourself what they mean.
  - Recite the points under each heading.
  - Check to see if you are right.
  - Recite summaries.
  - Reread the summaries.
  - Review once or twice before your tests.
  - Recite the information you must know for a test.

TAKING NOTES

Note taking helps you understand and remember. Your notes give you important information for reviewing. They should be clear and short and outline the most important parts.

- Read the assignment before the lecture.
- Look up unfamiliar terms.
- Listen for answers to material you do not understand.
- Ask questions in class.
- Keep separate sections for your classes.
- Use a new page for each lecture.
- Date your notes and number the pages.
- Use symbols and abbreviations (e.g., TPR, B/P, $\bar{c}$, $\bar{s}$; see medical terminology).
- Use phrases or words, not sentences, if possible.
- Put notes in your own words.
- Develop a code for your notes (e.g., ? = not clear; ! = important; * = assignment; Q = question; C = your own comments).
- Look for clues of important information:
  - Material on blackboard
  - Visual aids such as slides and overheads
  - Repeated information
  - Questions the instructor asks the class
- Go over notes as soon as possible after class and check them for errors.
- Be sure you understand your notes.
- Review your notes within 24 hours to help you remember

See the figure on page xv on taking notes for results.

PREPARING FOR TESTS AND QUIZZES

Taking tests and quizzes requires preparation. The preparation begins when you enter your class.

- Do your work daily.
- If you do not understand, ask.
- Take clear notes.
- Review daily.
- Test yourself.
- Study with others.
- Think about the instructor's point of view. What kinds of questions do you think will be asked?
- Go to the test with pencils, pens, and other needed supplies.
- Do not cram at the last minute.
- Go to class with a clear mind.

TAKING TESTS AND QUIZZES

When you are finally ready to take the test, follow these steps:

- Skim the whole test to help you know what is being asked and how it is organized.
- Be sure you understand the format. How do you answer? If you have questions, ask your instructor.
- Ask about items if you are not sure what is being asked.
- Budget your time. If a question is worth more points, give it more time.
- Do the easy items first.
- Begin working. Read carefully.
- Answer the question as it relates to class. For example, if you are asked about medical care in other cultures, answer from what you learned in class. Do not give information that you know but that was never discussed.

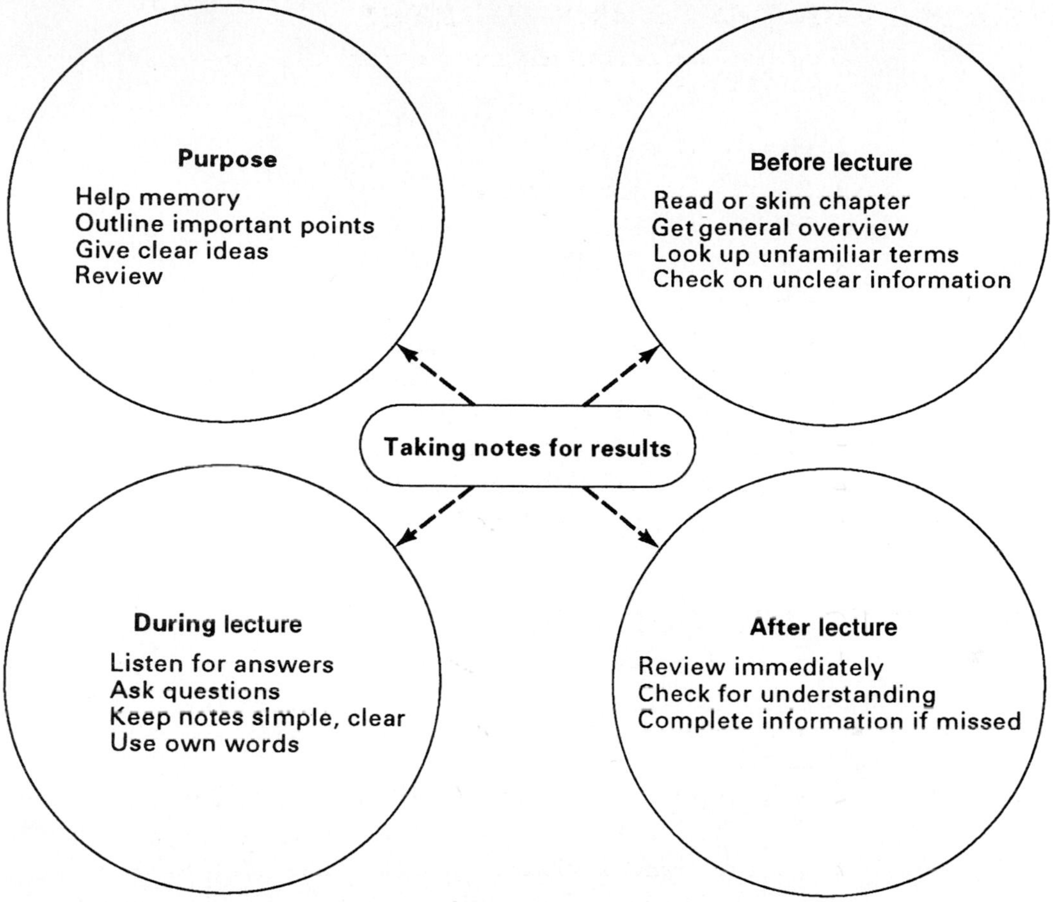

- Reread.
- Make changes or additions.
- Check to be sure you answered all the questions.
- Guess at items you are not sure of unless you are given other instructions.

Use these skills to help you be successful in your studies. Learn the information in your textbook carefully, and complete all assignments given in class and in your workbook. Effective study habits will help you become a successful health care worker.

• WORKSHEET 2

Identify nine scientists, and explain what they contributed to medicine (18 points).

1. ______________________________
____
2. ______________________________
____
3. ______________________________
____
4. ______________________________
____
5. ______________________________
____
6. ______________________________
____
7. ______________________________
____
8. ______________________________
____
9. ______________________________
____

There are 18 possible points in this worksheet.

• WORKSHEET/ACTIVITY 3

Talk to an older person about diseases that affected past generations and that are no longer a primary threat. Ask them to describe how they tried to prevent illness caused by those same diseases. Write notes about your dialogue and prepare to report briefly to your classmates.

There are 20 possible points in this worksheet/activity.

• WORKSHEET/ACTIVITY 4

Choose one era in the history of health care, and write a short paper to explain how health care technology changed during that period (10 points). Use information learned in class, do research in the library, and/or use the Internet for your report. Follow these guidelines when preparing your report:

- Type, word-process, or write neatly in ink.
- Use 8.5-by-11-inch paper.
- Use correct spelling and grammar.

There are 10 points in this worksheet/activity.

• WORKSHEET/ACTIVITY: 5

In a small group of students, discuss the advances in medicine in the twentieth century. Answer the following questions during your discussion. Use information from your essay, class discussion, the textbook, and other classroom resources (25 points).

1. How did medical care for the injured and ill change from the time when patients were cared for in monasteries and homes?

____

____

____

2. Are these changes better for the patient?

____

____

____

3. Are more people cared for at home today than in the recent past?

____

____

____

4. How has the discovery of microorganisms affected research for AIDS, tuberculosis, and other serious diseases?

____

____

____

5. What do you feel are the greatest advances made in the twentieth century?

____

____

____

There are 25 points in this worksheet/activity.

• WORKSHEET/ACTIVITY: 6

Bring to class an article from a newspaper, magazine, or Internet Web site that discusses current medical research. Give a report about the article to the class (25 points).

There are 25 points in this worksheet/activity.

Then compare value 1 against value 3, 1 against 4, and so on. Circle the important value in each pair. When you have completed column A, do the same with the other columns, using the grid.

Values Grid

Columns	A	B	C	D	E	F	G	H	I
	1 2								
	1 3	2 3							
	1 4	2 4	3 4						
	1 5	2 5	3 5	4 5					
	1 6	2 6	3 6	4 6	5 6				
	1 7	2 7	3 7	4 7	5 7	6 7			
	1 8	2 8	3 8	4 8	5 8	6 8	7 8		
	1 9	2 9	3 9	4 9	5 9	6 9	7 9	8 9	
	1 10	2 10	3 10	4 10	5 10	6 10	7 10	8 10	9 10

3. When you finish comparing your values, total the times you circled each number.

Count the number of 1s, 2s, and 3s, and so on that are circled. Enter the totals for each value here.

1. ____ **2.** ____ **3.** ____ **4.** ____ **5.** ____ **6.** ____ **7.** ____ **8.** ____ **9.** ____ **10.** ____

4. Recopy your original list below.

5. Fill in the prioritized values list, beginning with the value that you circled most often.

6. Have your values changed? Are you surprised by the results? Knowing your work values will help you decide on a satisfying career.

Values

Original List	Prioritized List
1. ____________________	**1.** ____________________
2. ____________________	**2.** ____________________
3. ____________________	**3.** ____________________
4. ____________________	**4.** ____________________
5. ____________________	**5.** ____________________
6. ____________________	**6.** ____________________
7. ____________________	**7.** ____________________
8. ____________________	**8.** ____________________
9. ____________________	**9.** ____________________
10. ____________________	**10.** ____________________

There are 40 points in this worksheet/activity.

• WORKSHEET/ACTIVITY 2

From the following list, choose the 15 abilities that bring you the greatest satisfaction and that you would like to use in a job.

____ Accepting others
____ Adjusting things
____ Advising, coaching
____ Appreciating beauty
____ Arranging, scheduling
____ Assembling, producing
____ Assigning tasks
____ Assisting others to see themselves
____ Attention to detail
____ Budget preparation, financial planning
____ Building, constructing
____ Calculating
____ Cataloging
____ Clerical ability
____ Collecting things
____ Comparing
____ Compiling
____ Composing
____ Conveying warmth
____ Coordinating, organizing
____ Counseling
____ Creating products
____ Cultivating, growing
____ Curing, nursing
____ Decorating
____ Delegating responsibility
____ Demonstrating
____ Designing
____ Developing rapport, relationship building
____ Discovering, detecting
____ Distributing, delivering
____ Drafting, making layouts
____ Dramatizing, acting
____ Drawing, illustrating
____ Ear for languages, accents
____ Empathizing
____ Encouraging, raising others' self-esteem
____ Estimating
____ Evaluating
____ Experimenting, testing
____ Explaining
____ Finding shortcuts
____ Finger or manual dexterity
____ Generating ideas
____ Identifying, defining
____ Imagining, fantasizing
____ Influencing, persuading, selling
____ Informing, teaching, training
____ Installing
____ Lifting, pushing, balancing
____ Listening
____ Maintaining
____ Managing
____ Measuring
____ Mechanical reasoning
____ Memory for detail
____ Molding, shaping
____ Money management
____ Motivating
____ Musical ability
____ Numerical ability
____ Observing, examining, monitoring

____ Offering support, serving others
____ Operating tools or machinery
____ Ordering, purchasing
____ Organizing, putting in order
____ Organizing outdoor activities
____ Photography
____ Physical coordination, agility
____ Planning, developing programs, formulating ideas
____ Precision working
____ Preparing reports
____ Public speaking
____ Questioning
____ Record keeping
____ Rehabilitating
____ Repairing, fixing
____ Researching
____ Responding to feelings
____ Retrieving
____ Reviewing, screening
____ Risk taking
____ Sensitivity to others' needs
____ Setting up equipment
____ Sports ability
____ Supervising
____ Taking inventory
____ Talking easily with strangers
____ Teamwork
____ Tending animals
____ Transcribing
____ Troubleshooting
____ Verbal ability
____ Visualizing
____ Writing ability

There are 15 points in this worksheet/activity.

• WORKSHEET/ACTIVITY 3

Choose a career that interests you, and use Unit 2 of this chapter in your textbook and other resources to answer the following questions (25 points).

- What is the name of the career?
- What type of work is done in this career?
- What personal qualities and abilities are needed for success in this career?
- What are the educational requirements? High school graduation? Four years of college?
- Is licensure, certification, or registration required?
- What are the working conditions?
- Are there advancement opportunities?
- What wages and benefits are usually offered?
- What is the job outlook for the future?
- Where can you get further information about the career?
- Are at least seven of the abilities you marked on Worksheet 2 needed for this career?

There are 25 possible points in this worksheet.

• WORKSHEET/ACTIVITY 4

Interview an employee who works in an occupation that interests you. You may do the interviews by phone, by mail, by e-mail, or in person. Make contact ahead of time to obtain consent for the interview. Here are some sample questions that you might ask (100 points).

- How did you select this occupation?
- What are the educational requirements?
- What are the opportunities for advancement?
- What do you like about your job?
- What are the hours? Do you have any control over your work schedule?
- Is there job security?
- Are you satisfied with the salary you receive?
- Is the job structured, or is there flexibility?
- Do you feel that you are respected in your position?
- What are your major responsibilities in the job?

There are 100 possible points in this worksheet/activity.

• WORKSHEET/ACTIVITY 5

Visit a career center or library, and answer the following questions on a separate sheet of paper (100 points).

1. What materials are available to help you learn about specific careers?
2. Use the microfiche to research one career that interests you, and write a brief discussion of what you found out about the occupation.

There are 100 possible points in this worksheet/activity.

• WORKSHEET/ACTIVITY 6

Write a paper titled "What I Learned About Selecting a Career" (75 points). Include the following in your paper:

- How interests affect career choice.
- How abilities affect career choice.
- How work values affect career choice.
- What you have learned about your interests, abilities, and work values and how they will affect your career choice.

Follow these guidelines when preparing your report:

- Use 8.5-by-11-inch paper.
- Type, word-process, or write neatly in ink.
- Use correct spelling and grammar.

There are 75 possible points in this worksheet/activity.

• WORKSHEET/ACTIVITY 7

A portfolio contains documents that show your knowledge of a subject. A vocational portfolio shows the abilities, knowledge, and skills that you have

Clues

Across

2. Relating to the treatment of disease or injury.
3. Involving penetration of the body during a test.
6. Able to transfer electrical current.
7. Pertaining to the hand.
9. The way an individual walks.
10. A type of sterilizer.
11. A fluid that protects against a given disease.
13. A worker who is knowledgeable about the details of a particular job.
15. A degree given by a college or university after the successful completion of four years of study.
17. The method used to make the environment, the worker, and the patient as germ-free as possible.
19. A written direction for preparing and giving treatment.
21. An assistant or helper.
24. To cause a body part to be immovable.
25. The therapeutic rubbing, kneading, or stroking of the body.
27. A program in which students study with a professional to develop skills they have learned in a classroom.
30. The plural of datum.
32. A school that trains people with special aptitudes in specific trades or occupations.
34. The act of eliminating foreign or harmful elements.
35. An aide or a helper.
36. Taking the first step; thinking and acting without being told.
37. A natural or acquired talent or ability.
38. To examine, judge, appraise, or estimate.

Down

1. A knifelike tool with a broad, flat blade.
4. Equality in substance, degree, value, force, or meaning.
5. Relating to the determination of the nature of a disease or injury by examination.
8. The qualities one needs to be successful in a certain type of job.
12. A specialist in the study of a technical field.
14. The number of patients in a hospital.
16. A change or adjustment to meet a need.
18. A procedure involving a warm, waxy liquid that becomes hard as it cools; frequently used to ease the pain of arthritis in the hands.
20. Skill in using one's hands.
22. Physical therapy.
23. The traits or qualities of one's nature.
26. Limitation.
28. A scholarship or grant awarded to a graduate student in a college or university.
29. Repeating the same thing over and over.
31. Authorized, licensed, or certified.
33. To become aware of through any of the senses.

There are 38 possible points in this worksheet.

• WORKSHEET 2

Compare the services performed by the therapeutic, diagnostic, information, and environmental services (12 points).

Department	Service	Contribution to Team Goal for Patient
Example:		
Nursing	Therapeutic	Treats patient by performing procedures
______	__________	______________________________
		______________________________
______	__________	______________________________
		______________________________
______	__________	______________________________
		______________________________

There are 12 possible points in this worksheet.

• WORKSHEET 3

Identify one health occupation in each of the health services (diagnostic, therapeutic, information, and environmental), and explain why it is found in that service (16 points).

Occupation	Service	Duty
Example:		
Electrocardiography tech	Diagnostic	Tests to help determine the condition of the heart in order to make a diagnosis
1. ________________	________	______________________
		______________________
		______________________
2. ________________	________	______________________
		______________________
		______________________
3. ________________	________	______________________
		______________________
		______________________
4. ________________	________	______________________
		______________________
		______________________

There are 16 possible points in this worksheet.

• WORKSHEET/ACTIVITY 4 JOB SHADOWING CONTRACT

Student Name: ______________________________

Class Title: ____________________ **Time:** ____________________

Job Shadowing Assignment: ______________________________

Street Address: ______________________________

City: ______________________________

Date(s): ______________ **Time(s):** ______________

Purpose: To observe a work setting in an occupational area of interest as part of the student decision-making process leading to vocational training.

Student Agrees to:

- Dress in clothes/uniform as described by the instructor.
- Communicate in an ethical, professional manner, reflecting the values described in Chapter 3 of this text.
- Be an interested observer, without interrupting the work process.
- Arrive at the assignment on time and leave the site at the end of the assigned time.
- Complete a written report describing the job shadowing experience.

Signatures:

Student: ______________________________

Instructor: ______________________________

• WORKSHEET/ACTIVITY 6

Create a skit that represents the assigned legal term. Your classmates must be able to identify the term you are acting out.

There are 15 points in this worksheet/activity.

• WORKSHEET/ACTIVITY 7

If assigned a clinical site (for job shadowing or internship) locate the policy and procedure book(s). Find and read the policy and procedure for handwashing. Write your interpretation of the policy and procedure, explaining the steps to follow when washing your hands.

There are 15 points in this worksheet/activity.

• WORKSHEET/ACTIVITY 5

Write a one-paragraph paper explaining how understanding cultural beliefs affects you as a health care worker (200 points). Follow these guidelines when preparing your report:

- Use 8.5-by-11-inch paper.
- Type, word-process, or write neatly in ink.
- Use correct spelling and grammar.

There are 200 possible points in this worksheet/activity.

• WORKSHEET 6

Conduct an Internet search for information on one or more topics covered in Chapter 4 related to meeting your needs and the needs of others. For example:

- Language, religion, medical practices, or feasts and celebrations of any culture or nationality
- Nutrition
- Exercise
- Biofeedback

When you have identified some good information, print it out for your portfolio. Prepare a brief, one-paragraph explanation of why you chose to print out and keep the information you did. Why did you consider that Web site a trustworthy source of information? Why did you think other Web sites were not so good? Be prepared to explain to your classmates your thoughts on doing research on the Internet.

There are 100 possible points in this worksheet.

• WORKSHEET/ACTIVITY 3

1. Explain why communication is important (1 point).

____

____

____

____

____

2. Name four elements that influence our relationship with others (4 points).

   a. ____

   b. ____

   c. ____

   d. ____

3. List three barriers to communication (3 points).

   a. ____

   b. ____

   c. ____

There are 8 possible points in this worksheet/activity.

• WORKSHEET/ACTIVITY 4

This communication game will help you:

- Discover that words mean different things to different people.
- Identify words that indicate clear directions.

Note to instructor: In groups of two, have students sit back to back. Give each student an identical set of colored squares, circles, triangles, and so on. Have one student put the pieces down one by one to create a design. Ask that student to describe the design clearly enough so that the other student will replicate it exactly. No questions may be asked! How well did the communication go? Are the designs alike? Were directions exact and clear? Change the communicator and receiver, and repeat the activity.

There are 10 possible points in this worksheet/activity.

• WORKSHEET 5

Directions: Mark each statement below by placing a check (✓) in the true or false column indicating your feelings about the statement.

Assertiveness Inventory

TRUE	FALSE	STATEMENT
		1. I know what my good points are and I tell others what they are.
		2. I like to make myself look good and sometimes tell others unrealistic stories to make me look better than I am.
		3. Defending myself and expressing my feelings makes me feel uncomfortable.
		4. Sometimes I make other people feel unimportant, afraid, or stupid.
		5. I let others get their way because I don't like to make a scene.
		6. I usually feel that my views and feelings are not important to others.
		7. Others' rights are not important to me.
		8. I am careful not to abuse or be cruel when telling others that I do not agree with them.
		9. I usually take as much as I can from others even when it is unfair.
		10. I receive compliments and thank the other person for the comment.
		11. It is easier to say yes than no, even when I'd really like to say no.
		12. Other people tell me I make unreasonable requests of them.
		13. I defend my rights, and I let others do the same.
		14. I usually try to be the center of conversation.
		15. I don't like to ask others to do things.
		16. I start and carry on conversations without discomfort.
		17. It is difficult for me to tell others what my good points are.
		18. I usually do not insist that my rights be respected.
		19. I usually ask for what is mine.
		20. I listen to criticism without acting defensive.
		21. When I am angry or criticizing others, I tend to assault them physically or verbally to get my point across.
		22. It is easy for me to say positive things about others.
		23. When I know I'm right it doesn't matter if I hurt someone's feelings.
		24. When I get my way in a conversation I usually feel good, but later I feel guilty.

To evaluate your Assertiveness Inventory, do the following (24 points):

1. On the chart below, place a circle around the number of each statement you marked *true*.
2. Add the number of circles in each column. *(If all numbers in a column are circled, the total will be 8.)*
3. The column with the highest number indicates your preferred form of communication.

	UNASSERTIVE	ASSERTIVE	AGGRESSIVE
	3	1	2
	5	8	4
	6	10	7
	11	13	9
	15	16	12
	17	19	14
	18	20	21
	24	22	23
Total			

There are 24 possible points in this worksheet.

• WORKSHEET 6

1. List three elements necessary for communication to take place (3 points).
   - **a.** ______
   - **b.** ______
   - **c.** ______

2. Describe three things that a good listener does (3 points).
   - **a.** ______
   - **b.** ______
   - **c.** ______

3. Differentiate between verbal and nonverbal communication (10 points).

______
______
______
______
______

There are 16 possible points in this worksheet.

• WORKSHEET 7

1. Explain what it means when you are asked to smile when you answer the phone (1 point). ______

______

______

______

2. What will you say when you answer the phone (1 point)? ______

______

______

______

3. When you take a message, what information must you include (4 points)?

 a. ______

 b. ______

 c. ______

______

 you let the caller hang up first (1 point)? ______

______

______

______

ts in this worksheet.

• WO

ere you will be divided into groups of three. e conversation, while the third person will obse the role-play the observer will give *helpful feedback* s activity will help you:

- Identify
- Create ideas a ur telephone communication skills.

There are 25 possible poi t/activity.

Chapter 6 Medical Terminology

UNIT 1

Pronunciation, Word Elements, and Terms

• OBJECTIVES

When you have completed this unit, you will be able to do the following:

- Define roots, prefixes, and suffixes.
- Define the word elements listed.
- Match medical terms with their correct meanings.
- Divide medical terms into elements.
- Combine word elements to form medical terms.

• DIRECTIONS

1. Read this unit.
2. Complete Worksheet/Activity 1, as assigned.
3. Complete Worksheets 2 through 4 as assigned.
4. When you are confident that you can meet each objective listed above, ask your instructor for the unit evaluation.

• EVALUATION METHODS

- Worksheets/activities
- Class participation
- Written evaluation

• WORKSHEET/ACTIVITY 1

Use index cards to make flash cards to help you learn the prefixes, roots, and suffixes listed in the text. Write each word element on one side of a card, and write its meaning on the other side. Review the cards whenever you have a minute (such as when standing in line or waiting for a ride). Work with your classmates, quizzing each other until you know all of the word elements and their meanings. Learn 12 elements each day. Before going to bed each night, quiz yourself on the 12 elements that you learned that day (1 point for each card).

• WORKSHEET 2

1. Fill in the blanks with the appropriate answer (6 points).
   - a. *ch* sounds like K.
   - b. *ps* sounds like S.
   - c. *pn* sounds like n.
   - d. *c* sounds like S when it comes before *e, i,* and *y.*
   - e. *g* sounds like j when it comes before *e, i,* and *y.*
   - f. *i* sounds like eye when added to the end of the word to form a plural.
2. How are medical terms formed (1 point)? They have a root, combining vowel, + suffix
3. List three types of word elements (3 points).
   - a. Root/Prefix
   - b. combining vowel
   - c. Suffix
4. The element at the beginning of a medical term is known as a prefix (1 point).
5. The element that is the subject of a medical term is known as a root (1 point).
6. The element found at the end of a medical term is called a suffix (1 point).
7. Combined vowels are used to help make medical terms easier to say + prevent confusion (1 point).
8. Commonly used combined vowels are (a) O and (b) i and sometimes (c) y and (d) u (4 points).
9. Learning word elements gives you the tools necessary to create hundreds of medical terms (1 point).
10. Use the text to help you put the correct word elements together to form medical terms for the following (10 points).
    - bradicardio a. Slow heart condition brady
    - unintercosto b. Pertaining to between the ribs uninter
    - hemiplegia c. Paralysis of half the body hemi

viscerasclerosis sclerosis
d. Condition of hardening of the arteries
carcinoma e. Cancerous tumor carcin
gastritis f. Inflammation of the stomach itis
renosis g. Condition of the kidney ren
acromegaly h. Enlarged extremities megaly
hysterectomy i. Surgical removal of the uterus ectomy
trachiotomy j. Incision of the trachea otomy

11. Write the meaning next to the following medical terms (10 points).

a. Epigastric upper stomach pretaining to
b. Esophagitis esophagus inflamation
c. Melanoma black tumor
d. Laparotomy incision of the stomach
e. Postpartum pertaining to after labor
f. Thoracentesis thorac puncture
g. Rhinoplasty nose repair surgically
h. Dermocyanosis condition of the skin
i. Craniotomy brain surgrey
j. Hepatitis inflamation of the liver

12. Divide the following medical terms into elements (10 points).

a. Acromegaly acro/megal/y
b. Antifebrile anti/febr/ile
c. Bradycardia brady/cardia
d. Carcinoma carci/noma
e. Dentalgia dental/gia
f. Gastroenteritis gastro/enter/itis
g. Hemiplegia hemi/plegia
h. Intracostal intra/cost/al
i. Osteoarthritis osteo/arthr/itis
j. Pericarditis peri/cardi/itis

There are 49 possible points in this worksheet.

• WORKSHEET 3

Go onto the Internet and look at the various free resources that could help you with medical terminology. You may use search engines or go to various health care publishers' Web sites. Look at the textbooks you use for Web addresses as a beginning.

Look up the same terms on different sites and compare what they say. Print out some examples and be ready to tell your classmates which are the best resources and why.

There are 100 possible points in this worksheet.

• WORKSHEET 4

1. Change the following words from singular to plural. Define each word.

Singular	Plural	Definition
a. Stratum	__________	__________
b. Retinoblastoma	__________	__________
c. Decubitus	__________	__________
d. Disease	__________	__________
e. Vena cava	__________	__________
f. Allergy	__________	__________
g. Metastasis	__________	__________

There are 14 possible points in this worksheet.

UNIT 2 Medical Abbreviations

• OBJECTIVES

When you have completed this unit, you will be able to do the following:

- Recognize and define abbreviations that are commonly used by health care workers.
- Replace terms with abbreviations.

• DIRECTIONS

1. Read this unit.
2. Complete Worksheet/Activity 1.
3. Complete Worksheets 2 and 3 as assigned.
4. Prepare responses to each item listed in the Chapter Review—Your Link to Success at the end of this Chapter.
5. When you are confident that you can meet each objective listed above, ask your instructor for the unit evaluation.

• EVALUATION METHODS

- Worksheets/activities
- Class participation
- Written evaluation

• WORKSHEET/ACTIVITY 1

Using index cards, make flash cards to help you learn the abbreviations listed in the text. Write each abbreviation on one side of a card, and write its meaning on the other side. Review the cards whenever you have a minute (such as when standing in line or waiting for a ride). Work with your classmates, quizzing each other until you know all of the abbreviations and their meanings. Learn 12 abbreviations each day. Before going to bed each night, quiz yourself on the 12 elements you learned that day (1 point for each card).

• WORKSHEET 2

Fill in the correct medical term for each of the following abbreviations (50 points).

1. cath.	__________	**27.** B/P	__________
2. am, AM	__________	**28.** fx	__________
3. bid, BID	__________	**29.** IV	__________
4. hs	__________	**30.** spec.	__________
5. lab	__________	**31.** ROM	__________
6. hyper	__________	**32.** po	__________
7. CPR	__________	**33.** pc	__________
8. w/c	__________	**34.** qid, QID	__________
9. qhs	__________	**35.** Pt, pt	__________
10. $\bar{q}$	__________	**36.** q_2h	__________
11. amt.	__________	**37.** dc, d/c	__________
12. I & O	__________	**38.** post	__________
13. qod, QOD	__________	**39.** $\overline{ss}$	__________
14. CA	__________	**40.** OPD	__________
15. $\bar{c}$	__________	**41.** postop, PostOp	__________
16. prn	__________		
17. bm, BM	__________	**42.** BR, br	__________
18. O_2	__________	**43.** CBC	__________
19. ax	__________	**44.** stat	__________
20. $\bar{s}$	__________	**45.** c/o	__________
21. wt	__________	**46.** dx	__________
22. ht	__________	**47.** cc	__________
23. amb	__________	**48.** liq.	__________
24. BRP	__________	**49.** H_2O	__________
25. OOB, oob	__________	**50.** noct, noc.	__________
26. NPO	__________		

There are 50 possible points in this worksheet.

• WORKSHEET 3

Fill in the correct medical term for each of the following abbreviations (10 points).

1. adm ____________________
2. amb ____________________
3. cath. ____________________
4. lab ____________________
5. CPR ____________________
6. B/P ____________________
7. ROM ____________________
8. NPO ____________________
9. prn ____________________
10. I & O ____________________

There are 10 possible points in this worksheet.

Chapter 7 Medical Math

UNIT 1

Math Review

• OBJECTIVES

When you have completed this unit, you will be able to do the following:

- Add and subtract whole numbers, fractions, mixed numbers, decimals, and percentages.
- Multiply and divide whole numbers, fractions, mixed numbers, decimals, and percentages.
- Convert:
  - Decimals to percentages
  - Percentages to decimals
  - Fractions to percentages
  - Percentages to fractions

• DIRECTIONS

1. Complete Worksheet 1, Pretest, in the Student Workbook.
2. Read "Introduction to the Math Review" and complete Worksheet 2.
3. Read the information following the Addition and Subtraction headings.
4. Complete Worksheet 3.
5. Read the information following the Multiplication heading.
6. Complete Worksheet/Activity 4.
7. Read the information under the Division heading.
8. Complete Worksheet 5.
9. Read the information following Decimals, Percentages, and Fractions headings.

10. Complete Worksheet 6.
11. When you are confident that you can meet each objective for this unit, ask your instructor for the unit evaluation.

• EVALUATION METHODS

- Pretest
- Worksheets/Activities
- Class participation
- Written evaluation

• WORKSHEET 1, PRETEST (100 POINTS)

Write the following numbers using commas and decimals in the correct places (5 points).

NUMBER	YOUR ANSWER
1. 9345	
2. 10345	
3. 100345	
4. 9345 40/100	
5. 1234567	

Add commas and decimals to the following numbers, then write their description as you would describe them to another person.

6. 9345

7. 10345

8. 100345

9. 9345 4/100

10. 19345 4/100

Calculate the following (show your work).

Addition

11. 3 + 9 =

12. 8 + 4 =

13. 4 + 5 =

14. 12 + 27 =

15. 54 + 72 =

16. 62 + 5 =

17. 15 + 15 =

18. 186 + 204 =

19. 549 + 222 =

20. 1,008 + 89,345 =

Subtraction

21. 9 – 3 =

22. 8 – 4 =

23. 5 – 4 =

24. 27 – 12 =

25. 62 – 5 =

26. 15 – 15 =

27. 204 – 186 =

28. 549 – 222 =

29. 89,345 – 1,008 =

30. 100,000 – 84,694 =

Multiplication

31. 8 × 4 =

32. 3 × 3 =

33. 12 × 6 =

34. 27 × 9 =

35. 58 × 18 =

36. 165 × 10 =

37. 2,222 × 93 =

38. 624 × 1,000 =

39. 5,524 × 320 =

40. 8,350 × 600 =

Division

21. 6 ÷ 2 =

22. 12 : 3 =

23. 42 ÷ 7 =

24. 25 ÷ 5 =

25. 72 ÷ 9 =

26. 240 ÷ 10 =

27. 3,232 ÷ 32 =

28. 960 ÷ 60 =

29. 8,250 ÷ 150 =

50. 5,200 ÷ 16 =

Percentages

Band-aids are packaged in 100 per box. You had four full boxes when you started work yesterday. At the end of the day, you had two full boxes left.

51. What percentage of them were used yesterday? ______________________

52. What percentage is still left? ______________________

There are 100 sample bottles of cough medicine in the cupboard.

53. If you give 25 bottles away, how many will you have left? ______________

54. What percentage is left in the cupboard? ______________________

55. What percentage was given away? ______________________

56–100. Fill in the blank spaces on the following multiplication table.

	1	2	3	4	5	6	7	8	9	10
1										
2										
3										
4										
5										
6										
7										
8										
9										
10										

There are 100 possible points in this worksheet/pretest.

• WORKSHEET 2

Write the place values for each of the digits in the number below. One answer has been completed for you (2,222.22) (20 points).

2	, 2	2	2	. 2	2
1. ______	2. ______	3. ______	4. ______	5. tenths	6. ______

Write the following numbers using commas and decimals in the correct places.

NUMBER	ANSWER	NUMBER	ANSWER
7. 8492		**11.** 2536	
8. 654 3/10		**12.** 5558555	
9. 92184		**13.** 2645	
10. 108627		**14.** 32323	

15. Describe a whole number. ______

16. Describe a nonwhole number. ______

17. Describe a mixed number. ______

18. Describe a percentage. ______

19. Write a percentage sign. ______

20. Describe the value of a zero in front of a whole number. ______

There are 20 possible points in this worksheet.

• WORKSHEET 3

Add the following numbers, show your work (26 points).

1. 8 + 7 =

2. 9 + 6 + 2 =

3. 23 + 35 =

4. 36 + 72 + 18 =

5. 555 + 398 + 421 =

6. 746 + 843 + 341 =

7. 9,742 + 23 + 1,008 + 6,842 =

8. 43 + 5,432 + 987 + 8,764 =

9. 8,765 + 964 + 1,053 + 3,338 =

10. 10,079 + 365 + 5,432 + 89,935 =

Subtract the numbers in the following problems (show your work for each).

11. 9 – 6 =

12. 8 – 3 =

13. 12 – 3 =

14. 24 – 13 =

15. 555 – 72 =

16. 693 – 545 =

17. 1,003 – 946 =

18. 1,233 – 895 =

19. 9,843 – 6,979 =

20. 6,321 – 93 =

Show your work as you subtract, and check your answers, in the following:

21. 145 – 68 =

22. 913 – 43 =

23. 26 – 10 =

24. 960 – 96 =

25. 872 – 154 =

26. 1,000 – 347 =

There are 26 possible points in this worksheet.

• WORKSHEET/ACTIVITY 4

Learn the multiplication table from your text, and then fill in the following table by multiplying the top row of numbers against the numbers in the column at the left. Place the correct answer in the square that intersects with the numbers being multiplied. See example below (100 points)

Example: five times five:

	1	2	3	4	5	6
1						
2						
3						
4						
5					25	
6						

	1	2	3	4	5	6	7	8	9	10
1										
2										
3										
4										
5										
6										
7										
8										
9										
10										

Make flash cards by putting each problem represented in the multiplication table on the front side of a card and the answer on the back of the card. Use the cards to review multiplication. Ask a classmate to quiz you using the cards.

There are 150 possible points in this worksheet/activity.

• WORKSHEET 5

Calculate the following (15 points).

1. 225 ÷ 5 =

2. 486 ÷ 3 =

3. 240 ÷ 8 =

4. 8,289 ÷ 9 =

5. 1,060 ÷ 5 =

6. 3,826 ÷ 8 =

7. 4,832 ÷ 8 =

8. 2,222 ÷ 4 =

9. 6,324 ÷ 3 =

10. 7,248 ÷ 8 =

11. 963.54 ÷ 9 =

12. 339.28 ÷ 4 =

13. 637.42 ÷ 7 =

14. 2,967.40 ÷ 5 =

15. 8,954.73 ÷ 9 =

There are 15 possible points in this worksheet.

• WORKSHEET 6

Convert the following decimals to percentages (24 points).

1. .33 = _____%
2. .46 = _____%
3. .75 = _____%
4. .13 = _____%
5. .50 = _____%
6. .96 = _____%

Convert the following percentages to decimals.

7. 100% = _______
8. 20% = ________
9. 64% = _______
10. 85% = _______

Convert the following percentages into fractions.

11. 33% =
12. 13% =
13. 3% =
14. 8% =
15. 833% =
16. 1,025% =

Calculate percentages of the following.

17. 20% of 100 =
18. 25% of 100 =
19. 30% of 50 =
20. 3% of 65 =
21. 28% of 1,000 =
22. 15% of 25,000 =
23. 65% of 90 =
24. 7.25% of 8 =

There are 24 possible points in this worksheet.

UNIT 2 The Metric System

• OBJECTIVES

When you have completed this unit, you will be able to do the following:

- Match vocabulary words with their correct meanings.

- State the metric unit of measure used to determine length, distance, weight, and volume.
- Use metric terms to express 100 and 1,000 units of measure.
- Use metric terms to express 0.1, 0.01, and 0.001 units of measure.
- List four basic rules to follow when using the metric system.
- Identify metric measures of length and volume.
- Convert ounces to cubic centimeters/milliliters, pounds to kilograms, and ounces to grams.

• DIRECTIONS

1. Read this unit.
2. Complete Worksheet 1.
3. Complete Worksheet/Activity 2.
4. Complete Worksheet 3.
5. Complete Worksheets/Activities 4 through 5.
6. When you are confident that you can meet each objective for this unit, ask your instructor for the unit evaluation.

• EVALUATION METHODS

- Worksheets/Activities
- Class participation
- Written evaluation

• WORKSHEET 1

Match each definition or abbreviation in column B to the correct word in column A (12 points). One answer is used more than once.

Column A	*Column B*
____ **1.** Abbreviation	**a.** International System of Units
____ **2.** Convert	**b.** A shortened form of a word
____ **3.** Decimal	**c.** A number containing a decimal point
____ **4.** Metric system	**d.** To transform; to change into another form
____ **5.** Meter	**e.** L
____ **6.** Gram	**f.** m
____ **7.** Liter	**g.** d
____ **8.** Kilo	**h.** g
____ **9.** Hecto	**i.** c
____ **10.** Deci	**j.** k
____ **11.** Centi	**k.** h
____ **12.** Milli	

There are 12 possible points in this worksheet.

• WORKSHEET/ACTIVITY 2

1. Ask your teachers for containers and rulers marked in standard and metric units to help you visualize these measures.
2. What is the metric measure for

   a. Length ______________ **c.** Distance ______________

   b. Weight ______________ **d.** Volume ______________

There are 5 points in this worksheet/activity.

• WORKSHEET 3

1. Write each item below in the space next to the correct measure (8 points).

length and distance	weight	0.01 of a unit
100 units	1,000 units	0.1 of a unit
volume	0.001 of a unit	

______________ **a.** Meter

______________ **b.** Gram

______________ **c.** Liter

______________ **d.** Kilo

______________ **e.** Hecto

______________ **f.** Deci

______________ **g.** Centi

______________ **h.** Milli

2. Use metric terms to express the following (5 points):

   1,000 units ______________________________

   100 units ______________________________

   1/10 or 0.1 of a unit ______________________________

   1/100 or 0.01 of a unit ______________________________

   1/1,000 or 0.001 of a unit ______________________________

3. List four basic rules for using the metric system (4 points).

   a. ______________________________

   b. ______________________________

   c. ______________________________

   d. ______________________________

There are 17 possible points in this worksheet.

• WORKSHEET 4

1. There are ______________________________ ml/cc in 1 ounce.
2. To determine the number of ml/ccs in a container marked with ounces, multiply ______________________________.
3. 8 oz. of water = ______________________________ ml/cc.
4. 6 oz. of soup = ______________________________ ml/cc.
5. 16 oz. of juice = ______________________________ ml/cc.
6. 1 lb = ______________________________ k.
7. 1 k = ______________________________ lb.
8. To convert pounds to kilograms, multiply the number of pounds by______.
9. To convert kilograms to pounds, multiply the number of kilograms by ____.
10. Convert 110 lbs. to kilograms. 110 × __________ = __________ (1 point).
11. Convert 50 k to pounds. 50 × __________ = __________(1 point).
12. Convert the following (4 points):
    - **a.** 300 lbs. to kilograms ______________________________
    - **b.** 150 lbs. to kilograms ______________________________
    - **c.** 20 kg to pounds ______________________________
    - **d.** 85 kg to pounds ______________________________
13. To convert ounces to grams, multiply ___ 3 the number of ounces (1 point).
14. To convert grams into ounces, divide 30 into the ______________ (1 point).
15. Convert the following (4 points):
    - **a.** 8 oz. to grams ______________________________
    - **b.** 16 oz. to grams ______________________________
    - **c.** 30 g to ounces ______________________________
    - **d.** 120 g to ounces ______________________________

There are 21 possible points in this worksheet.

• WORKSHEET/ACTIVITY 5

Practice weighing your classmates and convert their weight from pounds to kilograms. Practice measuring your classmates and convert from feet to inches and feet to meters. Practice measuring water in centimeters and liters. Convert to ccs.

There are 30 points in this worksheet/activity.

UNIT 3

The 24-Hour Clock/Military Time

• OBJECTIVES

When you have completed this unit, you will be able to do the following:

- Recognize time on a 24-hour clock.
- Express 24-hour time/military time verbally and in writing.
- Convert Greenwich time to 24-hour time.

• DIRECTIONS

1. Read this unit.
2. Complete Worksheet 1.
3. Complete Worksheet/Activity 2.
4. When you are confident that you can meet each objective listed above, ask your instructor for the unit evaluation.

• EVALUATION METHODS

- Worksheet
- Class participation
- Written evaluation

• WORKSHEET 1

1. Define *Greenwich time* (1 point). ______________________________

   ____
2. Define *24-hour time/military time* (1 point). ______________________________

   ____
3. Military time is always expressed in how many digits (1 point)?
4. To determine how 5:00 P.M. is expressed in military time, add __________ to 0500 (1 point).
5. Write the correct military time for each of the following Greenwich times (6 points). ______________________________
   - **a.** 3:00 A.M. ______________________________
   - **b.** 9:00 A.M. ______________________________
   - **c.** 12:00 noon ______________________________
   - **d.** 6:00 P.M. ______________________________
   - **e.** 12:00 midnight ______________________________
   - **f.** 12:30 A.M. ______________________________

6. Write the Greenwich time for each of the following military times (6 points).

a. 0130____________________

b. 0500____________________

c. 1700____________________

d. 1430____________________

e. 0045____________________

f. 0000____________________

There are 16 possible points in this worksheet.

• WORKSHEET/ACTIVITY 2

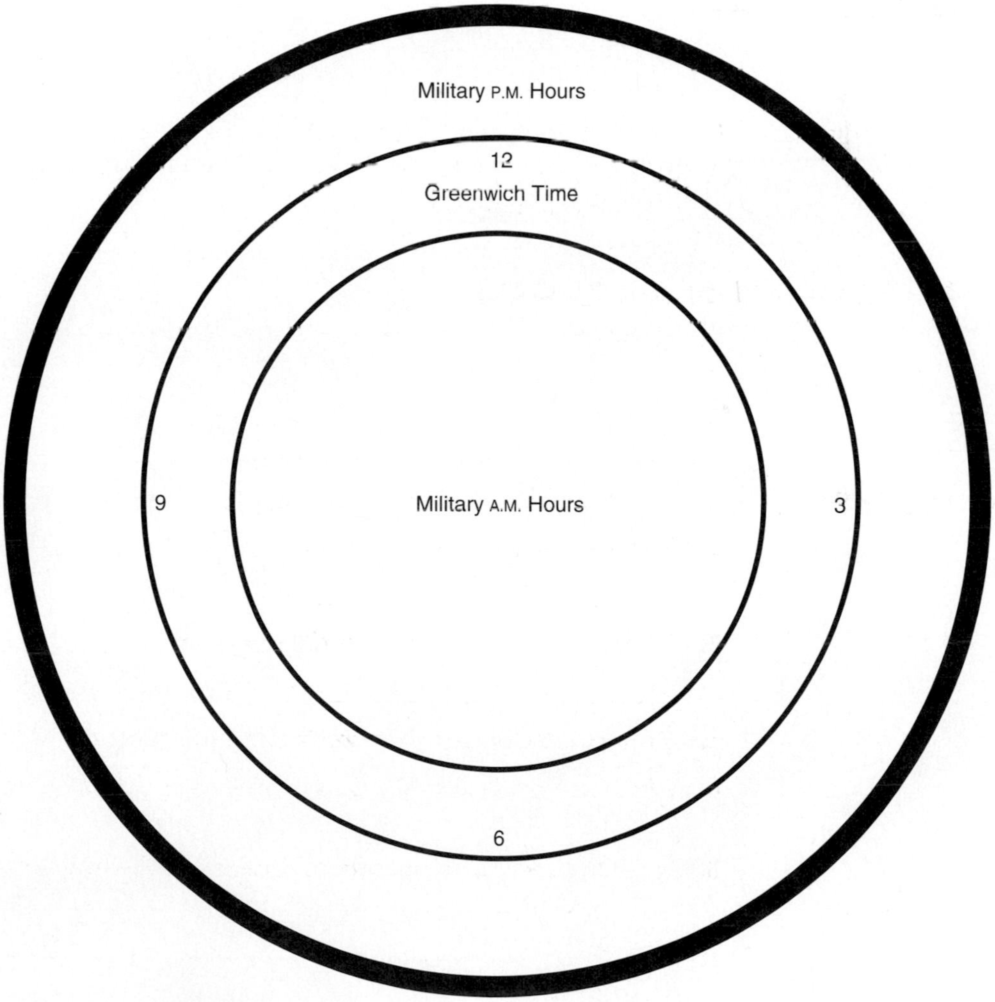

Directions: Fill in the clock diagram with the correct Greenwich and military times. The 3:00, 6:00, 9:00, and 12:00 are reference times in the Greenwich circle to help guide you.

There are 20 points in this worksheet/activity.

Chapter 8 Your Body and How It Functions

UNIT 1

Overview of the Body

• OBJECTIVES

When you have completed this unit, you will be able to do the following:

- Match vocabulary words with their correct meanings.
- List seven cell functions.
- Identify three main parts of the cell and explain their functions.
- Describe the relationship between cells, tissues, organs, and systems of the body.
- Identify terms relating to the body.
- Label a diagram of the body cavities.
- Explain why health care workers must have a basic knowledge of body structures and how they function.

• DIRECTIONS

1. Complete Worksheet 1 before beginning the reading.
2. Read this unit.
3. Complete Worksheet 2.
4. Ask your instructor for directions to complete Worksheet/Activity 3.
5. Complete Worksheets 4 through 6.
6. When you are confident that you can meet each objective listed above, ask your instructor for the unit evaluation.

Laura Zack

• EVALUATION METHODS

- Worksheets/Activities
- Class participation
- Written evaluation

• WORKSHEET 1

Match each definition in column B with the correct vocabulary word in column A (14 points).

Column A

d 1. Cell
b 2. Cell membrane
e 3. Composed
g 4. Connective tissue
f 5. Cytoplasm
n 6. Epithelial
c 7. Function
i 8. Microscopic
k 9. Nucleus
l 10. Nutrients
m 11. Reproduction
j 12. Sacral region
a 13. Structure
h 14. Tissue

Column B

a. The form in which the body is made.
b. A thin, soft layer of tissue that surrounds the cell and holds it together.
c. The action or work of tissues, organs, or body parts.
d. The smallest structural unit in the body that is capable of independent functioning.
e. Formed by putting many parts together.
f. Jellylike liquid that carries on the activities of the cell.
g. Tissue specialized to bind together and support other tissues.
h. A group of cells of the same type that act together to perform a specific function.
i. Too small to be seen by the eye but large enough to be seen through a microscope.
j. The area where the sacrum is located.
k. The part of a cell that is vital for its growth, metabolism, reproduction, and transmitted characteristics.
l. Food.
m. The process that takes place in animals to create offspring.
n. Pertaining to the covering of the internal and external organs of the body.

There are 14 possible points in this worksheet.

• WORKSHEET 2

1. Label the three main parts of a basic cell (3 points).

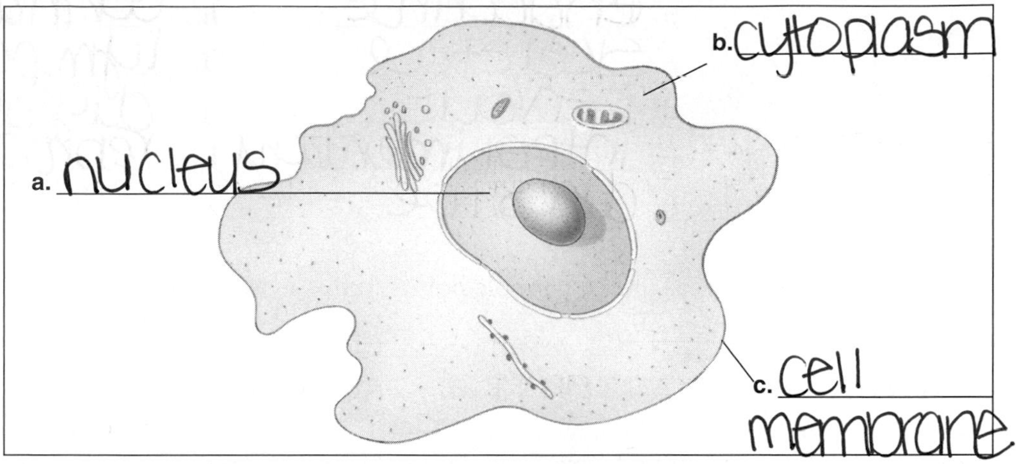

2. Name the three main parts of a cell, and explain the function of each (6 points).

Cell Part	Function
a. nucleus	Part of the cell vital for growth, metabolism, reproduction
b. cytoplasm	jelly like liquid where the activities of the cell occur
c. cell membrane	outer covering of the cell; lets stuff in + keeps stuff out

3. Explain how cells, tissues, organs, and systems form a body (5 points).

The cells come together to make tissues, Like tissues become organs, + those form the body.

4. List the five primary kinds of tissues found in the body (5 points).

a. nerve
b. epithelial
c. connective
d. blood
e. muscle

5. Name the eleven body systems that will be discussed in this chapter (11 points).

a. respiratory
b. endocrine
c. skeletal
d. nervous
e. integumentary
f. digestive
g. glandular
h. urinary
i. lympathetic
j. digestive
k. reproductive

There are 30 possible points in this worksheet.

• WORKSHEET/ACTIVITY 3

Study the new terms in Unit 1. Prepare to participate in a spelling bee by learning to spell and define the new terms in this unit. Your instructor will assign points for this activity.

• WORKSHEET 4

Match each statement in column B with the correct word in column A (15 points).

Column A	*Column B*
f 1. Superior	a. Contains the heart, lungs, and large blood vessels.
c 2. Inferior	b. Near the surface or front of the body.
b 3. Ventral or anterior	c. Below or lower.
i 4. Dorsal or posterior	d. Near the head.
d 5. Cranial	e. Near the center or midline of the body.
k 6. Caudal	f. Above or in a higher position.
e 7. Medial	g. Nearest the point of attachment.
h 8. Lateral	h. Away from the midline.
g 9. Proximal	i. Near the back of the body.
j 10. Distal	j. Farthest from the point of attachment.
n 11. Cranial cavity	k. Encloses the spinal cord.
L 12. Spinal cavity	l. Tail end or sacral region.
a 13. Thoracic cavity	m. Contains the stomach, most of the intestines, the kidneys, liver, gallbladder, pancreas, and spleen.
m 14. Abdominal cavity	n. Houses the brain.
o 15. Pelvic cavity	o. Contains urinary bladder, rectum, and parts of the reproductive system.

There are 15 possible points in this worksheet.

• WORKSHEET 5

Label the cavities of the body on the following diagram. Then indicate which are the ventral cavities and which are the dorsal cavities by writing *V* or *D* in spaces 6 and 7 (7 points).

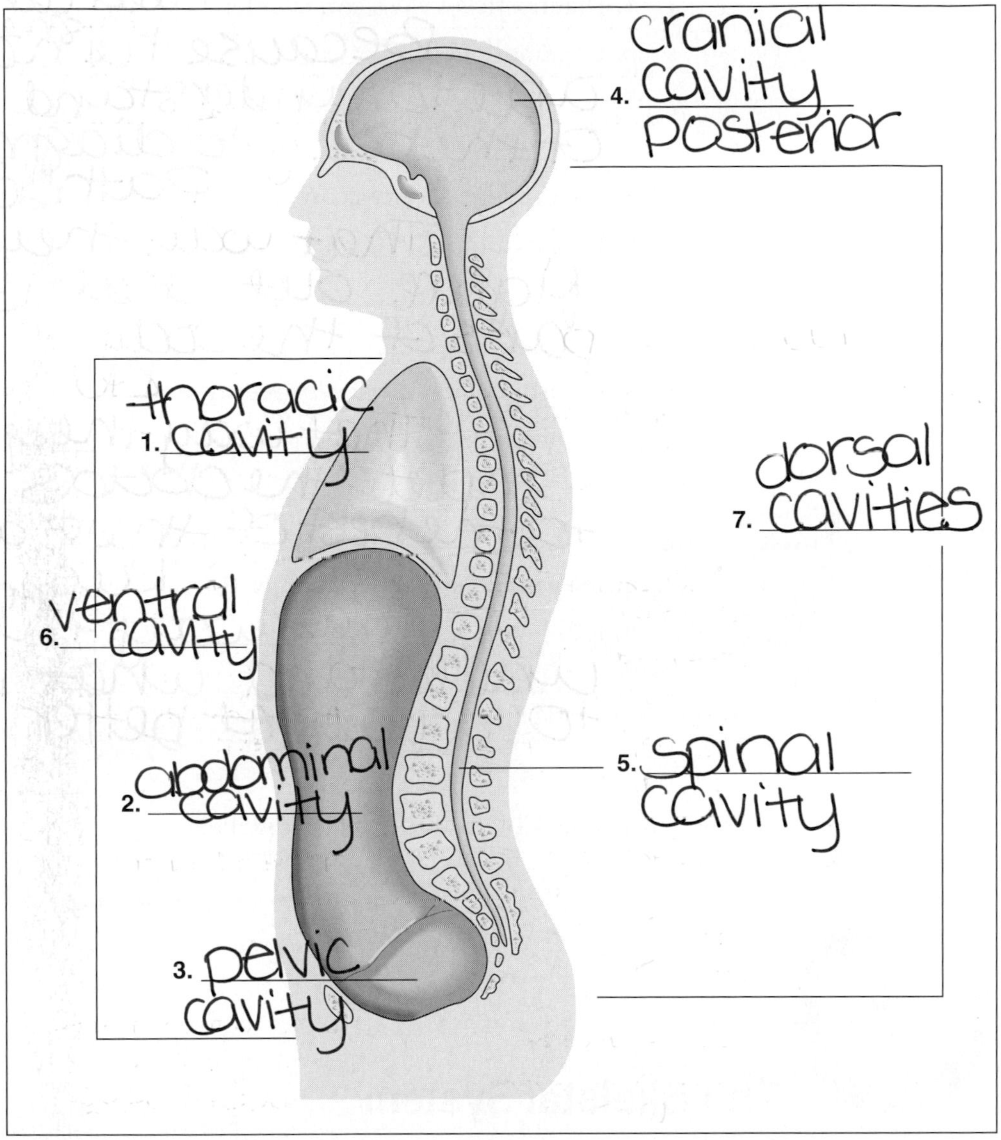

There are 7 possible points in this worksheet.

• WORKSHEET 6

Select one career from each health service area, and explain why a worker in that service must have a basic knowledge of body structures and how they function (8 points).

1. **a.** Diagnostic services career title: Medical Doctor
   b. Explanation: Because he/she needs to be able to understand all parts of the body to diagnose correctly
2. **a.** Therapeutic services career title: Pathologist
   b. Explanation: That way they can figure out what is affecting parts of the body.
3. **a.** Environmental services career title: RN
   b. Explanation: That way they can complete the doctors orders to the best of their ability
4. **a.** Informational services career title: Nursing Assistant
   b. Explanation: That way they can understand what is happening to a patient better

There are 8 possible points in this worksheet.

UNIT 2

The Skeletal System

• OBJECTIVES

When you have completed this unit, you will be able to do the following:

- Match vocabulary words with their correct meanings.
- Label a diagram of major bones in the body.
- Select from a list the functions of bones.
- Name the long, short, flat, and irregular bones of the body.
- Identify immovable, slightly movable, and freely movable joints of the body.
- Identify common disorders of the skeletal system.

- Label a diagram of four types of bone fractures.
- Explain why health care workers must have a basic knowledge of the skeletal system and how it functions.

• DIRECTIONS

1. Complete Worksheet 1 before beginning the reading.
2. Read this unit.
3. Complete Worksheets 2 through 4 as assigned.
4. Complete Worksheet 5 after your instructor discusses this unit in class.
5. Ask your instructor for directions to complete Worksheets/Activities 6 and 7.
6. When you are confident that you can meet each objective listed above, ask your instructor for the unit evaluation.

• EVALUATION METHODS

- Worksheets/Activities
- Class participation
- Written evaluation

• WORKSHEET 1

Match each definition in column B with the correct vocabulary word in column A (15 points).

Column A

d 1. Appendicular
c 2. Axial
g 3. Brittle
e 4. Calcify
j 5. Cartilage
a 6. Components
n 7. Concave
i 8. Conception
b 9. Embryo
k 10. Flexible
l 11. Lateral
f 12. Osseous
h 13. Penetrates
m 14. Porous
o 15. Spontaneous

Column B

a. Parts or elements of a whole.
b. Living human being during the first eight weeks of development in the uterus.
c. Pertaining to the central structures of the body.
d. Pertaining to any body part added to the axis.
e. To harden by forming calcium deposits.
f. Bonelike.
g. Fragile, easy to break.
h. Enters or passes through.
i. Occurs when the male sperm fertilizes the female ovum and a new organism begins to develop.
j. Tough connective tissue.
k. Able to bend easily.
l. Relating to the sides or side of.
m. Filled with tiny holes.
n. Curved inward; depressed; dented.
o. Occurring naturally without apparent cause.

There are 15 possible points in this worksheet.

• WORKSHEET 2

Label the bones of the skeletal system shown on the diagram (31 points).

1. skull
2. orbit
3. sternum
4. xiphoid process
5. lumbar vertebra
6. coastal cartilage
7. Illium
8. symphysis pubis
9. fibula
10. tibia
11. patella
12. femur
13. coccyx
14. sacrum
15. radius
16. ulna
17. elbow
18. numerus
19. ribs
20. scapula
21. mandible
22. maxilla
23. clavicle
24. Carpals
25. metacarpals
26. phalanges
27. calcaneus
28. metarsals
29. phalanges
30. tarsals
31. ischium

There are 31 possible points in this worksheet.

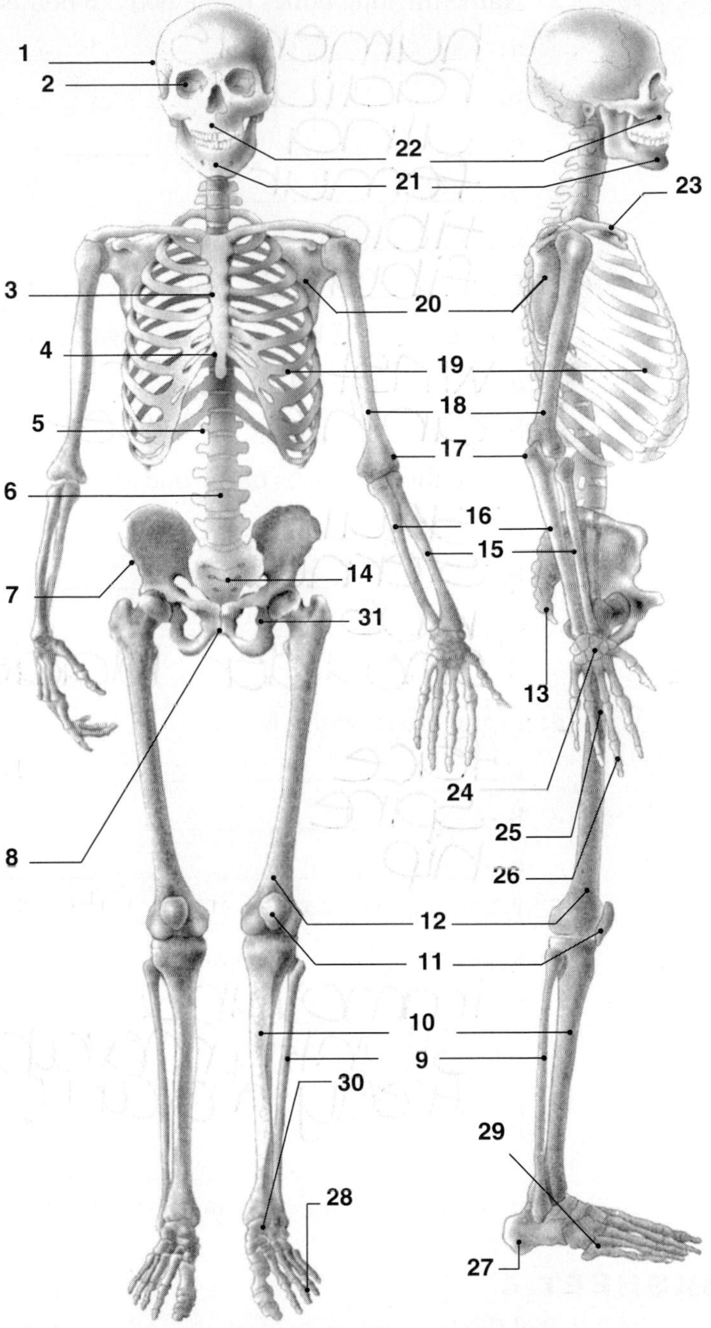

• WORKSHEET 3

1. List the four functions of bones (4 points).
   a. To serve as a framework
   b. To protect internal structure, such as brain
   c. To produce blood cells
   d. To allow flexibility when muscles move them.

2. Name the long bones of the body (6 points).
   a. humerus
   b. radius
   c. ulna
   d. femur
   e. tibia
   f. fibula
3. Name the short bones of the body (2 points).
   a. wrist + hand
   b. ankle + feet
4. Name the flat bones of the body (4 points).
   a. skull
   b. sternum
   c. ribs
   d. shoulder blade
5. Name the irregular bones of the body (3 points).
   a. face
   b. spine
   c. hip
6. Define *joint* (1 point).
7. Name three types of joints (3 points).
   a. immovable
   b. slightly movable
   c. freely movable

There are 23 possible points in this worksheet.

• WORKSHEET 4

Label the fractures shown on the following diagram (4 points).

a. simple transverse
b. compound
c. comminuted
d. greenstick

There are 4 possible points in this worksheet.

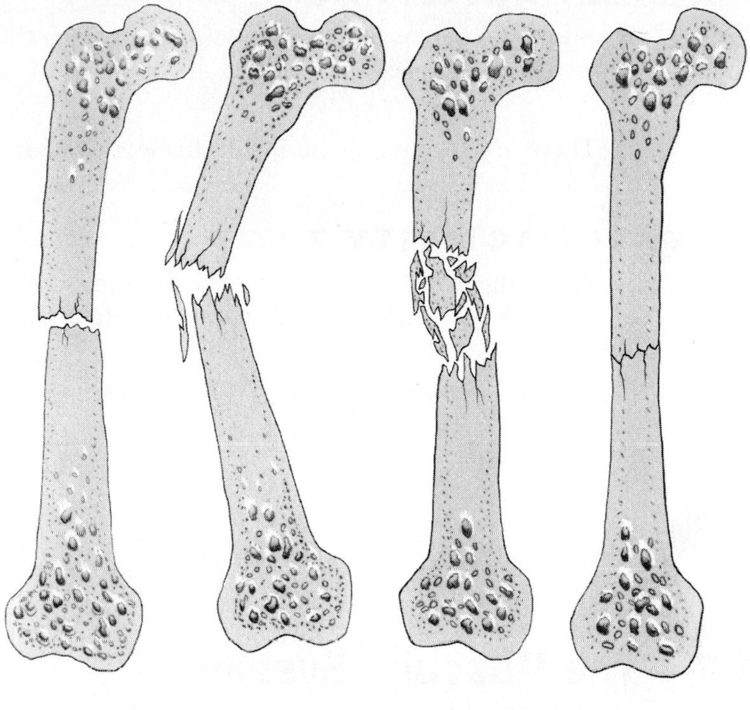

• WORKSHEET 5

Select two careers from different health services areas, and explain why a worker in that service must have a basic knowledge of the skeletal system and how it functions (6 points).

1. a. Name of health care service: ______
   b. Career title: Orthopedist
   c. Explanation: needs to know in order to help pain in patients

2. a. Name of health care service: ______
   b. Career title: cast technian
   c. Explanation: That way they know where to put the cast exactly

There are 6 possible points in this worksheet.

• WORKSHEET/ACTIVITY 6

Study the new terms in Unit 2 and memorize the bones of the body and their locations. Be prepared to label the bones of the body on a skeleton.

There are 10 possible points in this worksheet/activity.

• WORKSHEET/ACTIVITY 7

Learn the joints of the body, their locations, and their functions. Be prepared to identify, label, and explain the movement of each joint of the body.

There are 10 possible points in this worksheet/activity.

UNIT 3

The Muscular System

• OBJECTIVES

When you have completed this unit, you will be able to do the following:

- Match vocabulary words with their correct meanings.
- Explain the difference between muscle and bone functions.
- List three major functions of the muscles.
- Match common disorders of the muscular system with their descriptions.
- Match basic muscle movements to their correct names.
- Label a diagram of the muscular system.
- Describe how muscles provide support and movement.
- Explain why the health care worker's understanding of the muscular system is important.

• DIRECTIONS

1. Complete Worksheet 1 before beginning the reading.
2. Read this unit.
3. Complete Worksheets 2 through 5 as assigned.
4. When you are confident that you can meet each objective listed above, ask your instructor for the unit evaluation.

• EVALUATION METHODS

- Worksheets
- Class participation
- Written evaluation

• WORKSHEET 1

Match each definition statement in column B with the correct vocabulary word in column A (8 points).

Column A

e 1. Axis
g 2. Contract (v.)
a 3. Deteriorate
h 4. Digestion
f 5. Elastic
b 6. Involuntary
c 7. Trauma
d 8. Voluntary

Column B

~~a.~~ To break down.
~~b.~~ Not under control.
~~c.~~ Damage to the body caused by an injury, wound, or shock.
~~d.~~ Under the control of the person.
~~e.~~ A center point.
~~f.~~ Easily stretched.
~~g.~~ To shorten; to draw together.
~~h.~~ Process of breaking down food mechanically and chemically.

There are 8 possible points in this worksheet.

• WORKSHEET 2

1. List the three main functions of muscles (3 points).
   a. Produce heat
   b. Produce movement
   c. maintain posture
2. Write each word listed below in the space next to the statement that best defines it (6 points).

   ~~adduct~~ ~~flex~~ ~~rotate~~
   ~~abduct~~ ~~extended~~ ~~sphincter~~

   a. ~~adduct~~ abduct To move a body part away from the midline.
   b. sphincter Circular muscle that controls an opening.
   c. adduct To move a body part toward the midline.
   d. rotate To turn a body part on its axis.
   e. extended To straighten a body part by moving it away from the body.
   f. flex To bend a body part toward the body.
3. Write the name of the correct muscular system disorder beside each of the definitions below (4 points).
   a. Disease that progressively deteriorates muscle tissue muscular dystrophy
   b. Trauma to the muscle, usually caused by a violent contraction muscle strain
   c. Muscle pain muscle strain
   d. Tear of the muscle tissue torn muscle

There are 13 possible points in this worksheet.

• WORKSHEET 3

Label the parts of the muscular system on the following diagram (19 points).

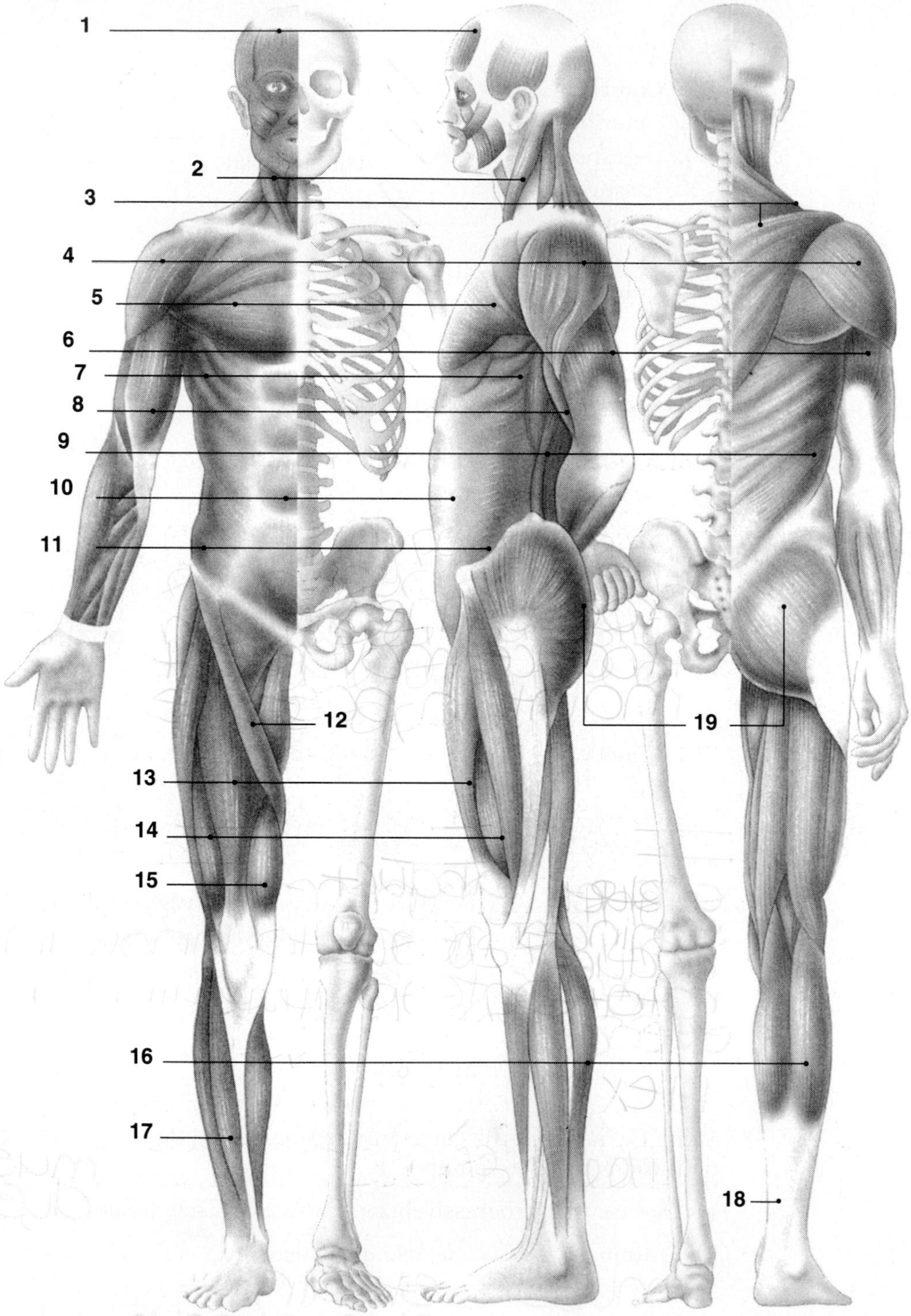

1. frontalis
2. sternocleidomastoid
3. trapezius
4. deltoid
5. pectoralis
6. triceps
7. ~~anterior biceps~~ serratus
8. anterior biceps
9. lattisimus
10. rectus abdominis
11. exterior obliques
12. sartorious
13. rectus femoris
14. vastus medialis
15. vastus lateralis
16. gastrocnemius
17. tibialis anterior
18. achilles tendon
19. gluteus maximus

There are 19 possible points in this worksheet.

• WORKSHEET 4

Fill in the crossword puzzle using the common disorders and terminology list from Unit 3 in your text (14 points).

▢ Indicates a space between two words.

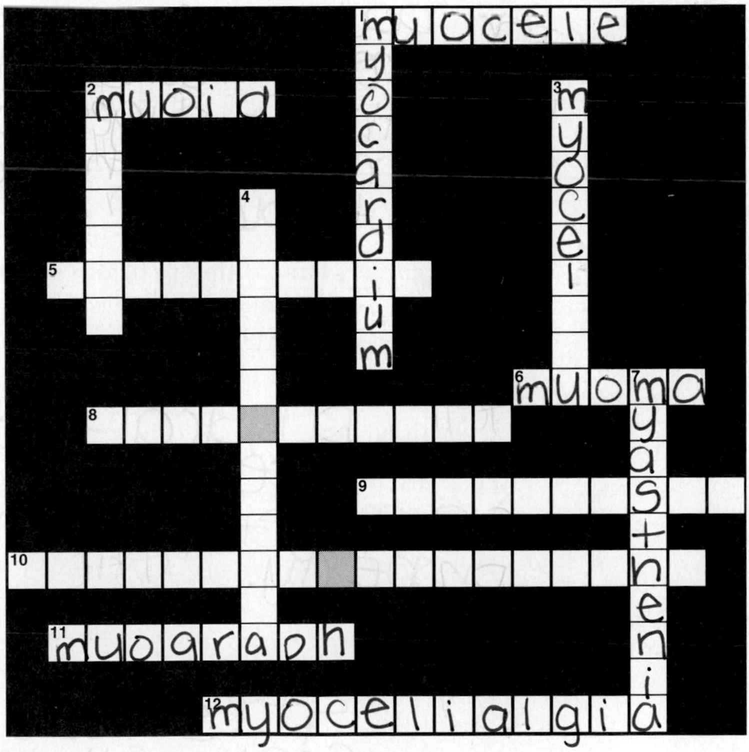

Clues

Across

1. Muscular protrusion (bulge) through a muscle.
2. Resembling muscle.
5. Inflammation of connective tissue.
6. Tumor containing muscle tissue.
8. Tear of the muscle tissue.
9. Weakness or partial paralysis of a muscle.
10. Disease that progressively deteriorates muscle tissue.
11. Beginning in the muscle.
12. Pain of the abdominal muscle.

Down

1. Heart muscle or cardiac muscle.
2. Muscle pain.
3. Record of muscle contractions.
4. Trauma to the muscle, usually caused by a violent contraction.
7. Muscle weakness.

There are 12 possible points in this worksheet.

• WORKSHEET 5

1. Describe how muscles provide support for the body (5 points). Muscles make all movement possible. Muscles move body parts, allowing for proper functioning, such as heartbeat, digestion of food, + movement of the body from place to place.
2. Describe how muscles allow movement (5 points). They allow for body parts to move allowing for proper functioning, such as heartbeat, digestion of food, + movement of the body from place to place.
3. Select two careers from different health service areas, and explain why a worker in that service must have a basic knowledge of the muscular system and how it functions (6 points).
   - **a.** Name of health care service:
   - **b.** Career title: physical therapist
   - **c.** Explanation: Needs to know so they can get patients moving properly.
   - **d.** Name of health care service:
   - **e.** Career title: sports medicine assitant
   - **f.** Explanation: Gets athletes moving properly + healing the right way.

There are 16 possible points in this worksheet.

UNIT 4

The Circulatory System

• OBJECTIVES

When you have completed this unit, you will be able to do the following:

- Match vocabulary words with their correct meanings.
- Name the major organs of the circulatory system.
- Label a diagram of the heart and blood vessels.
- Recognize functions of the circulatory system.
- Identify the common disorders of the circulatory system.
- List the parts of the circulatory system through which blood flows.
- Describe how the circulatory system supports life.
- Explain why the health care worker's understanding of the circulatory system is important.

• DIRECTIONS

1. Complete Worksheet 1 before beginning the reading.
2. Read this unit.
3. Complete Worksheets 2 through 5 as assigned.
4. When you are confident that you can meet each objective listed above, ask your instructor for the unit evaluation.

• EVALUATION METHODS

- Worksheets
- Class participation
- Written evaluation

• WORKSHEET 1

Fill in the crossword puzzle using the vocabulary words from Unit 4 in your text (12 points).

▢ Indicates a space between two words.

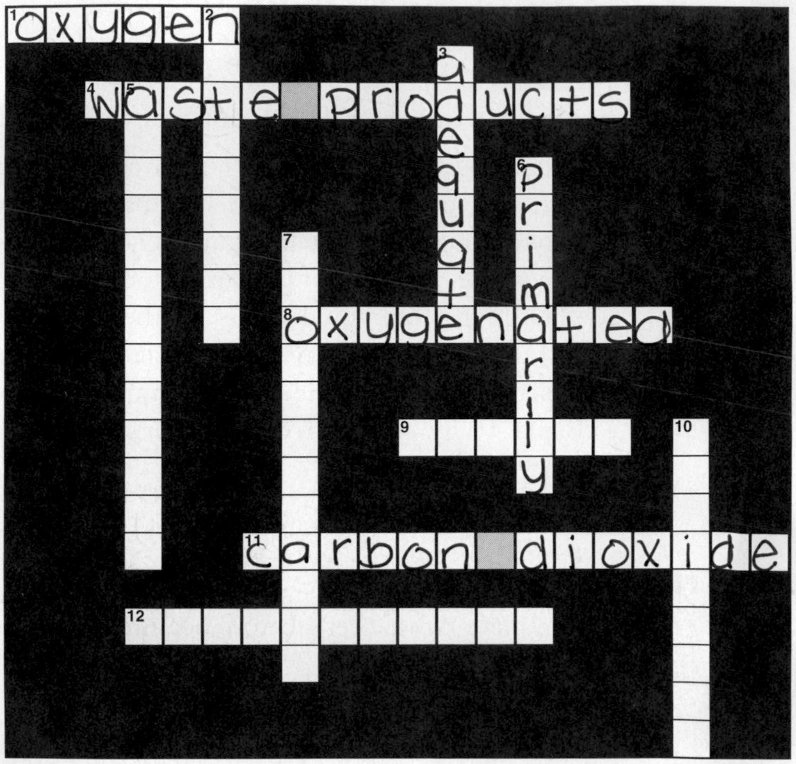

Clues

Across

1. Element in the atmosphere that is essential for maintaining life.
4. Elements that are unfit for the body's use and are eliminated from the body.
8. Containing oxygen.
9. Defective or imperfect.
11. A gas, heavier than air; a waste product from the body.
12. Arms, legs, hands, and feet.

Down

2. Food substances that supply the body with necessary elements for good health.
3. Enough, sufficient.
5. Things that are not usual, that differ from the standard.
6. For the most part; chiefly.
7. Lacking oxygen.
10. Pertaining to old age; over 65 years.

re 12 possible points in this worksheet.

• WORKSHEET 2

Label the parts of the circulatory system on the following diagram (16 points).

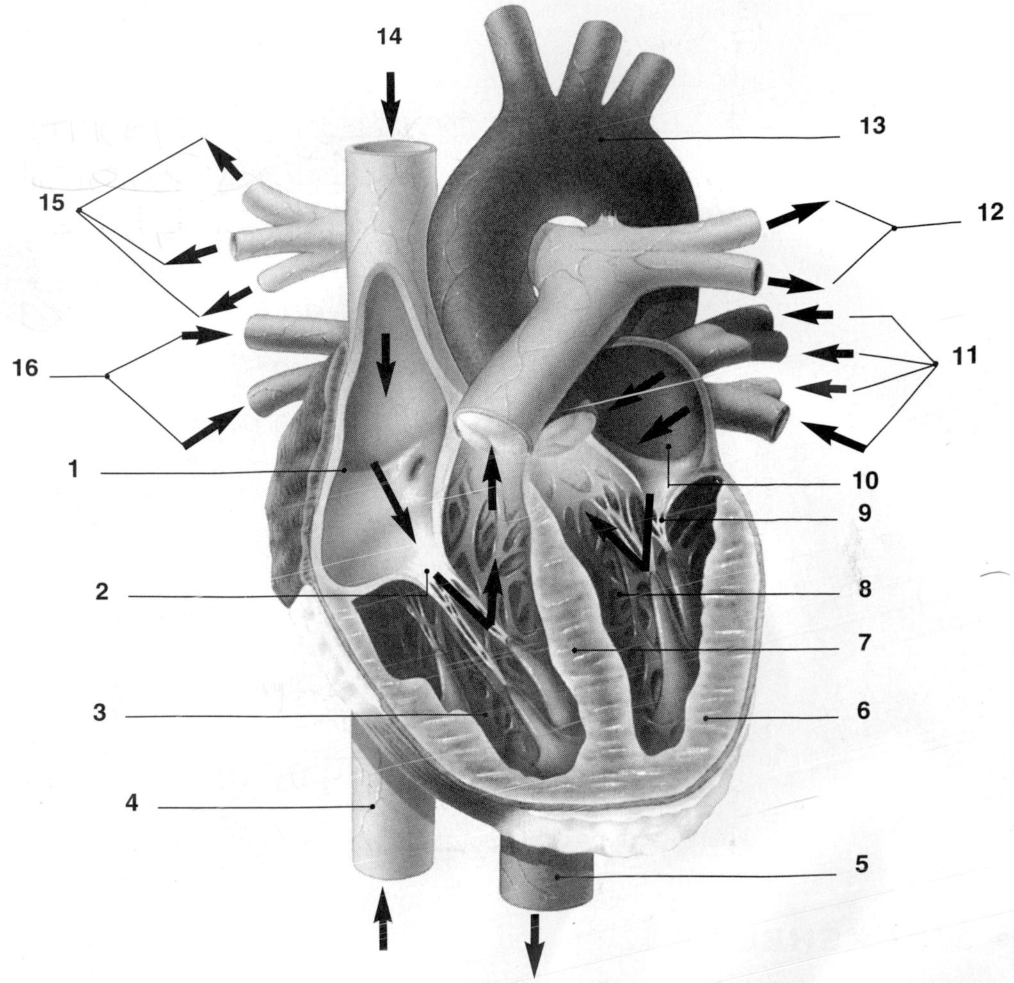

1. right atrium
2. coronary sinus
3. right ventricle
4. inferior vena cava
5. descending aorta
6. apex
7. interventricular ~~spe~~ septum
8. left ventricle
9. bisupsid valve
10. left atrium
11. left pulmonary vein
12. left pulmonary artery
13. aorta
14. superior vena cava
15. right plumonary
16. right plumonary artery

There are 16 possible points in this worksheet.

• WORKSHEET 3

Label the following diagram, indicating the names of vessels and showing the movement of oxygen (O_2) and carbon dioxide (CO_2) in the cells of body organs (5 points).

1. ______________________
2. ______________________
3. ______________________
4. ______________________
5. ______________________

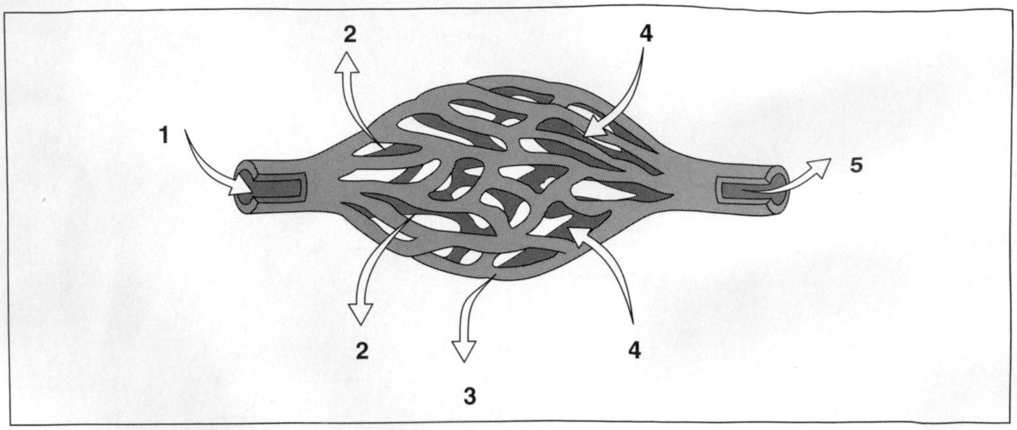

There are 5 possible points in this worksheet.

• WORKSHEET 4

List the parts of the circulatory system through which blood flows. Begin at the right atrium and return to the right atrium (20 points).

1. Right atrium
2. ______________________
3. ______________________
4. ______________________
5. ______________________
6. ______________________
7. ______________________
8. ______________________
9. ______________________
10. ______________________
11. ______________________
12. ______________________
13. ______________________
14. ______________________
15. ______________________
16. ______________________
17. ______________________
18. ______________________
19. ______________________
20. ______________________

There are 20 possible points in this worksheet.

• WORKSHEET 5

1. Describe how the circulatory system supports life (1 point.) ____________

2. Explain why your understanding of the circulatory system is important (1 point). ____________

There are 2 possible points in this worksheet.

UNIT 5

The Lymphatic System

• OBJECTIVES

When you have completed this unit, you will be able to do the following:

- Match vocabulary words with their correct meanings.
- Describe the general functions of the lymphatic system.
- Describe what lymph is.
- Match lymph vessels and organs to their function.
- Explain the difference between an antigen and an antibody.
- Identify common disorders of the lymphatic system.
- Describe how the lymphatic system helps provide immunity.

• DIRECTIONS

1. Complete Worksheet 1 before beginning the reading.
2. Read this unit.
3. Complete Worksheets 2 and 3 as assigned.
4. When you are confident that you can meet each objective listed above, ask your instructor for the unit evaluation.

• EVALUATION METHODS

- Worksheets
- Class participation
- Written evaluation

• WORKSHEET 1

Fill in the crossword puzzle using the vocabulary words and terminology list from Unit 5 in your text (11 points).

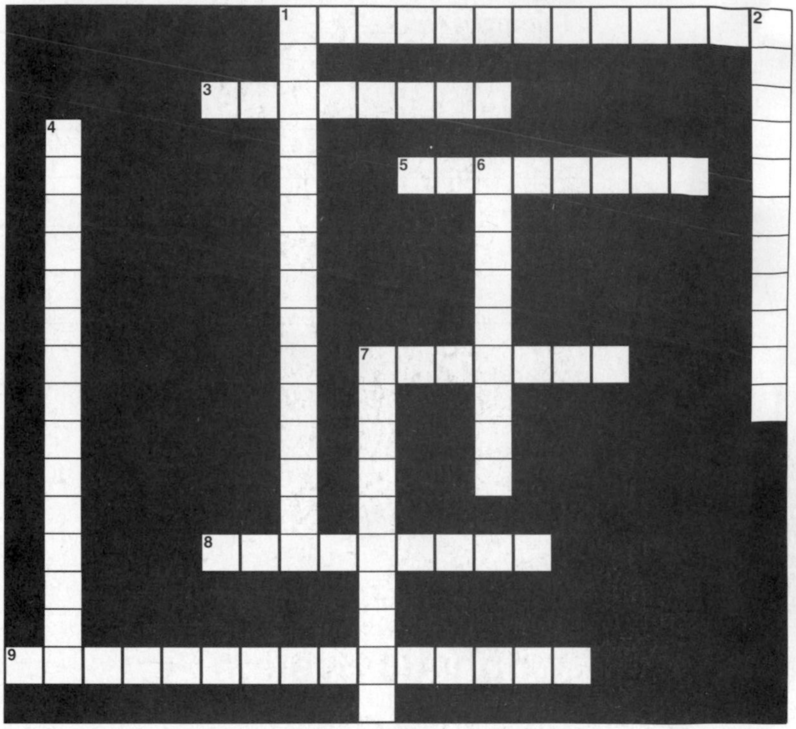

Clues

Across

1. Abnormally high number of lymphocytes in the blood.
3. Tumor made up of lymphatic tissue.
5. Absence of a spleen.
7. Foreign matter that causes the body to produce antibodies.
8. Cell that surrounds, eats, and digests microorganisms.
9. Surgical removal of the lymph nodes.

Down

1. Abnormally low number of lymphocytes in the blood.
2. Surgical removal of the spleen.
4. Enlargement of the lymph nodes.
6. Pertaining to an organism that lives in or on another organism, taking nourishment from it.
7. Substances made by the body to produce immunity to an antigen.

There are 11 possible points in this worksheet.

Laura Zack

• WORKSHEET 2

1. What other system does the lymphatic system work closely with (1 point)?
our defense system

2. What is the main function of the lymphatic system (4 points)?
   a. filters out organisms that cause disease
   b. produces white blood cells
   c. makes antibodies
   d. drains excess fluids+ proteins so that tissue doesn't swell up

3. Name the tissue fluid in the lymphatic system (1 point). ______

4. What does the lymphatic system protect the body against (1 point)?
harmful substances that cause disease

5. List the parts of the lymphatic system (10 points).
   a. lymph capillaries
   b. lymph vessels
   c. lymph nodes
   d. tonsils
   e. spleen
   f. thymus
   g. lacteals
   h. cisterna chyli
   i. thoracic duct
   j. right lymphatic duct

6. Write each word listed below in the space next to the statement that best describes it (8 points).

~~lymph capillaries~~	~~lymph~~	~~tonsils~~
~~thymus~~	~~lymphocytes~~	~~lymph nodes~~
~~lymph vessels~~	~~spleen~~	

spleen a. Help the body defend itself.
lymph nodes b. Lie along the lymph vessels.
capillaries c. Tubes that reach into the interstitial spaces of most body tissues.
~~spleen~~ d. Filters microorganisms and waste products from the blood. lymphocytes
vessels e. Have valves to help move the lymph from the tissues.
lymph f. Tissue fluid that is in a capillary.
thymus g. Stores lymphocytes that work with the lymphatic system to defend the body.
tonsils h. Filter tissue fluid, not lymph.

There are 25 possible points in this worksheet.

• WORKSHEET 3

1. Describe the difference between an antigen and an antibody (1 point).

2. Explain how the lymphatic system helps provide immunity (1 point).

3. Describe how you would have to live if your immune system did not protect you from bacteria (1 point).

There are 3 possible points in this worksheet.

UNIT 6

The Respiratory System

• OBJECTIVES

When you have completed this unit, you will be able to do the following:

- Match vocabulary words with their correct meanings.
- Label major organs of the respiratory system on a diagram.
- Describe the flow of oxygen through the body.
- Identify common disorders of the respiratory system.
- Describe how the respiratory system supports life.
- Explain why the health care worker's understanding of the respiratory system is important.

• DIRECTIONS

1. Complete Worksheet 1 before beginning the reading.
2. Read this unit.
3. Complete Worksheets 2 through 4 as assigned.
4. When you are confident that you can meet each objective listed above, ask your instructor for the unit evaluation.

• EVALUATION METHODS

- Worksheets
- Class participation
- Written evaluation

• WORKSHEET 1

Fill in the crossword puzzle using the vocabulary words and terminology list from Unit 6 in your text (21 points).

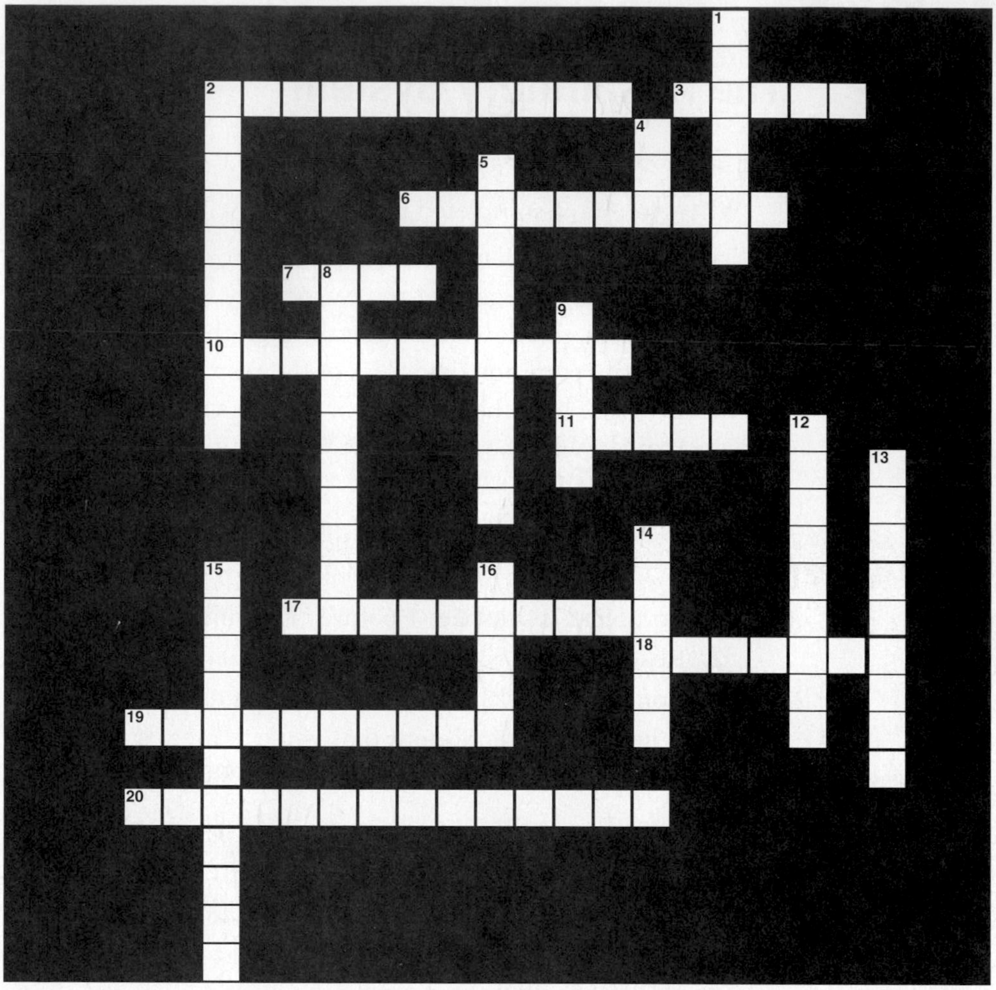

Clues

Across

2. Getting rid of.
3. Cessation of breathing.
6. Inflammation of the bronchial tubes.
7. Abbreviation for "eye, ear, nose, throat."
10. Process of breathing in air during respiration (see also 18).
11. Hairlike projections that move rhythmically on the inside lining of the bronchial tubes.
17. Process of breathing in air during respiration (see also 11).
18. Difficult or painful breathing.
19. Inflammation of the larynx.
20. Dilation of the bronchi.

Down

1. Lack of oxygen.
2. Process of forcing air out of the body during respiration (see also 9).
4. Abbreviation for "upper respiratory infection."
5. Things that contaminate the air.
8. Process of forcing air out of the body during respiration (see also 2).
9. Small bag or sac.
12. Rapid breathing.
13. Nosebleed.
14. To cause to be or become.
15. Between the ribs.
16. Nostrils.

There are 21 possible points in this worksheet.

• WORKSHEET 2

1. Label the parts of the respiratory system on the following diagram (10 points).

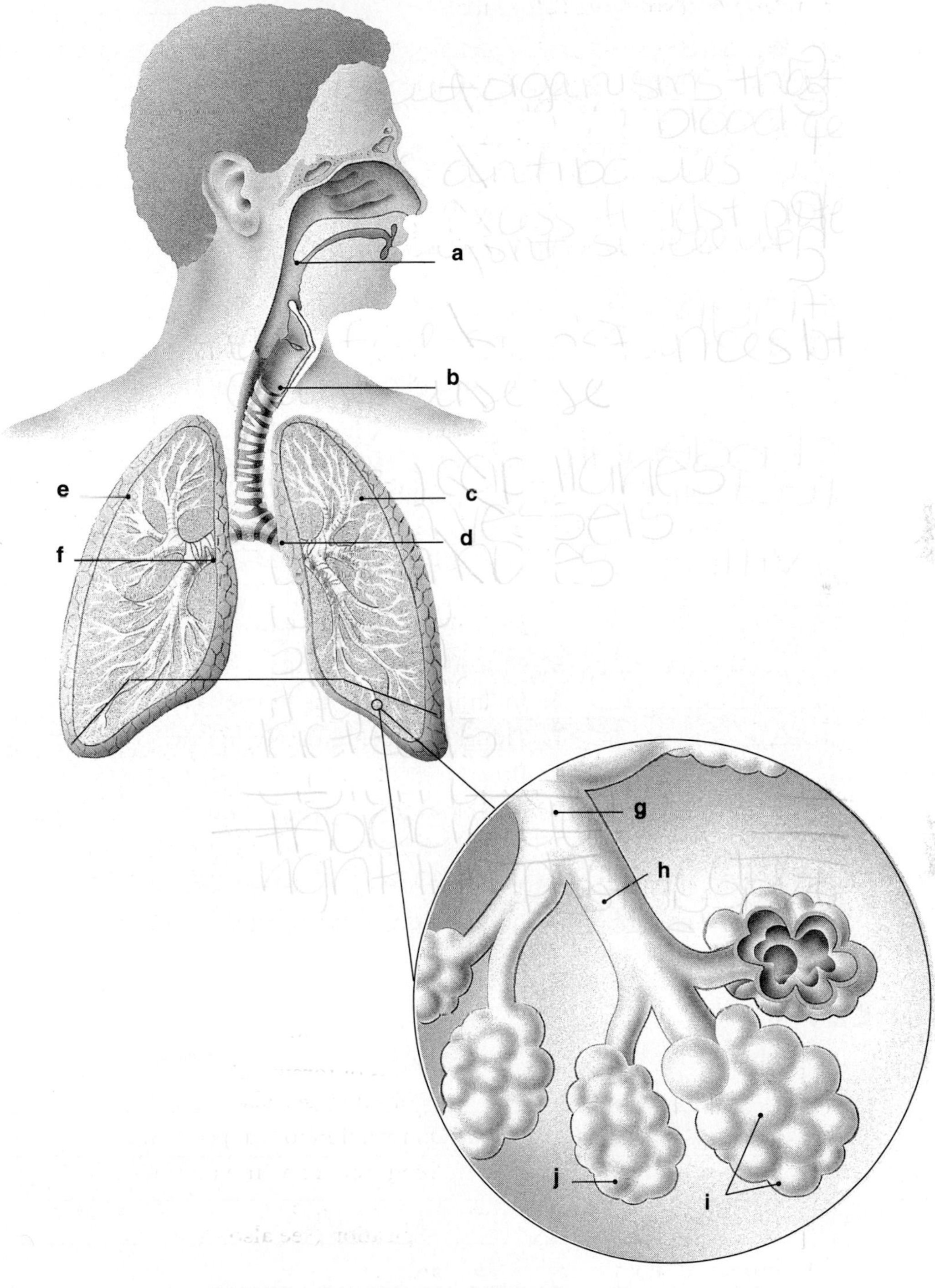

a. ______________	f. ______________
b. ______________	g. ______________
c. ______________	h. ______________
d. ______________	i. ______________
e. ______________	j. ______________

2. Describe the flow of oxygen through the body, starting with the nose or mouth and ending at the cell (10 points).

a.	nose or mouth	f.	________________
b.	________________	g.	________________
c.	________________	h.	________________
d.	________________	i.	________________
e.	________________	j.	________________

There are 20 possible points in this worksheet.

• WORKSHEET 3

Write the appropriate word for each of the following definitions (10 points).

________________ 1. Condition in which the alveoli become stretched and unable to force carbon dioxide out of the lungs.

________________ 2. Essential life-giving element.

________________ 3. Process of forcing air out of the body during respiration.

________________ 4. Condition in which the walls of the bronchial tubes become narrow and less air passes through.

________________ 5. Gaseous waste product of the cell.

________________ 6. Inflammation of the lungs.

________________ 7. Things that contaminate the air.

________________ 8. Breathing.

________________ 9. Infectious disease caused by the tubercle bacillus.

________________ 10. Process of breathing in air during respiration.

There are 10 possible points in this worksheet.

• WORKSHEET 4

1. Describe how the respiratory system supports life (1 point). __________

____

____

____

____

____

____

____

2. Explain why your understanding of the respiratory system is important (1 point). ____

____

____

____

____

____

____

____

There are 2 possible points in this worksheet.

UNIT 7 The Digestive System

• OBJECTIVES

When you have completed this unit, you will be able to do the following:

- Match vocabulary words with their correct meanings.
- Label a diagram of the digestive system and its accessory organs.
- Explain the functions of the digestive system.
- Recognize the function of organs associated with the digestive system.
- Match common disorders of the digestive system with their descriptions.
- Describe how the digestive system absorbs nutrients.
- Explain why the health care worker's understanding of the digestive system is important.

• DIRECTIONS

1. Complete Worksheet 1 before beginning the reading.
2. Read this unit.
3. Complete Worksheets 2 through 5 as assigned.
4. When you are confident that you can meet each objective listed above, ask your instructor for the unit evaluation.

• EVALUATION METHODS

- Worksheets
- Class participation
- Written evaluation

• WORKSHEET 1

Match each definition in column B with the correct vocabulary word in column A (9 points).

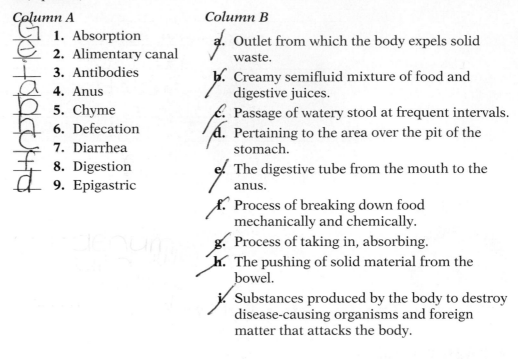

Column A	*Column B*
g 1. Absorption	a. Outlet from which the body expels solid waste.
e 2. Alimentary canal	b. Creamy semifluid mixture of food and digestive juices.
i 3. Antibodies	c. Passage of watery stool at frequent intervals.
a 4. Anus	d. Pertaining to the area over the pit of the stomach.
b 5. Chyme	e. The digestive tube from the mouth to the anus.
h 6. Defecation	f. Process of breaking down food mechanically and chemically.
c 7. Diarrhea	g. Process of taking in, absorbing.
f 8. Digestion	h. The pushing of solid material from the bowel.
d 9. Epigastric	i. Substances produced by the body to destroy disease-causing organisms and foreign matter that attacks the body.

Write each word listed below in the space next to the statement that best defines it (8 points).

liver	evacuated	insulin
minute (adj.)	feces	sphincter
peristalsis	secrete	

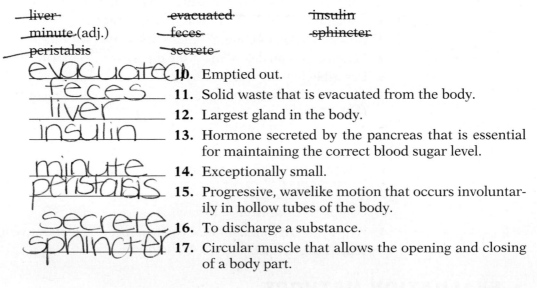

evacuated 10. Emptied out.

feces 11. Solid waste that is evacuated from the body.

liver 12. Largest gland in the body.

insulin 13. Hormone secreted by the pancreas that is essential for maintaining the correct blood sugar level.

minute 14. Exceptionally small.

peristalsis 15. Progressive, wavelike motion that occurs involuntarily in hollow tubes of the body.

secrete 16. To discharge a substance.

sphincter 17. Circular muscle that allows the opening and closing of a body part.

There are 17 possible points in this worksheet.

• WORKSHEET 2

Label the parts of the digestive system on the following diagram (23 points).

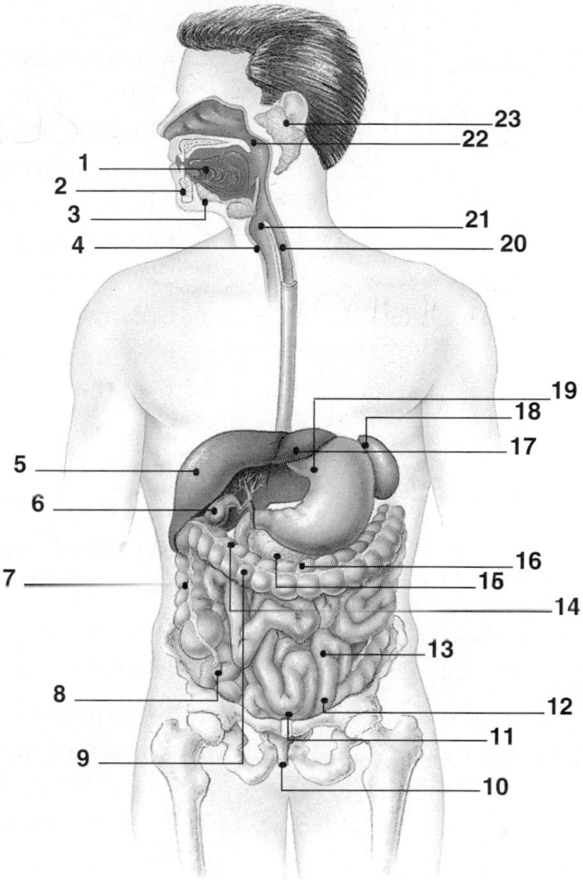

1. tongue
2. teeth
3. sublingual gland
4. trachea
5. liver
6. gallbladder
7. ascending colon
8. appendix
9. large colon
10. anus
11. rectum
12. sigmoid colon
13. small intestine
14. duodenum
15. pyloric sphincter
16. pancreas
17. cardiac sphincter
18. spleen
19. stomach
20. esophagus
21. larynx
22. pharynx
23. parotid gland

There are 23 possible points in this worksheet.

• WORKSHEET 3

Write the appropriate word next to each of the following statements (24 points).

__________ **1.** Process of changing food into a usable substance by the body.

__________ **2.** A passageway for food located at the back of the oral cavity.

peristalsis **3.** Rhythmic wavelike motion.

__________ **4.** Produces secretions that dissolve food and coat food with mucus.

__________ **5.** Long muscular tube that begins at the mouth and ends at the anus.

chyme **6.** Creamy semifluid mixture of food and digestive juices.

__________ **7.** Flap that covers the trachea.

__________ **8.** Where food enters the body.

duodenum **9.** First 10 to 12 inches of the small intestine.

rectum **10.** Last 6 to 8 inches of the alimentary canal.

__________ **11.** Receives food and water from the pharynx.

villi **12.** Minute projections that line the small intestine.

__________ **13.** Is attached to the small intestine and absorbs water.

__________ **14.** Ringlike muscle found at the far end of the stomach.

__________ **15.** Receives food and water from the esophagus.

__________ **16.** Portion of the alimentary canal where most absorption takes place.

__________ **17.** End of the alimentary canal.

__________ **18.** Produces pancreatic juices.

__________ **19.** Produces bile, heparin, and antibodies.

__________ **20.** Sac that stores bile.

__________ **21.** Condition that occurs when the cells of the liver become damaged.

__________ **22.** Inflammation of the pancreas.

__________ **23.** Inflammation of the liver.

__________ **24.** Presence of a stone in the gallbladder.

There are 24 possible points in this worksheet.

• WORKSHEET 4

1. Describe how the digestive system absorbs nutrients (1 point).__________

____

____

____

____

____

____

2. Explain why your understanding of the digestive system is important (1 point). ____

____

____

____

____

____

____

____

There are 2 possible points in this worksheet.

• WORKSHEET 5

Fill in the crossword puzzle using the terminology list from Unit 7 in your text (16 points).

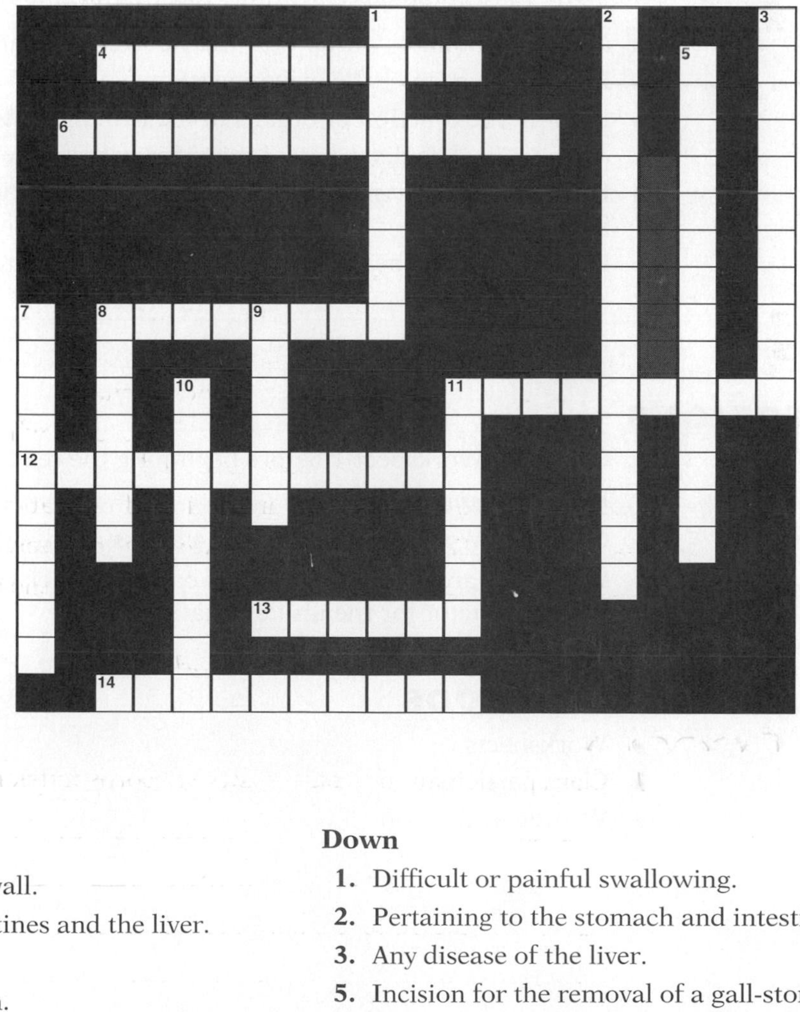

Clues

Across

4. Cyst of the intestinal wall.
6. Pertaining to the intestines and the liver.
8. Lack of appetite.
11. Opening into the colon.

Down

1. Difficult or painful swallowing.
2. Pertaining to the stomach and intestines.
3. Any disease of the liver.
5. Incision for the removal of a gall-stone.

12. Pertaining to the cheek and tongue.
13. Vomiting.
14. Hernia involving the intestine.

7. Process by which food is changed into energy for the body's use.
8. Without acid.
9. Substance that induces vomiting.
10. Gallbladder.
11. Inflammation of the colon.

There are 16 possible points in this worksheet.

UNIT 8 The Urinary System

• OBJECTIVES

When you have completed this unit, you will be able to do the following:

- Match vocabulary words with their correct meanings.
- Label a diagram of the urinary system.
- Identify the function of organs in the urinary system.
- Match common disorders of the urinary system with their descriptions.
- Describe how the urinary system removes liquid waste and eliminates it from the body.
- Explain why the health care worker's understanding of the urinary system is important.

• DIRECTIONS

1. Complete Worksheet 1 before beginning the reading.
2. Read this unit.
3. Complete Worksheets 2 through 4 as assigned.
4. When you are confident that you can meet each objective listed above, ask your instructor for the unit evaluation.

• EVALUATION METHODS

- Worksheets
- Class participation
- Written evaluation

• WORKSHEET 1

1. Define the following vocabulary words. Look in a medical dictionary for words that are not in your glossary (7 points).

   a. Nephron ______________________________

   b. Hemodialysis ______________________________

   c. Micturition ______________________________

   d. Urination______________________________

   e. Peritoneal cavity ______________________________

   f. Excrete______________________________

   g. Mechanism ______________________________

2. Write each word listed below in the space next to the statement that best defines it. Look in a medical dictionary (7 points).

waste product	dialysis	obstruction	edema
elimination	symptom	infuses	

   ______________ a. Any change in the body or its functions that indicates a disease.

   ______________ b. Flows into the body by gravity.

   ______________ c. Process of removing waste from body fluids.

   ______________ d. Process of getting rid of something.

   ______________ e. Blockage or clogging.

   ______________ f. Material that is unfit for the body's use and is eliminated from the body.

   ______________ g. Abnormal or excessive collection of fluid in the tissues.

There are 14 possible points in this worksheet.

• WORKSHEET 2

Label the parts of the urinary system on the following diagram (12 points).

1.	______________	7.	______________
2.	______________	8.	______________
3.	______________	9.	______________
4.	______________	10.	______________
5.	______________	11.	______________
6.	______________	12.	______________

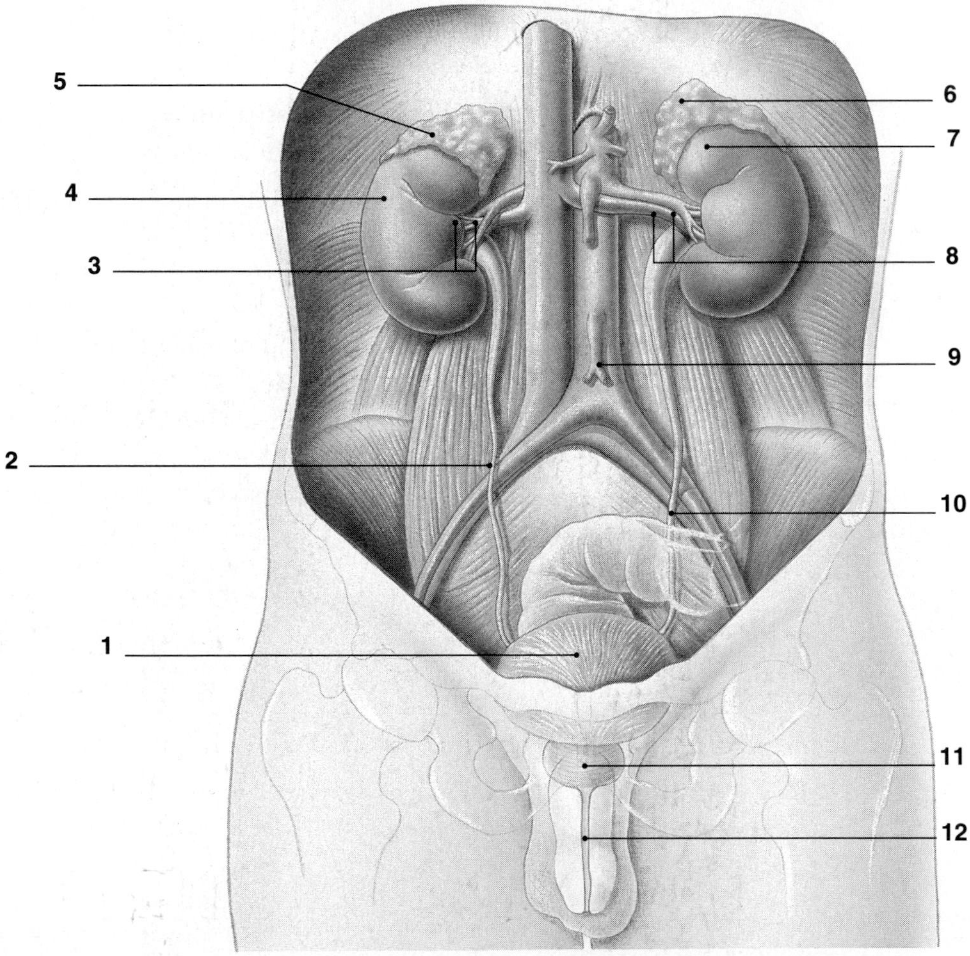

There are 12 possible points in this worksheet.

• WORKSHEET 3

Write the appropriate word next to each of the following statements (15 points).

urine 1. Liquid waste product of the body.
medulla 2. Inner part of the kidney.
nephritis 3. Inflammation of the kidney.
calculi 4. Kidney stones.
capsule 5. Sac surrounding the kidney.
edema 6. Abnormal or excessive collection of fluid in the tissue.
_______ 7. Inflammation of the urethra.
nephron 8. Chief filtering mechanism of the kidney.
Bowman's capsule 9. Cuplike capsule.
cystitis 10. Inflammation of the urinary bladder.
convoluted tubule 11. Tiny twisted tube of the nephron.
uremia 12. Accumulation of urine substances in the blood.
dialysis 13. Common treatment for kidney failure.
hydronephrosis 14. Expanded renal pelvis.
kidney or renal failure 15. Condition in which the nephron of the kidney is unable to filter waste.

There are 15 possible points for this worksheet.

• WORKSHEET 4

1. Describe how the urinary system removes liquid waste and eliminates it from the body (1 point). The nephron filters the waste, then the ureters carry urine from the kidneys to the urinary bladder. The uretha carries the urine outside of the body.

2. Explain why your understanding of the urinary system is important (1 point). That way if patients are having a problem going to the bathroom they can locate the problem or the source.

There are 2 possible points in this worksheet.

UNIT 9

The Glandular Systems

• OBJECTIVES

When you have completed this unit, you will be able to do the following:

- Match vocabulary words with their correct meanings.
- Label endocrine glands on a diagram.
- Identify the function of the endocrine glands.
- Identify common disorders of the endocrine glands.
- Explain the difference between the endocrine and exocrine glands.
- Describe the effects of the endocrine glands on the body.
- Explain why the health care worker's understanding of the glandular systems is important.

• DIRECTIONS

1. Complete Worksheet 1 before beginning the reading.
2. Read this unit.
3. Complete Worksheets 2 through 4 as assigned.
4. When you are confident that you can meet each objective listed above, ask your instructor for the unit evaluation.

• EVALUATION METHOD

- Worksheets
- Class participation
- Written evaluation

• WORKSHEET 1

Match each definition in column B to the correct vocabulary word in column A (6 points).

Column A

a 1. Duct
e 2. Hormone
d 3. Lacrimal
f 4. Sebaceous
b 5. Excrete
c 6. Metabolism

Column B

a. Narrow, round tube that carries secretions from a gland.
b. Throw off or eliminate as waste product.
c. Body's process of using food to make energy and use nutrients.
d. Pertaining to tears.
e. Protein substance secreted by an endocrine gland directly into the blood.
f. Pertaining to fatty secretions.

There are 6 possible points in this worksheet.

• WORKSHEET 2

Label the parts of the glandular system on the following diagram (9 points).

1. pineal
2. pituitary
3. parathyroids
4. thyroid
5. thymus
6. pancreas
7. adenals
8. ovanes
9. testes

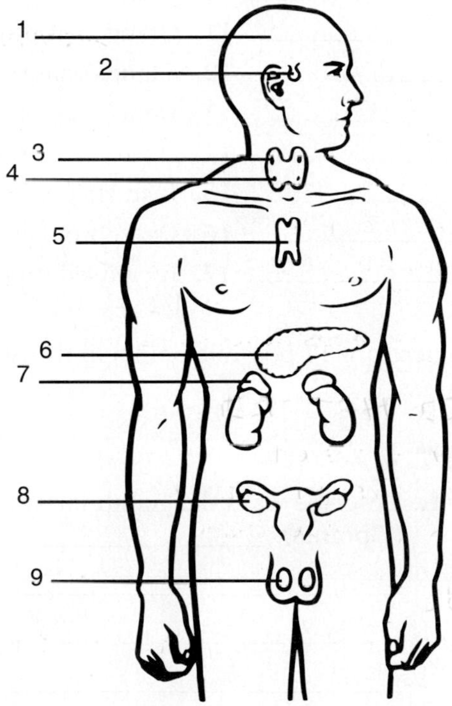

There are 9 possible points in this worksheet.

• WORKSHEET 3

Write the appropriate word next to each of the following statements (17 points).

_______________ 1. Fluids that are carried to a nearby organ or to the outside of the body.

_______________ 2. Glands that have ducts.

_______________ 3. Gland that produces thyroxin.

_______________ 4. Hormones that are carried to all parts of the body through the blood and lymph systems.

_______________ 5. Gland that produces adrenalin.

_______________ 6. Glands without ducts.

_______________ 7. Gland that produces parathyroid hormones.

_______________ 8. Gland that produces TSH, ACTH, FSH, LH, oxytocin, prolactin, and somatotropic hormones.

_______________ 9. Gland that produces insulin.

_______________ 10. Glands that produce estrogen and progesterone.

_______________ 11. Gland that produces corticoids.

_______________ 12. Glands that produce testosterone.

_______________ 13. Deficiency of sugar in the blood.

_______________ 14. Decreased production of the thyroid secretion.

_______________ 15. Insufficient amount of hormones from the adrenal glands.

_______________ 16. Overabundance of sugar in the blood.

_______________ 17. Increased production of the thyroid secretion.

There are 17 possible points in this worksheet.

• WORKSHEET 4

1. Describe ways the glandular systems help regulate body processes (7 points). ____

____

____

____

____

2. Explain why your understanding of the glandular systems is important (1 point). ____

____

____

____

____

There are 8 possible points in this worksheet.

UNIT 10

The Nervous System

• OBJECTIVES

When you have completed this unit, you will be able to do the following:

- Match vocabulary words with their correct meanings.
- Match and select the functions of various parts of the nervous system.
- Label diagrams of the eye and ear.
- Match common disorders of the nervous system with their correct names.
- Describe the influence of the nervous system on the body.
- Explain why the health care worker's understanding of the nervous system is important.

• DIRECTIONS

1. Complete Worksheet 1 before beginning reading.
2. Read this unit.
3. Complete Worksheets 2 through 6 as assigned.
4. When you are confident that you can meet each objective listed above, ask your instructor for the unit evaluation.

• EVALUATION METHODS

- Worksheets
- Class participation
- Written evaluation

• WORKSHEET 1

Write the appropriate word next to each of the following statements (5 points).

amplify 1. To increase or elevate a sound.

equilibrium 2. State of balance.

ossicles 3. Three small bones in the middle ear that amplify sound.

neuron 4. Nerve; includes the cell and the long fiber coming from the cell.

Stimuli 5. Elements in the external or internal environment that are strong enough to set up a nervous impulse.

Match each definition in column B with the correct vocabulary word in column A (9 points).

Column A	*Column B*
e 6. Cerebrum	a. Colored
g 7. Peripheral	b. Nerve that responds to stimuli.
h 8. CNS	c. Spreading in many directions; dispersing.
f 9. Ganglia	d. Action or movement due to a stimulus.
a 10. Pigmented	e. Portion of the brain that controls voluntary movements.
b 11. Receptor	f. Mass of nerve tissue composed of nerve cell bodies.
d 12. Response	g. Situated away from a central structure.
c 13. Scattering	h. Central nervous system.
i 14. Translate	i. To make understandable.

There are 14 possible points in this worksheet.

• WORKSHEET 2

Complete the following sentences.

1. The central nervous system includes the (a) brain and the (b) spinal cord (2 points).
2. The peripheral nervous system includes the (a) nerves and (b) ganglia outside the brain and spinal cord (2 points).
3. The nervous system is a system of nerve cells linked together to (a) receive stimuli and (b) respond to stimuli (2 points).
4. The nervous system works together in relay messages to the brain (1 point).
5. Each specialized neuron leads into a passage that delivers the message or stimuli to the areas in the brain that can (a) action and cause a (b) response (2 points).

There are 9 possible points in this worksheet.

• WORKSHEET 3

1. Label the parts of the eye on the following diagram (10 points).

a. ______________________ f. ______________________

b. ______________________ g. ______________________

c. ______________________ h. ______________________

d. ______________________ i. ______________________

e. ______________________ j. ______________________

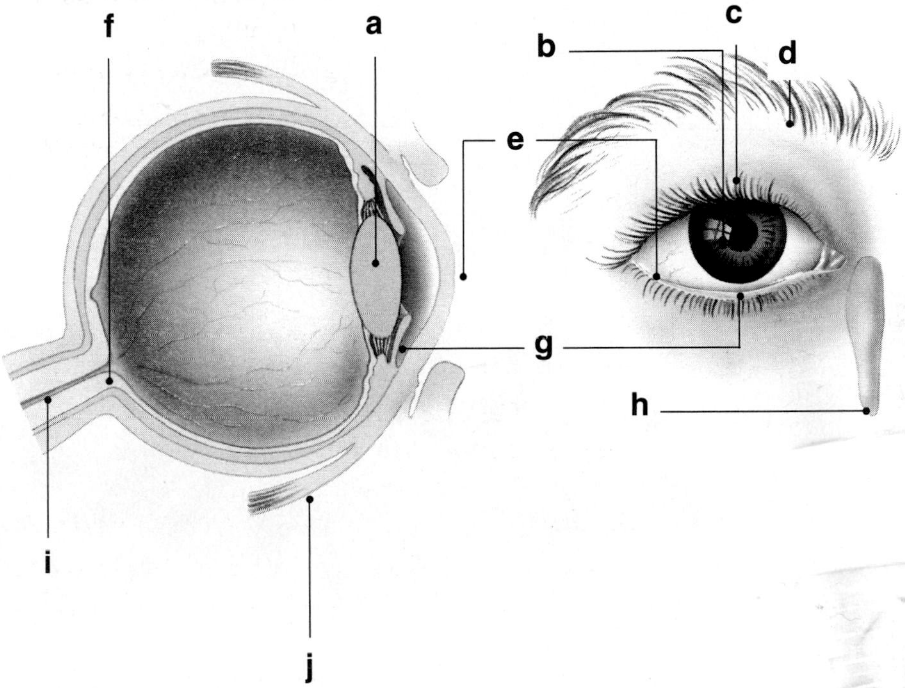

2. List three things that protect the eye (3 points).

a. ______________________

b. ______________________

c. ______________________

3. The white of the eye is the ________________ (1 point).

4. The heavily pigmented second coating of the eye is the ________________ (1 point).

5. The clear front portion of the sclera is the ________________ (1 point).

6. The innermost coating of the eye, which senses vision, is the ________________ (1 point).

7. The nerve that receives a picture and sends it to the brain for interpretation is the ________________ (1 point).

There are 18 possible points in this worksheet.

• WORKSHEET 4

1. Label the parts of the ear on the following diagram (11 points).

a. ______________________ g. ______________________
b. ______________________ h. ______________________
c. ______________________ i. ______________________
d. ______________________ j. ______________________
e. ______________________ k. ______________________
f. ______________________

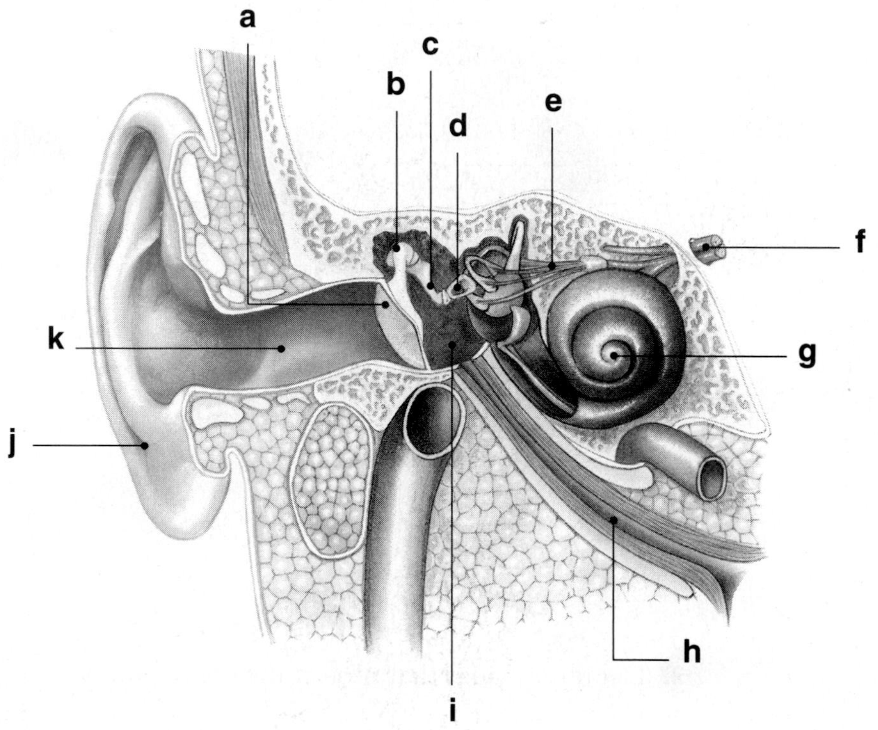

2. Name the three main parts of the ear (3 points).

a. ______________________
b. ______________________
c. ______________________

3. The middle ear contains (a) ________________ [number] bones called (b) ________________ (2 points).

4. The semicircular canals of the inner ear (a) ________________ sound waves to the (b) ________________ that allow us to (c) ________________ sound (3 points).

There are 19 possible points in this worksheet.

• WORKSHEET 5

1. Taste is sensed by receptors called receptors (1 point).
2. Name the four main tastes (4 points).
   a. Sweet c. Salty
   b. Sour d. bitter
3. The receptor that receives smells is called the olfactory epithelium (1 point).
4. Our special senses of sight, hearing, taste, and smell are limited to certain areas of the body. List the four general senses that are found throughout the body (4 points).
   a. pressure c. touch
   b. temperature d. Pain
5. Write the appropriate word for each of the following definitions (6 points).
   Glaucoma a. Clouding of the lens of the eye.
   Shingles b. Condition in which blisters appear on the nerves and cause a great deal of pain.
   otosclerosis c. Condition that causes deafness because the bones in the ear change.
   neuritis d. Inflammation of a nerve.
   conjunctivitis e. Inflammation of the eyelid lining.
   Cataract f. Condition that can cause deterioration of the optic nerve.

There are 16 possible points in this worksheet.

• WORKSHEET 6

1. Describe the influence of the nervous system on the body (7 points).
   The nervous system helps control the body. It lets us know if things are hot. It helps us move + get around better.
2. Explain why your understanding of the nervous system is important (1 point). Its important because you can then figure things out if a problem ar...

There are 8 possible points in this workshe...

UNIT 11

The Reproductive System

• OBJECTIVES

When you have completed this unit, you will be able to do the following:

- Match vocabulary words with their correct meanings.
- Label a diagram of the male and female reproductive systems.
- Match the various organs in the reproductive systems with their functions.
- Match common disorders of the reproductive system with their descriptions.
- Describe how the reproductive system affects the body.
- Explain why the health care worker's understanding of the reproductive system is important.

• DIRECTIONS

1. Complete Worksheet 1 before beginning the reading.
2. Read this unit.
3. Complete Worksheets 2 through 5 as assigned.
4. When you are confident that you can meet each objective listed above, ask your instructor for the unit evaluation.

• EVALUATION METHODS

- Worksheets
- Class participation
- Written evaluation

• WORKSHEET 1

Match each definition in column B with the correct vocabulary word in column A (7 points).

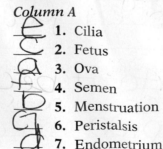

Column A

e 1. Cilia
c 2. Fetus
a 3. Ova
f 4. Semen
b 5. Menstruation
g 6. Peristalsis
d 7. Endometrium

Column B

a. Female reproductive cells that, when fertilized by the male, develop into a new organism.
b. Cyclic deterioration of the endometrium.
c. Infant developing in the uterus after the first three months until birth.
d. Interlining of the uterus.
e. Hairlike projections that move rhythmically.
f. Fluid from the testes, seminal vesicles, prostate gland, and bulbourethral glands that contains water, mucin, proteins, salts, and sperm.
g. Progressive, wavelike movement that occurs involuntarily in hollow tubes of the body.

Define the following words (6 points).

8. Estrogen female hormone
9. Mature becomes fully developed
10. Sex cell cells that allow reproduction to occur
11. Testosterone male hormone
12. Spermatozoa male sex cells
13. Projections ______

There are 13 possible points in this worksheet.

• WORKSHEET 2

1. Label the parts of the female reproductive system on the following diagram (10 points).

a. fundus of uterus
b. ovary
c. fallopian tube
d. ovum
e. sperm cell
f. broad ligament
g. uterus
h. cervix
i. vagina
j. bartholin's gland

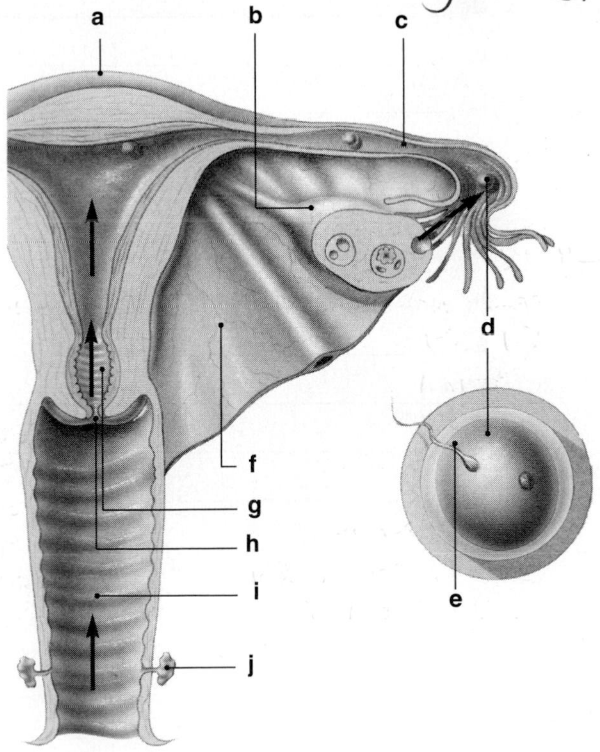

2. Write each organ listed below in the space next to the statement that best defines its function (5 points).

ovaries	fallopian tubes	fimbriae
uterus	vagina	

_____________ a. Houses and nourishes the fertilized ovum.

_____________ b. Houses the neck of the uterus and is known as the birth canal.

_____________ c. Produce ova and estrogen.

_____________ d. Function as passageways through which ova travel into the uterus.

_____________ e. Create a current that sweeps the ovum into the fallopian tube.

There are 15 possible points in this worksheet.

• WORKSHEET 3

1. Label the parts of the male reproductive system on the following diagram (14 points).

a. ____________________

b. ____________________

c. ____________________

d. ____________________

e. ____________________

f. ____________________

g. ____________________

h. ____________________

i. ____________________

j. ____________________

k. ____________________

l. ____________________

m. ____________________

n. ____________________

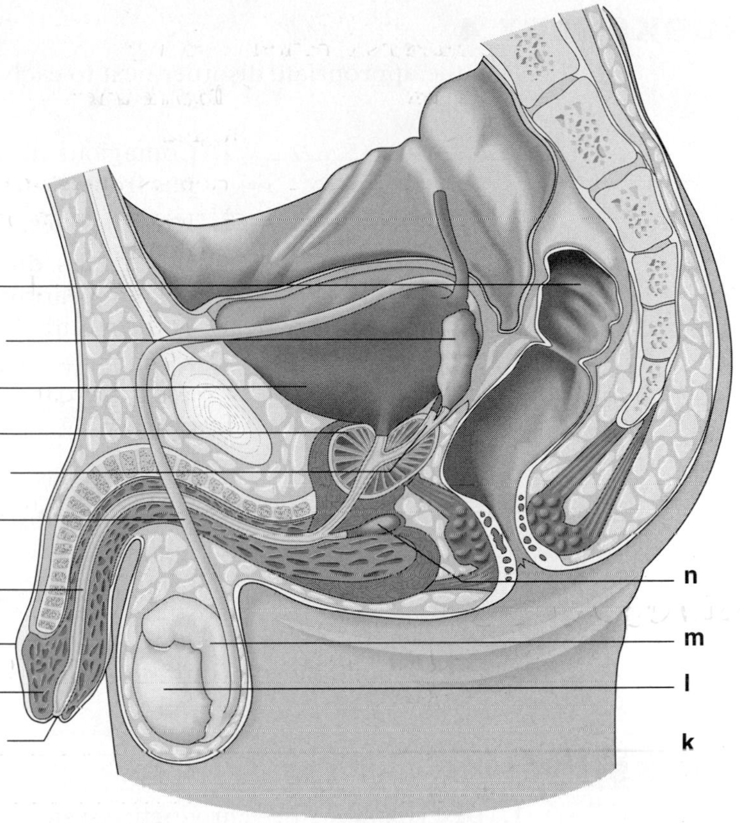

2. Write each organ listed below in the space next to the statement that best defines its function (6 points).

testes	epididymis	vas deferens
seminal vesicles	prostate gland	urethra

_______________ **a.** Produce a thick yellow secretion that adds to the volume of semen and nourishes the sperm.

_______________ **b.** Functions as a passageway for sperm.

_______________ **c.** Produces a secretion that maintains the mobility of sperm.

_______________ **d.** Serves as a passageway for sperm and urine.

_______________ **e.** Stores sperm until they mature.

_______________ **f.** Produce spermatozoa and testosterone.

There are 20 possible points in this worksheet.

• WORKSHEET 4

Write the appropriate disorder next to each of the following descriptions (8 points).

________________ 1. Contagious disease characterized by a discharge of pus from the urethra.

________________ 2. Hidden testes.

________________ 3. Contagious disease characterized by recurrent lesions appearing in the genital region and the mucosa of the mouth.

________________ 4. Nonbloody vaginal discharge usually caused by an infection.

________________ 5. Tightness of the foreskin.

________________ 6. Tumors in women that are usually benign.

________________ 7. Contagious disease characterized by lesions that may not appear for months.

________________ 8. Inflammation of the testes.

There are 8 possible points in this worksheet.

• WORKSHEET 5

1. Describe how the reproductive system affects the body (3 points).

____

____

____

____

____

____

____

2. Explain why your understanding of the reproductive system is important (1 point).

____

____

____

____

____

____

There are 4 possible points in this worksheet.

UNIT 12

The Integumentary System

• OBJECTIVES

When you have completed this unit, you will be able to do the following:

- Match vocabulary words with their correct meanings.
- Label a diagram of a cross section of skin.
- List the five main functions of skin.
- Identify three main layers of the skin.
- Match common disorders of the integumentary system with their descriptions.
- Describe how the integumentary system protects the body.
- Explain why the health care worker's understanding of the integumentary system is important.

• DIRECTIONS

1. Read this unit.
2. Complete Worksheets 1 and 2 as assigned.
3. Prepare responses to each item listed in the Chapter Review—Your Link to Success at the end of this chapter.
4. When you are confident that you can meet each objective listed above, ask your instructor for the unit evaluation.

• EVALUATION METHODS

- Worksheets
- Class participation
- Written evaluation

• WORKSHEET 1

1. Write each word listed below in the space next to the statement that best defines it (3 points).

epidermis sloughed subcutaneous

_______________ **a.** Under the skin.
_______________ **b.** Outer layer of skin.
_______________ **c.** Discarded; separated from.

2. Label the parts of the cross section of skin on the following diagram (14 points).

a. hair shaft
b. epidermis
c. dermis
d. subcutaneous fatty tissue
e. sweat gland
f. muscle
g. fatty lobule
h. deep fascia
i. artery
j. vein
k. hair root
l. nerve ending
m. sebaceous oil gland
n. sweat pore

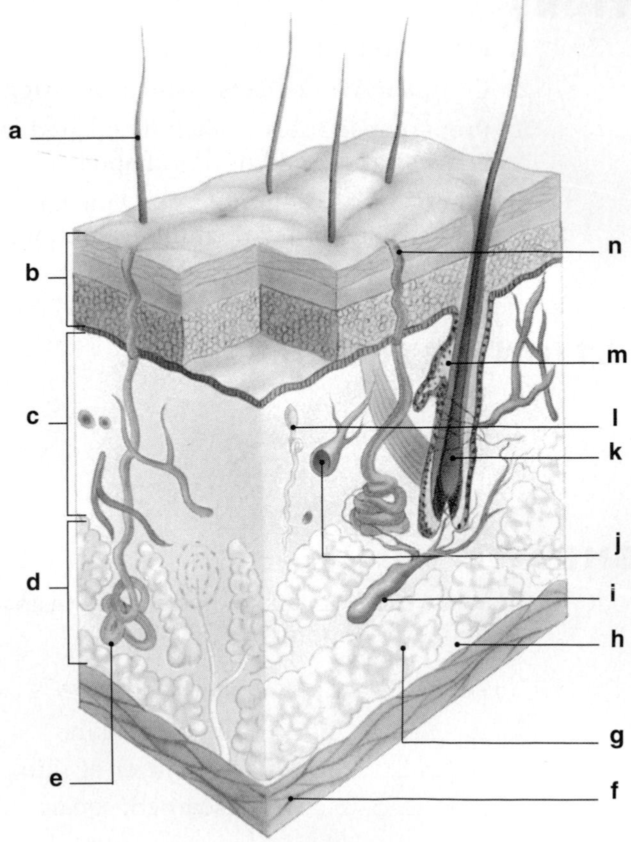

There are 17 possible points in this worksheet.

• WORKSHEET 2

1. Name the two kinds of glands that are present in the skin (2 points).

   a. sweat gland

   b. sebaceous gland

2. Name the kinds of tissues found in the skin (3 points).

   a. muscle

   b. dermis

   c. epidermis

3. List the five main functions of the skin (5 points).

   a. ______

   b. ______

   c. ______

   d. ______

   e. ______

4. List the three main layers of tissue (3 points).

   a. ______

   b. ______

   c. ______

5. Write the appropriate word next to each of the following statements (10 points).

   ______ a. Caused by a fungus; usually involves the toes and soles of the feet.

   ______ b. Refers to any skin condition.

   ______ c. Caused by bacteria entering the hair follicles or sebaceous glands.

   ______ d. Appears as itchy, reddened areas on the surface of the skin.

   ______ e. Waxlike in appearance.

   ______ f. Inflammation of the sebaceous gland.

   ______ g. Scaly skin.

   ______ h. Baldness.

   ______ i. Hives.

   ______ j. Hardened, thickened skin.

ere are 23 possible points in this worksheet.

Chapter 9 Human Growth and Development

UNIT 1

Development and Behavior

• OBJECTIVES

When you have completed this unit, you will be able to do the following:

- Match vocabulary words with their correct meanings.
- Identify three stages of development betwen conception and birth.
- List four common developments of growt in the first year of life and the age at which they usually occur.
- Define and describe characteristics of adlescent development.
- Interview a person between the ages of 5 and 80.
- Compare and contrast your life experienes to each stage described in this unit.
- Design a bulletin board representing oe stage of growth and development, including age-specific communicatio requirements.

• DIRECTIONS

1. Comp Worksheet 1 before reading this unit.
   is unit.
2. Rplete Worksheet 2 as assigned.
3. omplete Worksheets/Activities 3 through 6 as assigned.
4. When you are confident that you can meet each objectives listed abo your instructor for the unit evaluation.

• EVALUATION METHODS

- Worksheets/Activities
- Class participation
- Written evaluation

• WORKSHEET 1

Match each definition in column B with the correct vocabulary word in column A (11 points).

Column A	*Column B*
____ **1.** Adolescent	**a.** Lying on the stomach.
____ **2.** Continuum	**b.** Living human being during the first eight weeks of development in the uterus.
____ **3.** Coordination	**c.** Pertaining to the period of life between childhood and maturity.
____ **4.** Decade	**d.** Capable of living.
____ **5.** Embryo	**e.** Progression from start (birth) to finish (death).
____ **6.** Fetus	**f.** Period of 10 years.
____ **7.** Menstruation	**g.** Infant developing in the uterus after the first three months until birth.
____ **8.** Prone	**h.** Lying on the back.
____ **9.** Supine	**i.** Cyclic deterioration of the endometrium.
____ **10.** Viable	**j.** Any cell formed by the coming together of two reproductive (sex) cells.
____ **11.** Zygote	**k.** State of harmonized action.

There are 11 possible points in this worksheet.

• WORKSHEET 2

1. Identify the three stages of development between conception and birth (3 points).

   a. ______________________________

   b. ______________________________

   c. ______________________________

2. List four common developments of growth in the first year of life and the age at which they usually occur (8 points).

Developments of Growth	Age
a. ____________________	____________________
b. ____________________	____________________
c. ____________________	____________________
d. ____________________	____________________

3. List three characteristics of adolescent development (3 points).

a. ____

____

b. ____

____

c. ____

____

There are 14 possible points in this worksheet.

• WORKSHEET/ACTIVITY 3

Design a bulletin board representing one of the growth and development stages listed below (e.g., a collage of infants doing different activities, paired with their age, or photos of various ages depicting each developmental stage). Include age-specific communication requirements (100 points).

- Infant
- Toddler stage (18 months to 3 years)
- Preschool and elementary age (3 to 8 years)
- Preteen years or preadolescent years (8 to 13 years)
- Adolescent or teenage years (13 to 18 years)
- Young adult (18 to 20 years)
- Adulthood (20 and older)

There are 100 possible points in this worksheet/activity.

• WORKSHEET/ACTIVITY 4

Interview an individual between the ages of 50 and 80. Ask the following question, plus at least four more of your own (100 points).

Interviewee's name ____________________ Birth year ____________________

1. What was your daily life like, including family roles (mother's role, father's role, and children's role)?

Use the following worksheet as a guide for your interviews.

	Mother's Role	Father's Role	Children's Role
a. Before you were 20 years old?	______________	______________	______________
	______________	______________	______________
	______________	______________	______________
b. Between 20 and 40 years of age?	______________	______________	______________
	______________	______________	______________
	______________	______________	______________
c. Between 40 and 60 years of age?	______________	______________	______________
	______________	______________	______________
	______________	______________	______________

2. What were the clothing fads when you were in your teens?

a. Shoes ____

____

b. Hats ____

____

c. Coats ____

____

d. Length of women's skirts ____

____

e. Bathing suits ____

____

3. What were you doing the day . . .

a. Sputnik was launched? ____

____

b. Iran took hostages at the U.S. embassy? ____

____

c. The *Challenger* exploded? ____

____

d. President Kennedy was assassinated? ____

____

e. The Vietnam War ended? ____

____

4. What gave or gives you the most enjoyment . . .

   a. As a teenager? ______________________________

   b. In middle school? ______________________________

   c. Now? ______________________________

5. When did you first . . .

   a. Own a car? ______________________________

   b. Fly in an airplane?

   c. Own a television set? ______________________________

6. Can you tell me what an Edsel is?

7. What type of music was popular when you were in your teens? ______________________________

8. What was a common weekend like when you were a child?

9. What was your favorite activity, hobby, sport, and so on?

10. What was your first job? How old were you when you started? What was your starting salary?

There are 100 possible points in this worksheet/activity.

• WORKSHEET/ACTIVITY 5

Compare and contrast your life experience and that of the subject of your interview (500 points).

Age	My Experience	Interviewee's Experience
Example:		
16	I got my first job after school at a fast-food restaurant.	He worked on the farm after school, beginning in elementary school.

There are 500 possible points in this worksheet/activity.

• WORKSHEET/ACTIVITY 6

Using Worksheet 4 and additional research, develop a two- to five-minute skit or report depicting the 10-year time period assigned by your instructor. All group members must actively participate in the presentation. The presentation must give a picture of

- The time period
- Common leisure activities of the time
- Popular clothing styles (through pictures or wearing or describing the clothes of the time)
- Popular music or songs
- Comedians of the era
- News events
- Modes of transportation

There are 100 possible points in this worksheet/activity.

UNIT 2

Aging and Role Change

• OBJECTIVES

When you have completed this unit, you will be able to do the following:

- Match vocabulary words with their correct meanings.
- Identify six body systems and the common physical changes that occur with aging.
- Identify basic human needs that are met through work, environment, socialization, and family relationships.
- Write an "action plan" to assist another person in coping with changes due to aging.

• DIRECTIONS

1. Complete Worksheet 1 before beginning the reading.
2. Read this unit.
3. Complete Worksheets 2 through 5 as assigned.
4. When you are confident that you can meet each objective listed above, ask your instructor for the unit evaluation.

• EVALUATION METHODS

- Worksheets
- Class participation
- Written evaluation

• WORKSHEET/ACTIVITY 1

Select four or five individuals from among family, friends, and neighbors. Be sure to have a wide range of ages from children to the elderly. Interview them about their favorite pastimes, such as sports, music, dancing, gardening, and reading.

Think how aging and role changes have changed these activities and prepare a brief report for your classmates to identify any trends you have observed.

There are 50 possible points in this worksheet/activity.

• WORKSHEET 2

Fill in the crossword puzzle using the vocabulary words from Unit 2 (8 points).

Indicates a space between two words.

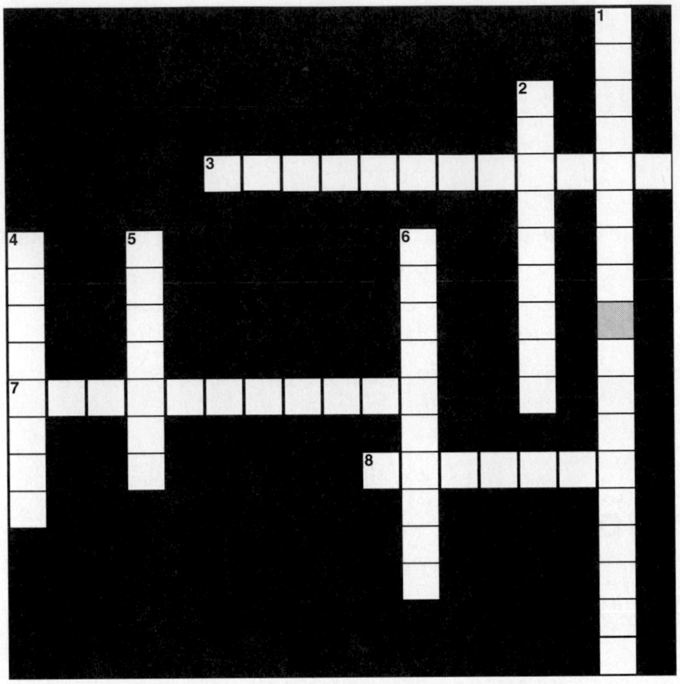

Clues

Across

3. Infrequent or difficult emptying of the bowel.
7. Surroundings we live in.
8. Elements in the environment that are strong enough to set up a nervous impulse.

Down

1. Air sacs in the lungs.
2. Keeping elements within the body that are normally eliminated.
4. Involuntary actions that occur when a nerve is stimulated.
5. Body's strength or energy.
6. Adjustment.

There are 8 possible points in this worksheet.

• WORKSHEET 3

1. List three changes that may occur in the nervous system with aging (3 points).

   a. ______________________________

   b. ______________________________

   c. ______________________________

2. List three disorders of the musculoskeletal system that are found in the elderly (3 points).

   a. ______________________________

   b. ______________________________

   c. ______________________________

3. The lungs become less (a) ____________ and the (b) ____________ membrane thickens; this makes (c) ____________ more difficult (3 points).

4. Arteries may become (a) ____________ and (b) ____________ (2 points).

5. Bladder ____________ may occur from retention of urine in the bladder (1 point).

There are 12 possible points in this worksheet.

• WORKSHEET 4

1. List four role changes that may occur in the elderly (4 points).

   a. ______________________________

   b. ______________________________

   c. ______________________________

   d. ______________________________

2. Give two ways an individual can adapt to the loss of family relationships (2 points).

   a. ______________________________

   b. ______________________________

3. What are two losses experienced when the work role is changed (2 points)?

   a. ______________________________

   b. ______________________________

4. Give two possible effects of change in environment (2 points).

   a. ______________________________

   b. ______________________________

There are 10 possible points in this worksheet.

• WORKSHEET 5

Complete the following action plan (25 points).

1. Name a person you know who is coping with the changes caused by aging.

   ____

2. List the changes you see in this person's daily life.

   ____

   ____

   ____

3. List things that might help this person cope with the changes you listed above.

   ____

   ____

   ____

4. Write a plan that could help this person cope with these changes.

   ____

   ____

Note: Always determine the other person's desire for assistance before trying to help him or her.

There are 25 possible points in this worksheet.

UNIT 3

Disabilities and Role Changes

• OBJECTIVES

When you have completed this unit, you will be able to do the following:

- Match vocabulary words with their correct meanings.
- Define *health.*
- List three examples of activities of daily living (ADL).
- Define *assistive or adaptive devices.*
- Identify ways to encourage independence.
- List eight birth defects.
- List 11 debilitating illnesses.
- Identify seven common changes that occur following the loss of body functions.
- State the goal of rehabilitation.
- Select a disability and summarize your feelings and expectations concerning:
  - What you think it would be like to live with that disability
  - The type of care you would expect
  - The way others respond to the disability

• DIRECTIONS

1. Complete Worksheet 1 before beginning the reading.
2. Read this unit.
3. Complete Worksheet/Activity 2 as assigned.
4. Complete Worksheet 3 as assigned.
5. Complete Worksheet/Activity 4 as assigned.
6. When you are confident that you can meet each objective for this unit, ask your instructor for the unit evaluation.

• EVALUATION METHODS

- Worksheets/Activities
- Class participation
- Written report
- Written evaluation

• WORKSHEET 1

Match each definition in column B with the correct vocabulary word in column A (22 points).

Column A

____ **1.** Passed from parent to child.
____ **2.** Impaired or abnormal functioning.
____ **3.** Deep sleep; unconscious state for a long period of time.
____ **4.** A number of symptoms occurring together.
____ **5.** Removal of a body part.
____ **6.** State of poisoning or becoming poisoned.
____ **7.** Shortage.
____ **8.** Moving forward, following steps toward an end product.
____ **9.** Causing weakness or impairment.
____ **10.** State of being confused about time, place, and identity of persons and objects.
____ **11.** Pertaining to the embryo.
____ **12.** Substance that causes a change to occur in other substances.
____ **13.** Events in a series.
____ **14.** Defect present at birth.
____ **15.** State of being weakened or deteriorated.
____ **16.** Pertaining to the nervous system.
____ **17.** To change, to become suitable.
____ **18.** Unsound or unhealthy state of being.
____ **19.** Condition of hardening of the arteries.
____ **20.** Fat.
____ **21.** Infections that occur when the immune system is weakened.
____ **22.** Belief in oneself.

Column B

a. Adapt
b. Amputation
c. Arteriosclerosis
d. Birth defect
e. Coma
f. Debilitating
g. Deficiency
h. Dysfunction
i. Embryonic
j. Hereditary
k. Impairment
l. Infirmity
m. Intoxication
n. Neurological
o. Opportunistic infections
p. Progressive
q. Self-esteem
r. Lipid
s. Syndrome
t. Episodes
u. Enzyme
v. Disorientation

There are 22 possible points in this worksheet.

• WORKSHEET/ACTIVITY 2

Work with your group to develop a verbal report on the disability assigned by your instructor (500 points).

1. Explain how daily life changes for those with your assigned disability.

2. List the types of jobs a person with this disability could do that would promote independence.

3. List the types of leisure activities a person with this disability could participate in.

4. List common attitudes about this disability.

5. Decide which part of the above information each person in the group will present to the class.

Student Name	Report Responsibility

There are 500 possible points in this worksheet/activity.

• WORKSHEET 3

1. List eight birth defects (8 points).
   a. ______
   b. ______
   c. ______
   d. ______
   e. ______
   f. ______
   g. ______
   h. ______
2. List 11 debilitating illnesses (11 points).
   a. ______
   b. ______
   c. ______
   d. ______
   e. ______
   f. ______
   g. ______
   h. ______
   i. ______
   j. ______
   k. ______
3. What is the goal of rehabilitation (1 point)? ______
   ______
   ______
4. Mark an *X* in the space next to the seven common changes that occur following the loss of body function (7 points).
   ______ **a.** Family
   ______ **b.** Eating habits
   ______ **c.** Animals
   ______ **d.** Elimination of waste
   ______ **e.** Ability to move
   ______ **f.** Communication skills
   ______ **g.** Sensory awareness
   ______ **h.** Ability to think and comprehend
   ______ **i.** Sexual activity

5. List three examples of activities of daily living (ADL) (3 points).

   a. ______________________________

   b. ______________________________

   c. ______________________________

6. What are assistive or adaptive devices (1 point)?______________________________

   ____

   ____

   ____

7. Mark an *X* in the space next to the ways that you can encourage independence in your patients (3 points).

   ______ a. Allow patients to help choose their clothing.
   ______ b. Always brush your patients' teeth for them.
   ______ c. Let patients do as many ADLs as possible.
   ______ d. Comb your patients' hair for them.
   ______ e. Do everything you can for your patients.
   ______ f. Help patients comb their hair.

8. Mrs. Wong is trying to comb her hair. She had a stroke two months ago and is still very slow. You have several more residents to care for and barely enough time to finish. What will you do, and why (2 points)?

   ____

   ____

   ____

9. Jaime Garcia is a young athlete. He was badly injured during a football game. He is very frustrated because he cannot move his right arm. He is trying to learn how to eat with his left hand. During breakfast, he throws the cereal across the room. What will you do, and why (2 points)?

   ____

   ____

There are 38 possible points in this worksheet.

• WORKSHEET/ACTIVITY 4

Select a disability, and summarize your feelings and expectations about the disability in a one-page paper (10 points).

- What do you think it would be like to live with the disability?
- What type of care would you expect if you had the disability?
- How would others respond to the disability?

Follow these guidelines when preparing your paper:

- Use 8.5-by-11-inch paper.
- Type, word-process, or write neatly in ink.
- Use correct spelling and grammar.

There are 10 possible points in this worksheet/activity.

UNIT 4

Psychological Stages in the Terminally Ill

• OBJECTIVES

When you have completed this unit, you will be able to do the following:

- Match vocabulary words with their correct meanings.
- Match the psychological stages of a long terminal illness with their names.
- Identify and discuss your feelings about terminal illness.
- Explain the philosophy of hospice care.

• DIRECTIONS

1. Complete Worksheet 1 before beginning the reading.
2. Read this unit.
3. Complete Worksheet 2.
4. Follow your instructor's directions to complete Worksheet/Activity 3.
5. When you are confident that you can meet each objective listed above, ask your instructor for the unit evaluation.

• EVALUATION METHODS

- Worksheets/Activities
- Class participation
- Written evaluation
- Written report

• WORKSHEET 1

Fill in the crossword puzzle using the vocabulary words from Unit 4 in your text (12 points).

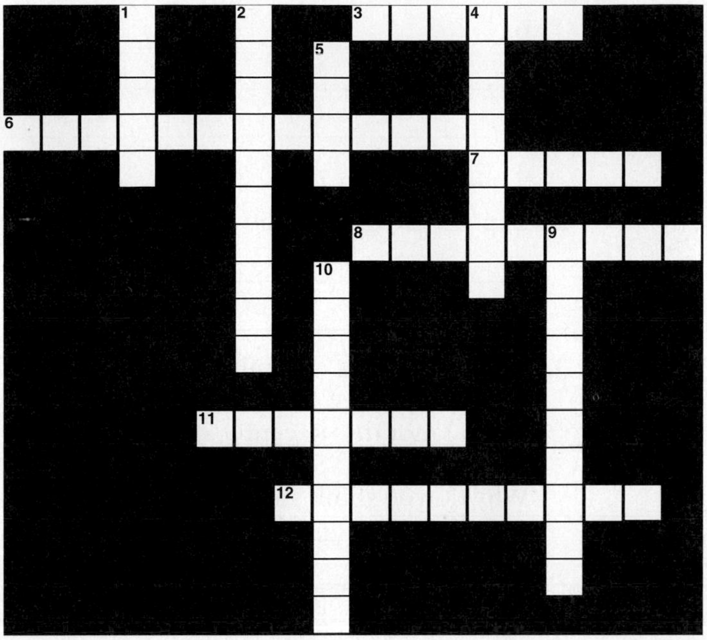

Clues

Across

3. Psychological stage one: unable to believe they are really going to die.

6. Pertaining to the mind.

7. Psychological stage two: mad because they are going to die.

8. About to happen.

11. Facility that helps the terminally ill live each day to the fullest.

12. Psychological stage three: admit they are dying but say they must live for a certain time or event.

Down

1. Psychological stage one: experience disbelief and amazement ("Not me!").

2. Theory; a general principle used for a specific purpose.

4. Limited in contact with others.

5 Psychological stage two: experience uncontrolled anger.

9. Psychological stage four: feel sadness, grief, and loss.

10. Psychological stage five: acknowledge that they are going to die.

There are 12 possible points in this worksheet.

• WORKSHEET 2

1. List the five psychological stages often experienced by the terminally ill, in the order in which they usually occur (5 points).

   a. ______________________________

   b. ______________________________

   c. ______________________________

   d. ______________________________

   e. ______________________________

2. Explain the philosophy of hospice (1 point).

   ____

   ____

3. Mrs. Nygun has a terminal illness. Until recently, she had been able to care for herself and was fairly independent. You have become friends over several months. Recently she became ill with pneumonia and unable to care for herself. She tells you to get away from her and calls you names. Why do you think she is so angry? Explain how you will respond to her and why (2 points). ______________________________

   ____

   ____

   ____

4. You are assigned Mr. Hong. He is near death. When you care for him, you notice that his breathing is very difficult. He feels cold to the touch, and he is losing control of body functions. How will you treat him? What do you think you might feel while caring for him (2 points)?

   ____

   ____

   ____

There are 10 possible points in this worksheet.

• WORKSHEET/ACTIVITY 3

Describe your experience with someone who is or was terminally ill. If you have no previous experience, describe what you think you might feel when you first learn of a terminal illness (10 points).

Follow these guidelines when preparing your paper:

- Use 8.5-by-11-inch paper.
- Type, word-process, or write neatly in ink.
- Use correct spelling and grammar.

There are 10 possible points in this worksheet/activity.

Chapter 10 Nutrition

UNIT 1

Basic Nutrition

• OBJECTIVES

When you have completed this unit, you will be able to do the following:

- Match vocabulary words with their correct meanings.
- Name the four functions of food.
- Name the five basic nutrients and explain how they maintain body function.
- Explain the USDA food pyramid.
- Compare your diet with the recommendations in the food pyramid.

• DIRECTIONS

1. Complete vocabulary Worksheet 1 in the Student Workbook.
2. Read this unit.
3. Complete Worksheet/Activity 2 as assigned.
4. Complete Worksheets 3 through 5 after your instructor discusses this chapter in class.
5. Ask your instructor for directions to complete Worksheets/Activities 6 and 7.
6. When you are confident that you can meet each objective listed above, ask your instructor for the unit evaluation.

• EVALUATION METHODS

- Worksheets/Activities
- Class participation
- Written evaluation

• WORKSHEET 1

Write each word listed below in the space next to the statement that best defines it (15 points).

vitality	nutrients	resistance
regulate	absorbed	protein
vitamins	minerals	essential
metabolism	stamina	hemoglobin
fecal	obesity	calories

_______________ **1.** Ability of the body to protect itself from disease.

_______________ **2.** Group of substances necessary for normal metabolism, growth, and body function.

_______________ **3.** Ability of an organism to go on living.

_______________ **4.** The body's process of using food to make energy and nutrients.

_______________ **5.** Substances that nourish the body.

_______________ **6.** Body's strength or energy.

_______________ **7.** To control or adjust.

_______________ **8.** Necessary.

_______________ **9.** Complex chemical in the blood; carries oxygen and carbon dioxide.

_______________ **10.** Extreme fatness; abnormal amount of fat on the body.

_______________ **11.** Taken up or received.

_______________ **12.** Inorganic elements that occur in nature; essential to every cell.

_______________ **13.** Complex compound found in plant and animal tissues; essential for heat, energy, and growth.

_______________ **14.** Units of measurement of the fuel value of food.

_______________ **15.** Pertaining to feces, a solid waste product.

There are 15 possible points in this worksheet.

• WORKSHEET/ACTIVITY 2

Make a poster identifying foods that supply different nutrients such as vitamins and their sources. Food pictures can be found in magazines or on the Internet, or you may draw them.

Number of points to be determined by your instructor.

• WORKSHEET 3

1. Name the four functions of food (4 points).

   a. ______________________ **c.** ______________________

   b. ______________________ **d.** ______________________

2. Name the five basic nutrients, and explain how they maintain body function (10 points).

	Basic Nutrients	How They Maintain Body Function
a.	______________________	______________________
		______________________
b.	______________________	______________________
		______________________
c.	______________________	______________________
		______________________
d.	______________________	______________________
		______________________
e.	______________________	______________________
		______________________

3. Describe the food pyramid, and explain why it is important (2 points).

   ____

   ____

   ____

There are 16 possible points in this worksheet.

• WORKSHEET 4

1. Following the example in this first question, keep a record (in question 2) of what you eat for two full days. At the end of each day, determine whether you had a balanced diet. If not, how could you have balanced it?

Example:

MEAL	FOOD EATEN	FOOD GROUP/SERVING AMOUNT
Breakfast	1 banana	2 servings fruit
	1 slice toast with jelly	1 serving bread and cereal
	½ cup milk	½ serving dairy
	coffee	zero
Lunch	fast-food hamburger:	
	3 oz. meat patty	1 serving meat
	bun	2 servings bread and cereal
	lettuce and tomato	½ serving fruit and vegetable
	20 french fries	2 servings vegetable
	8 oz. coke	zero
Snack	apple	1 serving fruit
Dinner	spaghetti with tomato sauce:	
	⅔ cup spaghetti	1 serving bread and cereal
	½ cup tomato sauce	1 serving fruit and vegetable
	Lettuce salad	1 serving vegetable
	1 cup milk	1 serving dairy
Snack	candy bar	zero

2. Total the number of servings from each food group in the food pyramid on your daily menu. Show how it is balanced, or what you could add to balance your diet.

   If you are an adult, you might add cheese and a glass of milk to lunch. A teen might add cheese to lunch and ice cream for an evening snack.

Day 1

MEAL	FOOD EATEN	FOOD GROUP/SERVING AMOUNT	FOODS NEEDED TO BALANCE DIET
Breakfast			
Lunch			
Dinner			
Snack			

Total ______________________________

To balance diet add: ______________________________

Day 2

MEAL	FOOD EATEN	FOOD GROUP/SERVING AMOUNT	FOODS NEEDED TO BALANCE DIET
Breakfast			
Lunch			
Dinner			
Snack			

Total ____________________

To balance diet add: ____________________

There are 50 possible points in this worksheet.

• WORKSHEET 5

1. Summarize what you learned from Worksheet 4 in the space below.

I Need to Eat More: | **I Need to Eat Less:**

____________________ ____________________

____________________ ____________________

____________________ ____________________

____________________ ____________________

____________________ ____________________

2. Write a realistic action plan to help you follow the food pyramid guidelines.

____

____

____

____

____

____

____

____

____

____

____

There are 25 possible points in this worksheet.

• WORKSHEET/ACTIVITY 6

Prepare a one-week menu for your family. Total the food group servings for each day and demonstrate whether the daily intake is balanced according to the food pyramid.

There are 100 points in this worksheet/activity.

• WORKSHEET/ACTIVITY 7

Your teacher will divide the class into groups and ask each group to identify food preferences of a specific ethnic group. Plan a two-day balanced menu which includes some of each group's ethnic food preferences.

There are 100 points in this worksheet/activity.

UNIT 2

Therapeutic Diets

• OBJECTIVES

When you have completed this unit, you will be able to do the following:

- Match vocabulary words with their correct meanings.
- List three factors that influence food habits.
- Select a correct therapeutic diet for physical disorders.

• DIRECTIONS

1. Complete Worksheet 1 before beginning the reading.
2. Read this unit.
3. Complete Worksheet 2 as assigned.
4. Complete Worksheet/Activity 3.
5. Complete the Learn by Doing assignment at the end of this unit.
6. Complete the Chapter Review—Your Link to Success at the end of this chapter.
7. When you are confident that you can meet each objective listed above, ask your instructor for the unit evaluation.

• EVALUATION METHODS

- Worksheets/Activities
- Class participation
- Written evaluation

• WORKSHEET 1

Write each word listed below in the space next to the statement that best defines it (14 points).

therapeutic	preferences	metabolic
edema	gastrointestinal	deficient
colitis	ileitis	diabetes mellitus
soluble	atherosclerosis	anorexia nervosa
hypertension	lactation	

____ **1.** Pertaining to all of the physical and chemical changes that take place in living organisms and cells.
____ **2.** Lacking something.
____ **3.** Pertaining to the treatment of disease or injury.
____ **4.** Able to break down or dissolve in liquid.
____ **5.** Priorities; first choices.
____ **6.** Condition of hardening of the arteries due to fat deposits that narrow the space through which blood flows.
____ **7.** Body's process of producing milk to feed newborns.
____ **8.** Swelling; abnormal or excessive collection of fluid in the tissues.
____ **9.** Inflammation of the ileum.
____ **10.** Pertaining to the stomach and intestine.
____ **11.** Inflammation of the colon.
____ **12.** Condition that develops when the body cannot change sugar into energy.
____ **13.** Loss of appetite with serious weight loss; considered a mental disorder.
____ **14.** High blood pressure.

There are 14 possible points in this worksheet.

• WORKSHEET 2

1. List three factors that influence food habits (3 points).

a. ______________________________

b. ______________________________

c. ______________________________

2. Name the therapeutic diet for each of the following (8 points). __________

a. For a patient having trouble chewing or swallowing: __________

b. To soothe the gastrointestinal system: __________

c. For a patient with anorexia nervosa: __________

d. To regulate the cholesterol in the blood: __________

e. To reduce salt intake: ______________________

f. To replace fluids lost by vomiting: ______________________

g. For a patient with diabetes mellitus: ______________________

h. For a patient with gallbladder and liver disease: ______________________

There are 11 possible points in this worksheet.

• WORKSHEET/ACTIVITY 3

Choose a therapeutic diet and make a poster depicting the foods in the diet. Tell why the diet is necessary.

There are 100 points in this worksheet/activity.

Chapter 11 Measuring Vital Signs

UNIT 1

Temperature, Pulse, and Respiration

• OBJECTIVES

When you have completed this unit, you will be able to do the following:

- Match vocabulary words with their correct meanings.
- Define *vital signs.*
- List fourteen factors that influence body temperature.
- Name the most common site at which to measure a temperature.
- Match the normal temperature to the site where it is measured.
- Measure temperature with a glass thermometer.
- Demonstrate how to measure oral, rectal, and axillary temperatures.
- Define *pulse.*
- Explain pulse oximetry.
- Identify sites where the pulse may be counted.
- Identify a normal adult pulse rate and a common method for counting a pulse.
- List six factors that influence the pulse rate.
- Demonstrate counting and recording a radial pulse accurately.
- Recognize two parts of a respiration.
- Relate types of abnormal respirations to their correct names.
- Select eight factors that affect respiration.
- Explain the importance of not being obvious when counting respirations.
- Demonstrate how to count and record respirations accurately.
- Explain the importance of each vital sign.

• DIRECTIONS

1. Complete Worksheet 1 before beginning the reading.
2. Read this unit.
3. Complete Worksheets 2 through 4 as assigned.
4. Complete Worksheet/Activity 5 as assigned.
5. Practice all procedures using skills check-off sheets in your workbook.
6. When you are confident that you can meet each objective listed above, ask your instructor for the unit evaluation.

• EVALUATION METHODS

- Worksheets/Activities
- Class participation
- Return demonstrations
- Written evaluation

• WORKSHEET 1

Fill in the crossword puzzle using the vocabulary words from Unit 1 in your text (1 point).

Indicates a space between two words.

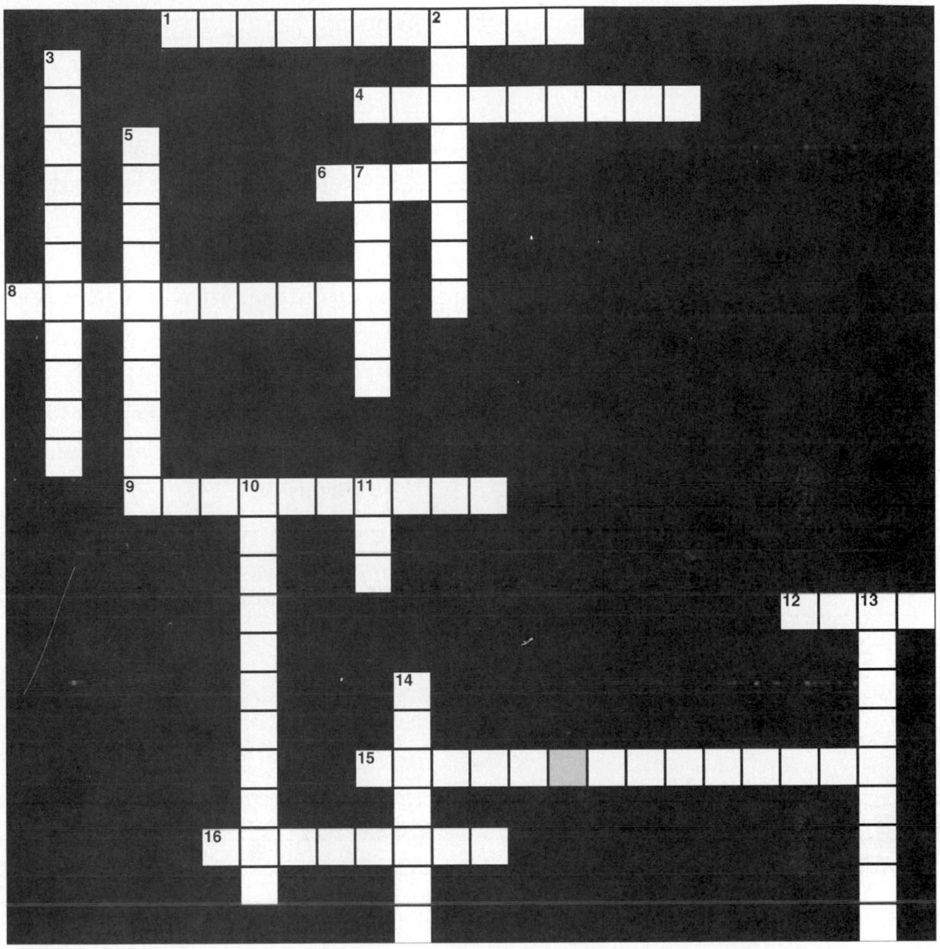

Clues

Across

1. Constant balance within the body.
4. The mixing together of oxygen and another element.
6. Referring to the mouth.
8. Measure of heat; abbreviated *F*.
9. Process of pushing air out of the lungs during respiration.
12. Pointed end of something.
15. Highest and lowest pressure against the walls of blood vessels.
16. Leaping; strong or forceful.

Down

2. Referring to the armpit.
3. Standard measure.
5. Large amount of bleeding.
7. Referring to the far end of the large intestine just above the anus.
10. Process of breathing in air during respiration.
11. Temperature, pulse, and respiration.
13. Process of eliminating waste material.
14. Measure of heat; abbreviated *C*.

There are 16 possible points in this worksheet.

• WORKSHEET 2

Write each word listed below in the space next to the statement that best defines it (9 points).

afebrile	Celsius	hypothermia
axillary	Fahrenheit	rectal
calibration	febrile	TPR

________________ **1.** Standard measure—e.g., each line on a thermometer or a ruler is a ________________.

________________ **2.** Measure of heat: abbreviated *F.*

________________ **3.** Referring to the far end of the large intestine just above the anus.

________________ **4.** Without fever.

________________ **5.** Condition in which the body temperature is below normal.

________________ **6.** Referring to the armpit.

________________ **7.** Temperature, pulse, and respiration.

________________ **8.** Measure of heat; abbreviated *C.*

________________ **9.** Feverish.

Fahrenheit Thermometers

10. Write the correct reading for each of the following thermometers (3 points).

a. ________________

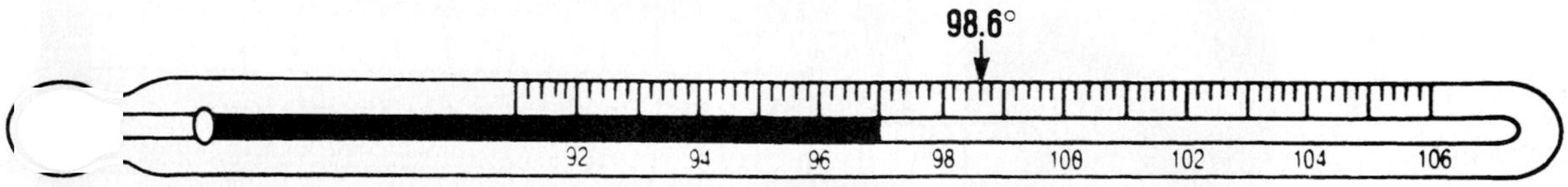

b. ________________

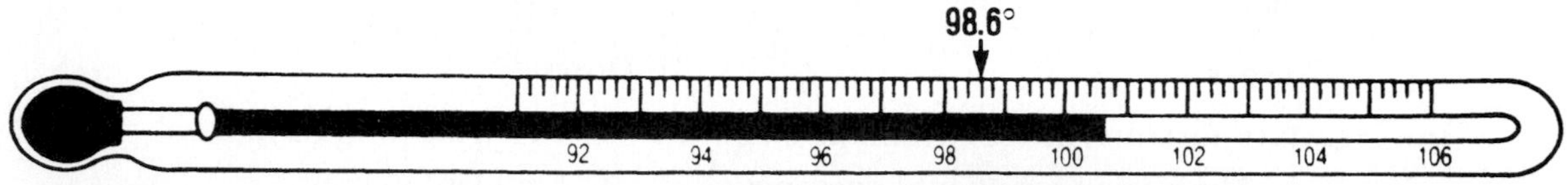

c. ________________

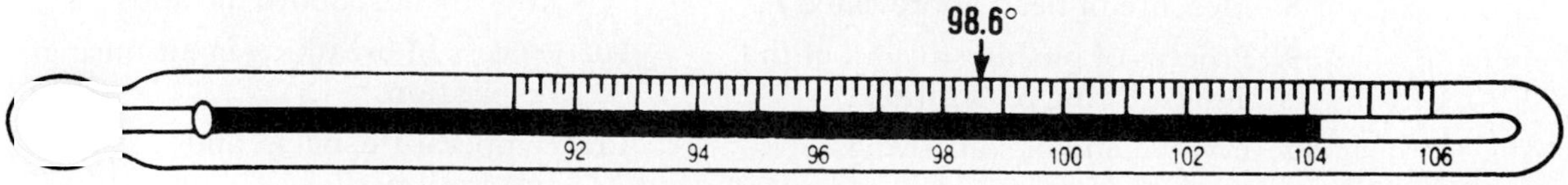

11. Draw a line to indicate where the mercury will end for the temperature listed just above the left end of each thermometer (4 points).

a. 98.6° F

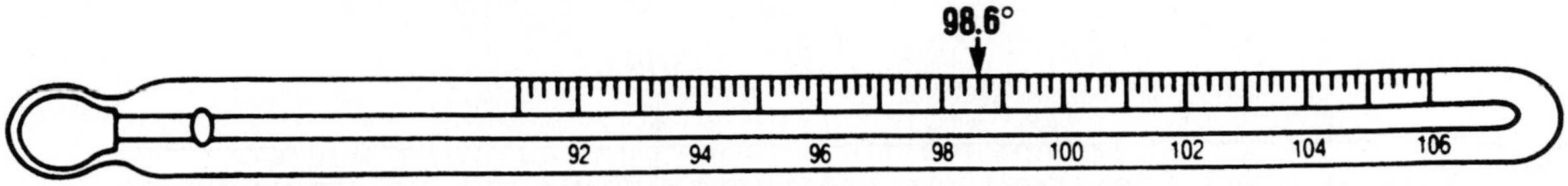

b. 99.2° F

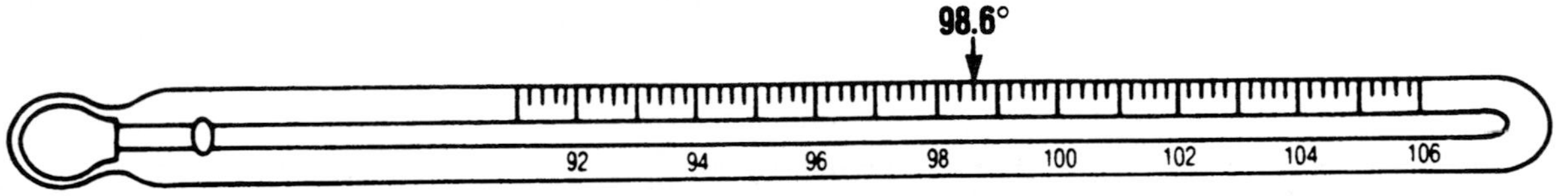

c. 101.8° F

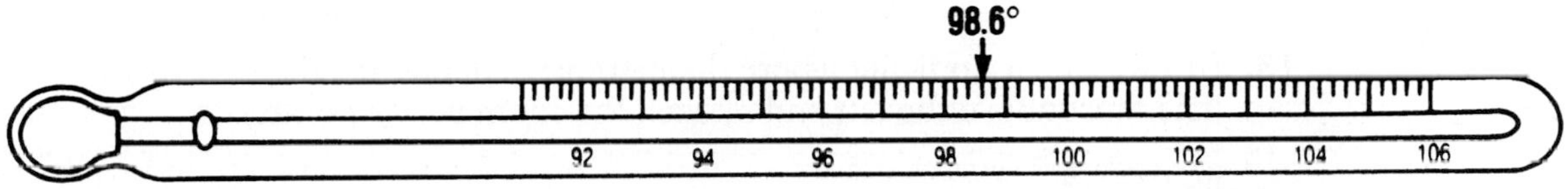

d. 103° F

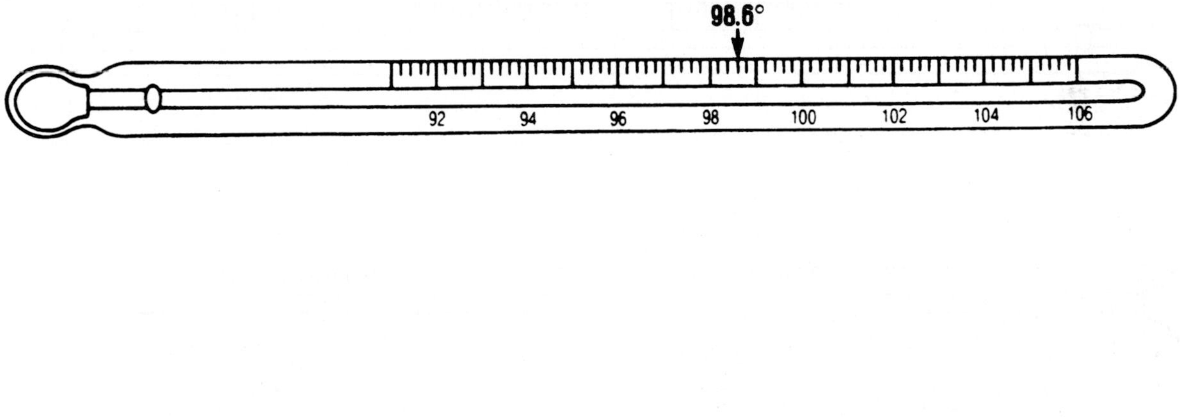

Celsius Thermometers

12. Write the correct reading for each of the following thermometers (2 points).

a. ____________________

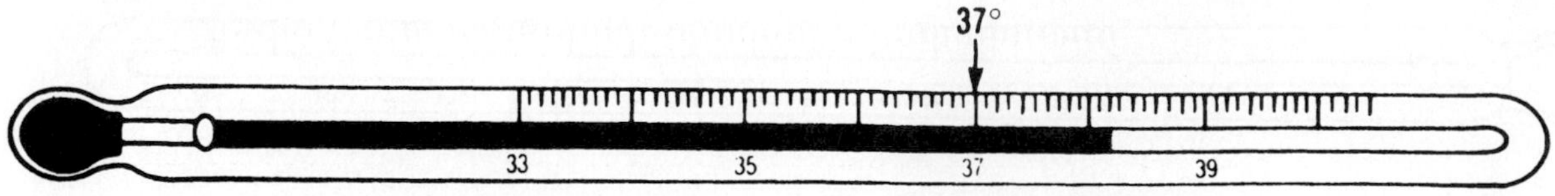

b. ____________________

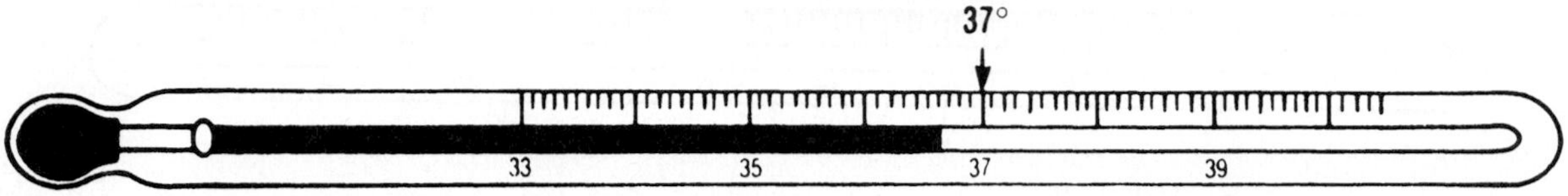

13. Draw a line to indicate where the mercury will end for the temperature listed just above the left end of each thermometer (3 points).

a. 37.2° C

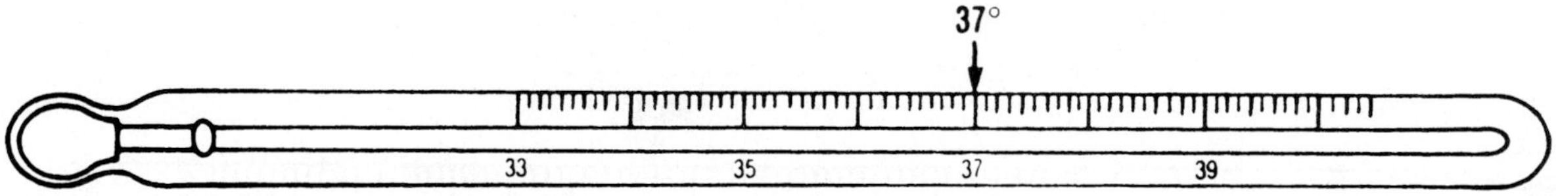

b. 39.4° C

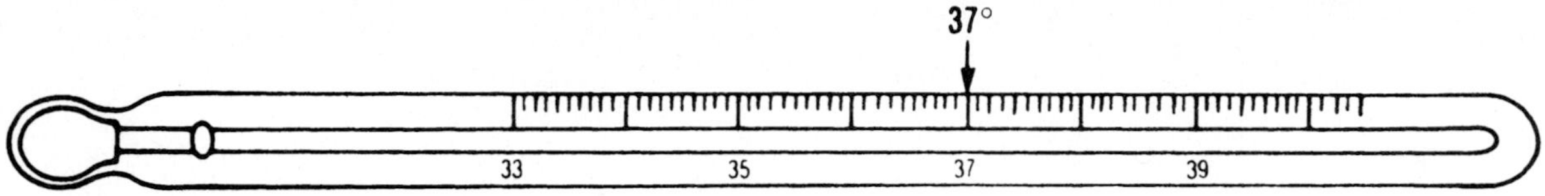

c. 38.6° C

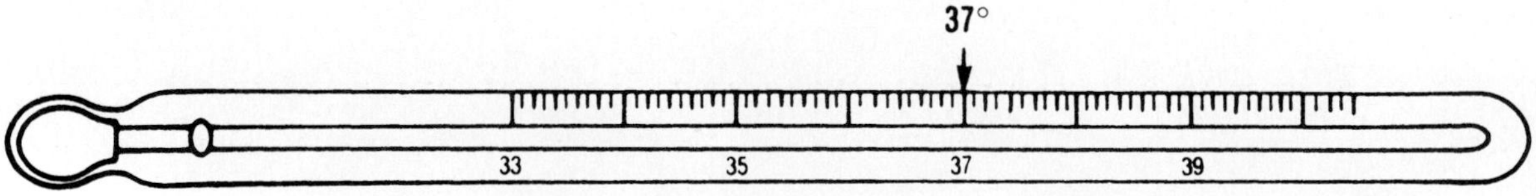

There are 21 possible points in this worksheet.

• WORKSHEET 3

1. Define the following words (6 points).

   a. Apex ______________________________

   b. Arrhythmia ______________________________

   c. Bounding ______________________________

   d. Bradycardia ______________________________

   e. Hemorrhage ______________________________

   f. Tachycardia ______________________________

2. Label the pulse points on the following diagram (7 points).

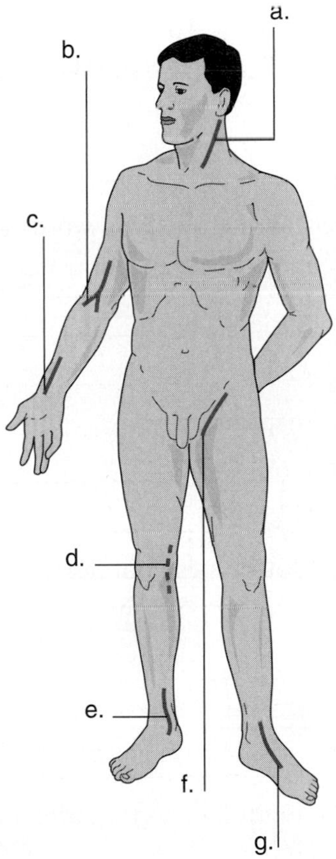

a. ______________________ e. ______________________

b. ______________________ f. ______________________

c. ______________________ g. ______________________

d. ______________________

3. Mark each of the following statements *T* for true or *F* for false (5 points).
   _______ a. The pulse rate indicates the number of times the heart beats in one minute.
   _______ b. When you take a pulse, you should use your thumb.
   _______ c. The apical pulse is the most common pulse that we take.
   _______ d. A normal pulse rate for an adult is 130 to 140.
   _______ e. A normal pulse rate for an adult is 60 to 80.
4. List six factors that affect the pulse rate (6 points).
   a. ____________________ d. ____________________
   b. ____________________ e. ____________________
   c. ____________________ f. ____________________
5. Define pulse oximetry (1 point).

There are 25 possible points in this worksheet.

• WORKSHEET 4

1. Define the following words (6 points).
   a. Cheynes-Stokes ____________________
   b. Apnea ____________________
   c. Rales ____________________
   d. Inspiration ____________________
   e. Expiration ____________________
   f. Dyspnea ____________________
2. List four types of abnormal respirations (4 points).
   a. ____________________
   b. ____________________
   c. ____________________
   d. ____________________
3. List eight factors that affect respiration (8 points).
   a. ____________________ e. ____________________
   b. ____________________ f. ____________________
   c. ____________________ g. ____________________
   d. ____________________ h. ____________________

There are 18 possible points in this worksheet.

• WORKSHEET/ACTIVITY 5

Ask people of various ages if you can practice counting their pulse and respirations. Complete the chart below with the appropriate information.

	Age	Pulse Rate	Note Characteristics of Pulse	Respiratory Rate	Note Characteristics of Respirations
1					
2					
3					
4					
5					
6					
7					
8					
9					
10					
11					

There are 25 points possible when you record the practice results of 5 people.
There are 50 points possible when you record the practice results of 11 people.

UNIT 2

Blood Pressure

• OBJECTIVES

When you have completed this unit, you will be able to do the following:

- Match vocabulary words with their correct meanings.
- Define *blood pressure.*
- Match descriptions of systolic and diastolic blood pressure.
- List four factors that increase blood pressure.
- List four factors that can reduce blood pressure.
- State the normal range of blood pressure.
- Demonstrate how to measure and record a blood pressure accurately.
- Explain how vital signs provide information about the patient's health.

• DIRECTIONS

1. Complete Worksheet 1 before beginning the reading.
2. Read this unit.
3. Complete Worksheets 2 through 3 as assigned.
4. Practice *all* procedures using the skills check-off sheets in your workbook.
5. Prepare responses to each item listed in the Chapter Review—Your Link to Success at the end of this chapter.
6. When you are confident that you can meet each objective listed above, ask your instructor for the unit evaluation.

• EVALUATION METHODS

- Worksheets
- Class participation
- Written evaluation
- Return demonstration

• WORKSHEET 1

Fill in the crossword puzzle using the vocabulary words from Unit 2 in your text (14 points).

Indicates a space between two words.

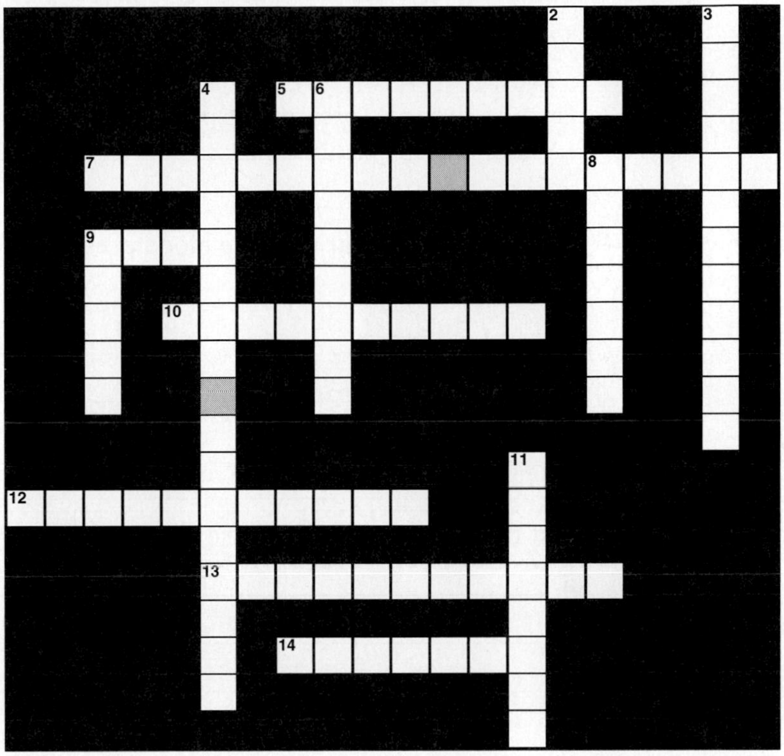

Clues

Across

5. Equipment needed to perform a task.
7. Lowest pressure against the blood vessels of the body.
9. Refers to pressure.
10. Measure of length.
12. Below normal blood pressure range.
13. Instrument used to amplify sound.
14. To swell or fill up with air.

Down

2. Standard scale for measurement.
3. High blood pressure.
4. First heart sound or beat heard when taking a blood pressure.
6. Feeling.
8. Refers to pulse.
9. Refers to measure.
11. Out of date.

There are 14 possible points in this worksheet.

• WORKSHEET 2

1. Define *blood pressure* (1 point).

   ____

   ____

2. Explain systolic pressure (1 point).

   ____

   ____

3. Explain diastolic pressure (1 point).

   ____

   ____

4. List five factors that increase blood pressure (5 points).

   a. ____

   b. ____

   c. ____

   d. ____

   e. ____

5. List four factors that decrease blood pressure (5 points).

   a. ____

   b. ____

   c. ____

   d. ____

   e. ____

6. List three types of blood pressure apparatus (3 points).

   a. ____

   b. ____

   c. ____

7. What is the normal range of blood pressure (1 point)? ______________

   ____

8. Define *hypertension* (1 point). ______________________

   ____

9. Define *hypotension* (1 point). ______________________

   ____

There are 19 possible points in this worksheet.

• WORKSHEET 3

Write the pressures indicated on the following diagrams in the spaces provided (6 points).

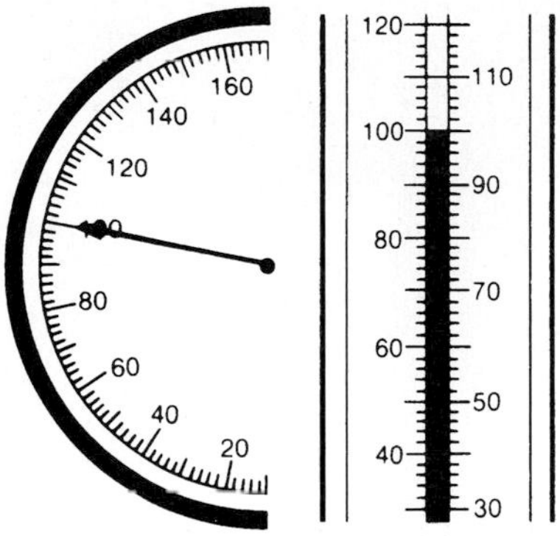

1. ______________________________

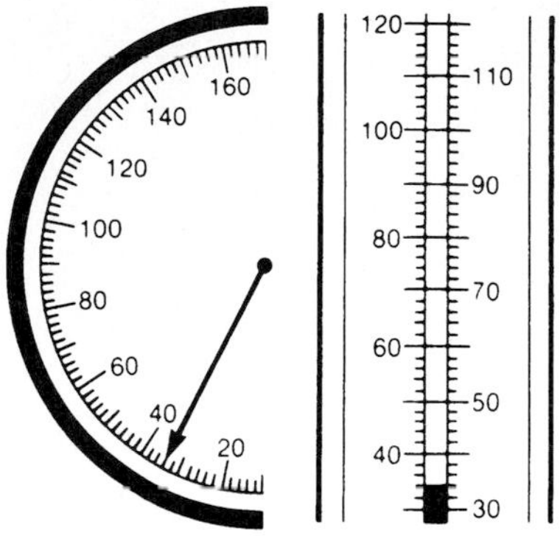

2. ______________________________

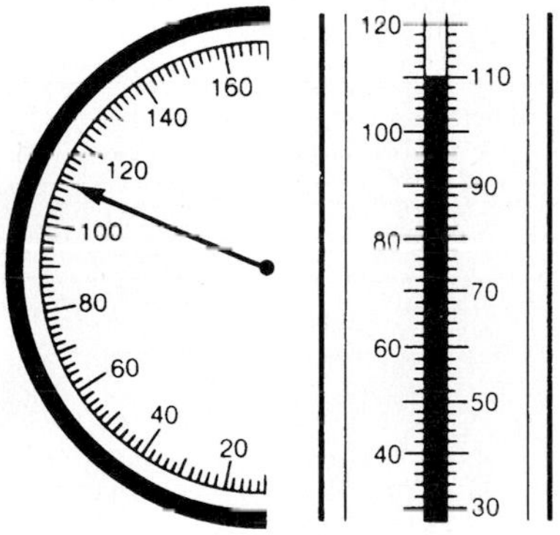

3. ______________________________

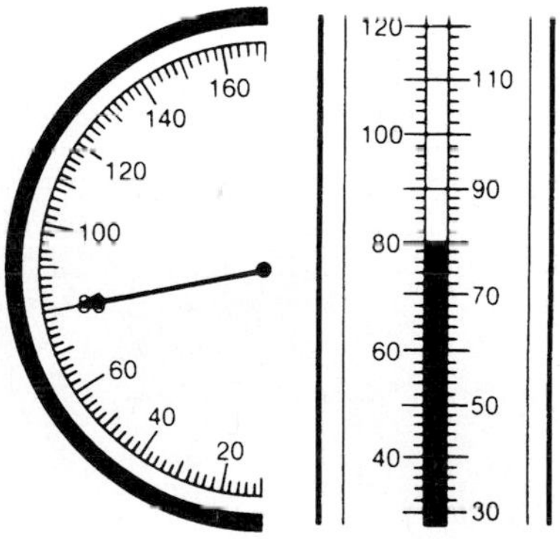

4. ______________________________

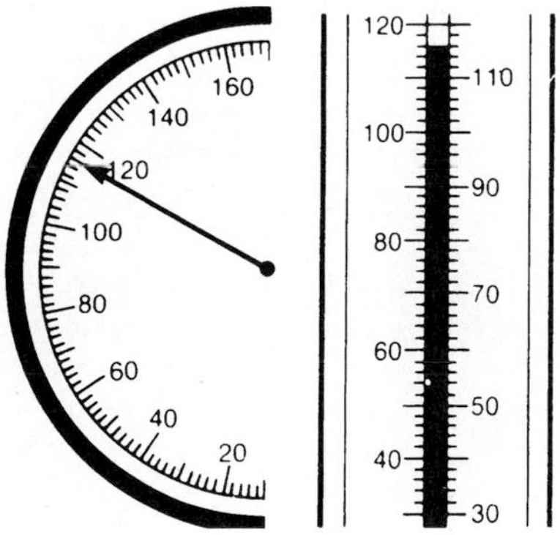

5. ______________________________

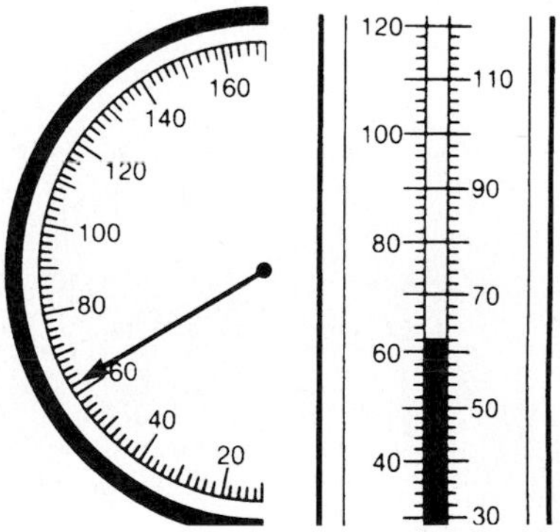

6. ______________________________

There are 6 possible points in this worksheet.

Check-off Sheet:

11-2 Measuring an Oral Temperature

Name ______________________________ **Date** __________

Directions: Practice this procedure, following each step. When you are ready to have your performance evaluated, give this sheet to your instructor. Review the detailed procedure in your textbook.

Procedure	Pass	Redo	Date Competency Met	Instructor Initials
Student must use Standard Precautions.	☐	☐	______	______
1. Wash hands.	☐	☐	______	______
2. Assemble equipment.*				
a. Clean oral thermometer	☐	☐	______	______
b. Alcohol wipes	☐	☐	______	______
c. Watch with second hand	☐	☐	______	______
d. Pad and pencil	☐	☐	______	______
e. Disposable thermometer cover	☐	☐	______	______
3. Identify client.	☐	☐	______	______
4. Explain what you are going to do.	☐	☐	______	______
5. Remove thermometer from container and apply disposable cover.	☐	☐	______	______
6. Check reading—94° F, or 35° C.	☐	☐	______	______
7. Ask patient if he or she has been smoking, eating, or drinking. If yes, wait 10 minutes before taking temperature.	☐	☐	______	______
8. Place thermometer under tongue.	☐	☐	______	______
9. Instruct client to hold with closed lips.	☐	☐	______	______
10. Leave in mouth for five minutes.	☐	☐	______	______
11. Remove from mouth.	☐	☐	______	______
12. Remove and discard disposable cover and wipe from stem to tip.	☐	☐	______	______
13. Read thermometer correctly.	☐	☐	______	______
14. Wash thermometer in cool water.	☐	☐	______	______
15. Put thermometer away.	☐	☐	______	______
16. Wash hands.	☐	☐	______	______
17. Record temperature correctly on pad.	☐	☐	______	______
18. Report any unusual observation immediately.	☐	☐	______	______

***Follow facility policy for wearing gloves.**

Check-off Sheet:

11-5 Counting a Radial Pulse

Name ______________________________ **Date** __________

Directions: Practice this procedure, following each step. When you are ready to have your performance evaluated, give this sheet to your instructor. Review the detailed procedure in your textbook.

Procedure	Pass	Redo	Date Competency Met	Instructor Initials
Student must use Standard Precautions.	☐	☐	______	______
1. Wash hands.	☐	☐	______	______
2. Assemble equipment.				
a. Watch with second hand	☐	☐	______	______
b. Pad and pencil	☐	☐	______	______
3. Identify client.	☐	☐	______	______
4. Explain what you are going to do.	☐	☐	______	______
5. Place fingers on radial artery—do not use thumb.	☐	☐	______	______
6. Count pulse (number of pulsations) for one minute.	☐	☐	______	______
7. Record pulse rate on pad immediately.	☐	☐	______	______
8. Wash hands.	☐	☐	______	______
9. Record pulse rate.	☐	☐	______	______
10. Report any unusual observation immediately.	☐	☐	______	______

Check-off Sheet:

11-7 Counting Respirations

Name ______________________________ **Date** __________

Directions: Practice this procedure, following each step. When you are ready to have your performance evaluated, give this sheet to your instructor. Review the detailed procedure in your textbook.

Procedure	Pass	Redo	Date Competency Met	Instructor Initials
Student must use Standard Precautions.	☐	☐	______	______
1. Wash hands.	☐	☐	______	______
2. Assemble equipment.				
a. Watch with second hand	☐	☐	______	______
b. Pad and pencil	☐	☐	______	______
3. Identify client.	☐	☐	______	______
4. Do not explain what you are going to do.	☐	☐	______	______
5. Relax fingers on pulse point.	☐	☐	______	______
6. Observe rise and fall of chest.	☐	☐	______	______
7. Count respirations for one minute.	☐	☐	______	______
8. Note regularity and depth.	☐	☐	______	______
9. Wash hands.	☐	☐	______	______
10. Record respiratory rate accurately.	☐	☐	______	______
11. Report any unusual observation immediately.	☐	☐	______	______

Check-off Sheet:

11-8 Measuring Blood Pressure

Name ______________________________ **Date** __________

Directions: Practice this procedure, following each step. When you are ready to have your performance evaluated, give this sheet to your instructor. Review the detailed procedure in your textbook.

Procedure	Pass	Redo	Date Competency Met	Instructor Initials
Student must use Standard Precautions.	☐	☐	______	______
1. Wash hands.	☐	☐	______	______
2. Assemble equipment.				
a. Alcohol wipes	☐	☐	______	______
b. Sphygmomanometer	☐	☐	______	______
c. Stethoscope	☐	☐	______	______
d. Pad and pencil	☐	☐	______	______
3. Identify client.	☐	☐	______	______
4. Explain what you are going to do.	☐	☐	______	______
5. Support patient's arm on firm surface.	☐	☐	______	______
6. Apply cuff correctly. (Refer to steps 4 and 5 in procedure "Palpating a Blood Pressure" in this unit of the text.)	☐	☐	______	______
7. Clean earpieces on stethoscope.	☐	☐	______	______
8. Place earpieces in ears.	☐	☐	______	______
9. Locate brachial artery.	☐	☐	______	______
10. Tighten thumbscrew on valve.	☐	☐	______	______
11. Hold stethoscope in place.	☐	☐	______	______
12. Inflate cuff to 170 mm.	☐	☐	______	______
13. Open valve. If systolic sound is heard	☐	☐		
immediately, reinflate cuff to 30mm Hg above systolic sound.	☐	☐	______	______
14. Note systolic at first beat.	☐	☐	______	______
15. Note diastolic.	☐	☐	______	______
16. Open valve and release air.	☐	☐	______	______
17. Record time and blood pressure reading correctly.	☐	☐	______	______
18. Wash hands.	☐	☐	______	______
19. Wash earpieces on stethoscope.	☐	☐	______	______
20. Put equipment away.	☐	☐	______	______
21. Record blood pressure in chart.	☐	☐	______	______
22. Report any unusual observation immediately.	☐	☐	______	______

• WORKSHEET 2

1. Write each word listed below in the space next to the statement that best defines it (4 points).

   bacteria viruses protozoa
   fungi

   ______________ **a.** Are smaller than bacteria.
   ______________ **b.** Cause amebic dysentery.
   ______________ **c.** Are a very low form of plant life.
   ______________ **d.** Causes strep throat.

2. List three ways that microorganisms affect the body and cause illness (3 points).

   a. ______________________________
   b. ______________________________
   c. ______________________________

3. List six conditions that affect the growth of bacteria (6 points).

   a. ______________________________
   b. ______________________________
   c. ______________________________
   d. ______________________________
   e. ______________________________
   f. ______________________________

4. Define *pathogen* and *nonpathogen* (2 points).

   ____
   ____

5. List two ways that microorganisms are spread, and give three examples of each (8 points).

Ways Microorganisms Spread	**Examples**
a. ______________	______________
	______________
	______________
b. ______________	______________
	______________
	______________

6. What two organisms always inhabit health care environments (2 points)?

   a. ______________________________
   b. ______________________________

7. List five ways the health care worker can prevent the spread of microorganisms (5 points).
   a. ______________________________
   b. ______________________________
   c. ______________________________
   d. ______________________________
   e. ______________________________

8. Explain the difference in signs and symptoms of generalized and localized infection (4 points). ______________________________

____

____

____

____

9. Explain why understanding microorganisms is important to health care workers (5 points). ______________________________

____

____

____

There are 39 possible points in this worksheet.

• WORKSHEET/ACTIVITY 3

Read about microorganisms in a reference book from the classroom or the library. Choose one microorganism, and write a two-to-three-page, double-spaced paper about it. Include the following in your paper:

- The microorganism's shape and size
- Its pattern of growth
- Whether it is aerobic or anaerobic
- How it affects the body (e.g., toxins, cell invasion, and so on)
- The symptoms it causes

Follow these guidelines when preparing your report:

- Use 8.5-by-11-inch paper.
- Type, word-process, or write neatly in ink.
- Use correct spelling and grammar.

There are 100 possible points in this worksheet.

20 points—format: introduction, body, summary
40 points—topic development
20 points—grammar
20 points—appearance, professional look

• WORKSHEET/ACTIVITY 4

Find a partner to work with. Take a sheet of paper each and divide the paper into three columns. List the infections that you have had in the first column and the signs and symptoms of those infections in the second column.

Switch papers and fill in the final column, which is a list of the possible causes of the infection.

When you are finished, switch back to your original paper and talk with your classmate about passing along infection. See if the known ways of getting an infection match with your recollection of how you may have gotten infected.

There are 10 possible points each in this worksheet/activity.

UNIT 2 Asepsis

• OBJECTIVES

When you have completed this unit, you will be able to do the following:

- Match terms related to medical asepsis with their correct meanings.
- Define *medical asepsis.*
- List five aseptic techniques.
- Demonstrate appropriate handwashing techniques.
- Explain the difference between *bactericidal* and *bacteriostatic.*
- List four reasons why asepsis is important.

• DIRECTIONS

1. Complete Worksheet 1 before beginning the reading.
2. Read this unit.
3. Complete Worksheet 2.
4. Practice the Handwashing Procedure P12-1 and ask your instructor to check your technique.
5. When you are confident that you can meet each objective listed above, ask your instructor for the unit evaluation.

• EVALUATION METHODS

- Worksheets
- Class participation
- Return demonstration
- Written evaluation

• WORKSHEET 1

Match each definition in column B with the correct vocabulary word in column A (10 points).

Column A

____ 1. Asepsis
____ 2. Exposed
____ 3. Aseptic technique
____ 4. Autoclaves
____ 5. Isolation
____ 6. Protective
____ 7. Disinfection
____ 8. Dysfunction
____ 9. Sterilized
____ 10. Standard Precautions

Column B

a. Methods used to make the environment, the worker, and the patient as germ-free as possible.
b. Abnormal functioning.
c. Standard procedures that protect patients, health care workers, and visitors from pathogens.
d. Process of freeing from microorganisms by physical or chemical means.
e. Sterilizers that use steam under pressure to kill all forms of bacteria on fomites.
f. Made free from all living microorganisms.
g. Sterile condition; free from all germs.
h. Guarding another from danger; providing a safe environment.
i. Condition of having limited contact with others.
j. Left unprotected.

There are 10 possible points in this worksheet.

• WORKSHEET 2

1. What is medical asepsis (1 point)? ____________________

____

2. What is a solution that slows the growth of microorganisms called (1 point)? ____________________

____

3. What is a solution that kills microorganisms called (1 point)? ____________________

____

4. Mark each of the following statements *T* for true or *F* for false (6 points).

______ **a.** Skin and hair can be sterilized.
______ **b.** Spores are killed when exposed to steam sterilization and high temperature.
______ **c.** Disinfection is a method of controlling the spread of infection.
______ **d.** There is only one kind of sterilization.
______ **e.** Proper handwashing helps control the spread of infection.
______ **f.** Handwashing is one of the most important controls of infection.

5. What does aseptic technique include (6 points)?

a. ______________________ d. ______________________

b. ______________________ e. ______________________

c. ______________________ f. ______________________

6. Explain why Standard Precautions are important (6 points).

____

____

____

7. What is a common household cleaner that is effective against microorganisms (1 point)? ______________________

____

8. What dilution do you use when preparing this cleaner for disinfecting (1 point)? ______________________

____

9. What method of sterilization destroys spore-forming bacteria (1 point)?

____

10. There are three types of sterilization. What are they (3 points)?

a. ____

b. ____

c. ____

11. List four major factors in the control of microorganisms (4 points).

a. ____

b. ____

c. ____

d. ____

12. You are carrying supplies down the hall. You notice you've dropped a towel. When you pick it up, it looks clean. What will you do, and why (2 points)? ______________________

____

____

There are 33 possible points in this worksheet.

UNIT 3

Standard Precautions

• OBJECTIVES

When you have completed this unit, you will be able to do the following:

- Name two primary levels of precautions identified in the guidelines developed by the Center for Disease Control (CDC).
- Identify three types of Transmission-based Precautions
- Demonstrate the correct procedure for entering and leaving an area where Transmission-based Precautions are followed.
- Differentiate between Standard Precautions and Transmission-based Precautions.

• DIRECTIONS

1. Read this unit.
2. Complete Worksheet 1.
3. Practice:
   - Applying personal protective equipment by following the steps in P12-2.
   - Removing personal protective equipment by following the steps in P12-3.
4. Complete the Chapter Review—Your Link to Success at the end of this chapter.
5. When you are confident that you can meet each objective listed above, ask your instructor for the unit evaluation.

• EVALUATION METHODS

- Worksheets
- Class participation
- Return demonstration
- Written evaluation

• WORKSHEET 1

Match the following statements with the appropriate terms listed at the left (8 points).

Terms	*Statements*
____ 1. Standard Precautions	a. Reduce the spread of pathogens 5 microns or smaller in size.
____ 2. Transmission-based Precautions	b. Reduce the risk of pathogen transmission through direct or indirect contact.
____ 3. Nosocomial	c. Hepatitis B Virus.
____ 4. Droplet Precautions	d. Primary strategy for successfully preventing hospital-acquired infections.
____ 5. Airborne Precautions	e. Hospital-acquired infection.
____ 6. Micron	f. Reduce the risk of transmission by a particle larger than 5 microns.
____ 7. Contact Precautions	g. Care for known or suspected patients infected with pathogens.
____ 8. HBV	h. One-millionth of a meter in size.

9. When should Standard Precautions be followed (1 point)? ____________

10. Why are Transmission-based Precautions necessary (1 point)? ____________

11. What is the difference between Transmission-based Precautions and Standard Precautions (6 points)? ____________

12. Which precautions require the room door to be closed (1 point)? ____________

13. When working with a client in Droplet Precautions, when do you put on a mask (1 point)? ____________

14. When working with a client in Contact Precautions, when do you take your gloves off (1 point)? ____________

15. Which of the three Transmission-based Precautions requires a private room with specific ventilation criteria (1 point)? ____________

16. Name the three Transmission-based Precautions (3 points).

    a. ____________

    b. ____________

    c. ____________

17. Name two primary levels of precautions identified in the guidelines developed by the Center for Disease Control (2 points).

    a. ____________

    b. ____________

There are 25 possible points in this worksheet.

Check-off Sheet:

12-1 Handwashing

Name ______________________ **Date** ________

Directions: Practice this procedure, following each step. When you are ready to have your performance evaluated, give this sheet to your instructor. Review the detailed procedure in your textbook.

Procedure	Pass	Redo	Date Competency Met	Instructor Initials
Student must use Standard Precautions.	☐	☐	________	________
1. Turn on water.	☐	☐	________	________
2. Regulate temperature.	☐	☐	________	________
3. Wet hands, with fingers pointed downward.	☐	☐	________	________
4. Apply soap to hands and wrists.	☐	☐	________	________
5. Rub hands in circular motion.	☐	☐	________	________
6. Interlace fingers, rub back and forth (add water when necessary to keep moist).	☐	☐	________	________
7. Use a nailbrush. If none is available, rub fingernails on palms of hands.	☐	☐	________	________
8. Rinse with fingers pointed down.	☐	☐	________	________
9. Dry hands with paper towel.	☐	☐	________	________
10. Turn off faucet with paper towel.	☐	☐	________	________
11. Leave area clean and neat.	☐	☐	________	________

Chapter 13 Patient and Employee Safety

UNIT 1

General Safety and Injury and Illness Prevention

• OBJECTIVES

When you have completed this unit, you will be able to do the following:

- Match vocabulary words with their correct meanings.
- Define *OSHA* and explain the agency's role in safety.
- Differentiate between IIPP, hazard communication, and exposure control.
- Name places to find information about hazards in a facility.
- Explain the health care worker's role in maintaining a safe workplace.
- Discuss the employer's role in maintaining a safe workplace.
- Identify fourteen general safety rules.
- Summarize the importance of safety in a health care environment.

• DIRECTIONS

1. Complete Worksheet 1 before beginning the reading.
2. Read this unit.
3. Complete Worksheets 2 and 3 as assigned.
4. Complete Worksheets/Activities 4 through 6 as assigned.
5. Complete Worksheets 7 and 8 as assigned.
6. When you are confident that you can meet each objective listed above, ask your instructor for the unit evaluation.

• EVALUATION METHODS

- Worksheets/Activities
- Class participation
- Written evaluation

• WORKSHEET 1

Define each of the following vocabulary words (10 points).

1. Abreast ______
2. Biohazard ______
3. Comply ______
4. Environment ______
5. Frayed ______
6. Implement ______
7. Horseplay ______
8. Malfunctioning ______
9. Mandates ______
10. Shock ______

There are 10 possible points in this worksheet.

• WORKSHEET 2

1. What is OSHA (1 point)? ______

   ______

2. Explain the agency's role in safety (3 points).

   a. ______

   ______

   b. ______

   ______

   c. ______

   ______

3. What does IIPP stand for (1 point)?

   ______

4. Every employer must establish an injury and illness prevention program. As an employee, you are responsible for understanding the injury and illness prevention program in your facility. What are your specific responsibilities (6 points)?

   a. ______
   b. ______
   c. ______
   d. ______
   e. ______
   f. ______

5. Explain the ergonomic program (1 point).

There are 12 possible points in this worksheet.

• WORKSHEET 3

1. Every employer must have a hazard communication program. Put an *X* next to the information that is mandated (6 points).

    ______ **a.** Chemicals or hazards in the environment
    ______ **b.** How to use the telephone in an emergency
    ______ **c.** Where chemicals or hazards are stored and used
    ______ **d.** How to interpret chemical labels and hazard signs
    ______ **e.** The names of the dangerous chemicals in the environment
    ______ **f.** Methods and equipment for cleaning chemical spills
    ______ **g.** Where important medications are stored
    ______ **h.** Personal protective equipment and its storage location
    ______ **i.** The hazard communication system
    ______ **j.** How to write an incident report

2. Define *biohazard* (1 point). ______________________________

    ____

3. What must the employee know about the hazard communication system (6 points)?

    a. ______________________________
    b. ______________________________
    c. ______________________________
    d. ______________________________
    e. ______________________________
    f. ______________________________

4. Explain the hazard communication program (1 point).

    ____

    ____

5. What is a material safety data sheet, or MSDS (1 point)?

    ____

    ____

6. Put an *X* next to the information that must be on a material safety data sheet (10 points). Refer to the MSDS in your textbook.

    ______ **a.** Spill or leak procedures
    ______ **b.** Special precautions
    ______ **c.** Table of contents
    ______ **d.** Product identification
    ______ **e.** How to use the product
    ______ **f.** Cost of product
    ______ **g.** Hazardous ingredients of mixtures
    ______ **h.** Physical data
    ______ **i.** Telephone number of the nearest fire department
    ______ **j.** Health hazard data

_______ **k.** Protection information and control measures
_______ **l.** Fire and explosion
_______ **m.** How to perform CPR
_______ **n.** Emergency and first aid procedures
_______ **o.** Name and address of your facility's director
_______ **p.** Reactivity data

7. Write the name of the section on an MSDS where you will find the following information (3 points).

a. How to clean up a spill _______________

b. How and where to store the product _______________

c. What protective wear to use when working with the product _______________

8. List the two hazard categories, and explain each one (4 points).

a. _______________

____

____

____

b. _______________

____

There are 32 possible points in this worksheet.

• WORKSHEET/ACTIVITY 4

Get together with three or four classmates and select a safety procedure or issue to demonstrate and explain to the class. For example, you might choose body mechanics and good posture for lifting, patient restraints, or ambulation devices. Have some demonstrate as others describe and explain the procedure and the issues involved.

There are 65 possible points in this worksheet/activity.

• WORKSHEET/ACTIVITY 5

1. Where should you look for hazard communications (5 points)?

a. _______________

b. _______________

c. _______________

d. _______________

e. _______________

2. Find all the places in your facility where safety information is available. List these places below (50 points).

____

____

3. When you find the material safety data sheets, choose two products and read the MSDSs for these products. Fill in the information below for each product (20 points).

	Product 1	Product 2
Product identification		
Health hazard data		
Protection information and control measures		
Spill or leak procedures		
Fire and explosion		
Hazardous ingredients of mixtures		
Emergency and first aid procedures		
Special precautions		
Reactivity data		
Physical data		

There are 75 possible points in this worksheet/activity.

• WORKSHEET/ACTIVITY 6

Read the labels on two products that are used in your facility. Use the information on the labels to answer the following questions.

1. What is the name of the product (2 points)?
   a. Product 1: ______________________
   b. Product 2: ______________________
2. Does the label tell you what precautions to take when using the product (2 points)?
   a. Product 1: ______________________
   b. Product 2: ______________________
3. What chemicals are listed on the label (2 points)?
   a. Product 1: ______________________
   b. Product 2: ______________________
4. What should you do if the product gets on your skin or in your eyes (2 points)?
   a. Product 1: ______________________
   b. Product 2: ______________________
5. How should you clean up a spill (2 points)?
   a. Product 1: ______________________
   b. Product 2: ______________________
6. What do you do if you breathe the fumes (2 points)?
   a. Product 1: ______________________
   b. Product 2: ______________________

7. What personal protective equipment do you need when using this product (2 points)?

   a. Product 1: ______________________________

   b. Product 2: ______________________________

8. Explain why the labeling of products is important (1 point). ______________________________

____

____

____

There are 15 possible points in this worksheet/activity.

• WORKSHEET 7

1. Explain what an exposure control program is (1 point). ______________________________

____

____

2. List three things the program includes (3 points).

   a. ______________________________

   b. ______________________________

   c. ______________________________

3. Differentiate between an IIPP, hazard communication, and exposure control (6 points). ______________________________

____

____

____

____

____

4. Explain the health care worker's role in maintaining a safe workplace (4 points). ______________________________

____

____

____

There are 14 possible points in this worksheet.

• WORKSHEET 8

1. Identify the 14 general safety rules by placing an *X* next to each one (14 points).

    ______ **a.** Do not use electrical cords that are frayed or damaged.
    ______ **b.** Run in an emergency.
    ______ **c.** Watch out for swinging doors.
    ______ **d.** Use handrails when using the stairs.
    ______ **e.** Report a shock you receive from equipment to your supervisor.
    ______ **f.** Horseplay is not tolerated.
    ______ **g.** Walk in the middle of the hall to avoid swinging doors.
    ______ **h.** Follow instructions carefully.
    ______ **i.** Wipe up spills only if you have time.
    ______ **j.** Do everything you are asked to do, and do not ask questions.
    ______ **k.** Report any injury to yourself or others to your supervisor immediately.
    ______ **l.** Always check labels.
    ______ **m.** Wipe up spills, and place litter in containers.
    ______ **n.** Follow Standard Precaution guidelines.
    ______ **o.** Report unsafe conditions to your supervisor immediately.
    ______ **p.** Walk! Never run in hallways.
    ______ **q.** Wait a day or two to report a minor injury; it may get better.
    ______ **r.** Walk on the right-hand side of the hall not more than two abreast.
    ______ **s.** Do not use malfunctioning equipment.
    ______ **t.** Avoid using handrails on stairs so you can securely hold items you are carrying.

2. Summarize the importance of safety in a health care environment. Explain how teamwork between the employer and the employee affects safety (6 points). ______________________________

    ____

    ____

    ____

    ____

There are 20 possible points in this worksheet.

UNIT 2

Patient Safety

• OBJECTIVES

When you have completed this unit, you will be able to do the following:

- Explain how to use ambulation devices, transporting devices, postural supports, and side rails safely.
- Match descriptions and principles associated with ambulation devices, transporting devices, postural supports, and side rails.
- Explain the importance of safety measures.
- Follow safe practice guidelines when caring for clients.

• DIRECTIONS

1. Read this unit.
2. Complete Worksheet 1.
3. When you are confident that you can meet each objective listed above, ask your instructor for the unit evaluation.

• EVALUATION METHODS

- Worksheet
- Class participation
- Written evaluation

• WORKSHEET 1

1. Complete the following sentences (4 points).

   a. Ambulation devices are used to ______________________________

   ____

   b. Transportation devices are used to ______________________________

   ____

   c. Postural supports are used to ______________________________

   ____

   d. Side rails are used to ______________________________

   ____

2. Write each word listed below in the space next to the example or principle that illustrates it (15 points).

ambulation devices postural supports transporting devices side rails

_______________ a. Wheelchair.
_______________ b. A release must be signed before you can leave them down.
_______________ c. These must have rubber tips covering areas that touch the floor.
_______________ d. Wheels must be locked when taking clients in or out of these devices.
_______________ e. Walker.
_______________ f. Small children always need them up.
_______________ g. Vest.
_______________ h. A doctor's order is required before they can be used.
_______________ i. They must be loosened every two hours.
_______________ j. They prevent clients from falling out of bed.
_______________ k. Gurney.
_______________ l. Always back these devices over indented or raised doorways.
_______________ m. Lock brakes except when moving.
_______________ n. Keep two fingers' width between these and the client's skin.
_______________ o. Check for breaks or cracks before using.

3. Explain the importance of safety measures (2 points). _______________
____
____

There are 21 possible points in this worksheet.

UNIT 3 Disaster Preparedness

• OBJECTIVES

When you have completed this unit, you will be able to do the following:

- Define vocabulary words.
- Identify what you are responsible for knowing and doing when a disaster occurs.
- List the three elements required to start a fire.
- Explain four ways to prevent fires.
- Summarize all safety requirements that protect the employee, student, patient, and employer.

• DIRECTIONS

1. Read this unit.
2. Complete Worksheet 1.
3. When you are confident that you can meet each objective listed above, ask your instructor for the unit evaluation.

• EVALUATION METHODS

- Worksheet
- Class participation
- Written evaluation

• WORKSHEET 1

1. Define the following vocabulary words (3 points).

   a. Observant ______________________________

   b. Cylinder ______________________________

   c. Potential ______________________________

2. List five examples of disasters (5 points).

   a. ______________________________

   b. ______________________________

   c. ______________________________

   d. ______________________________

   e. ______________________________

3. Identify what you are responsible for knowing and doing when a disaster occurs. Place an *X* next to your responsibilities (9 points).

   ______ **a.** Know who makes each type of fire extinguisher.
   ______ **b.** Know the floor plan of your facility.
   ______ **c.** Know what causes a tornado.
   ______ **d.** Know the magnitude of the earthquake.
   ______ **e.** Assess the situation and calm yourself.
   ______ **f.** Know the nearest exit route.
   ______ **g.** Do not place yourself in danger.
   ______ **h.** Know the name of the nearest fire station.
   ______ **i.** Remove those who are in immediate danger, if it is safe to do so.
   ______ **j.** Use the stairs, not the elevator.
   ______ **k.** Notify others of the emergency according to facility policy.
   ______ **l.** Know the location of the alarms and fire extinguishers.
   ______ **m.** Know your role as a health care worker when a disaster occurs.

4. List the three elements required to start a fire (3 points).

   a. ______________________________

   b. ______________________________

   c. ______________________________

5. Explain four ways to prevent a fire (4 points).
   a. ______
   b. ______
   c. ______
   d. ______
6. Summarize all safety requirements that protect the employee, student, patient, and employer (5 points).

There are 29 possible points in this worksheet.

UNIT 4

Principles of Body Mechanics

• OBJECTIVES

When you have completed this unit, you will be able to do the following:

- Define vocabulary words.
- Define *body mechanics.*
- List six rules of correct body mechanics.
- List six principles of body mechanics.
- Demonstrate the correct lifting and moving of objects.

• DIRECTIONS

1. Read this unit.
2. Complete Worksheet 1.
3. When you are confident that you can meet each objective listed above, ask your instructor for the unit evaluation.

• EVALUATION METHODS

- Worksheet
- Class participation
- Written evaluation

• WORKSHEET 1

1. Define the following vocabulary words (3 points).
   a. Efficiency ______
   b. Gravity ______
   c. Crouch ______

2. Define *body mechanics* (1 point). ______________________________

____

3. List the six principles of body mechanics (6 points).

   a. ______________________________

   b. ______________________________

   c. ______________________________

   d. ______________________________

   e. ______________________________

   f. ______________________________

4. List the six rules of correct body mechanics, and explain why you think each one is important (12 points).

   a. ______________________________

   ____

   b. ______________________________

   ____

   c. ______________________________

   ____

   d. ______________________________

   ____

   e. ______________________________

   ____

   f. ______________________________

   ____

There are 22 possible points in this worksheet.

UNIT 5

First Aid

• OBJECTIVES

When you have completed this unit, you will be able to do the following:

- Match vocabulary words with their correct meanings.
- Demonstrate the procedures for:
  - Mouth-to-mouth breathing
  - Obstructed airway
  - Serious wounds
  - Preventing shock
  - Splints
  - Slings
  - Bandaging

• DIRECTIONS

1. Complete Worksheets 1 through 4 as assigned.
2. Practice and then demonstrate the following procedures as your instructor directs you:
   - Rescue breathing
   - Obstructed airway in a conscious victim
   - Obstructed airway in an unconscious victim
   - Stopped breathing in an infant
   - Obstructed airway in a conscious infant
   - Obstructed airway in an unconscious infant
3. Read Serious Wounds through Preventing Shock.
4. Complete the Learn by Doing assignments at the end of this reading.
5. Complete Worksheet 5 as assigned.
6. Practice and then demonstrate the following procedures as your instructor directs you:
   - How to treat serious wounds
   - Identify pressure points on a diagram
   - Preventing shock
7. Read Poisoning through Treating Burns.
8. Complete the Learn by Doing assignment at the end of this reading.
9. Complete Worksheets 6 and 7 as assigned.
10. Practice and demonstrate the following procedures as your instructor directs you:
    - Treating a conscious poison victim
    - Treating an unconscious poison victim
    - Treating burns

11. Read Non-life-threatening Situations through the end of this unit.
12. Complete the Learn by Doing assignments at the end of this reading.
13. Complete Worksheet 8 as assigned.
14. Practice and demonstrate the following procedures as your instructor directs you:
    - Applying a splint
    - Applying a triangular sling
    - Triangular bandaging of a head wound
    - Circular bandaging of a small leg or arm wound
    - Spiral bandaging of a large wound
    - Bandaging of an ankle or foot wound
15. Prepare responses to each item listed in the Chapter Review—Your Link to Success at the end of this chapter.
16. When you are confident that you can meet each objective for this unit, ask your instructor for the unit evaluation.

• EVALUATION METHODS

- Worksheets
- Class participation
- Written evaluation

• WARNINGS

- Do not make mouth-to-mouth contact with your classmate during practice.
- Remember to only pretend to do abdominal thrusts on a real person.

• WORKSHEET 1

1. Place each word listed below in the space next to the statement that best defines it (6 points).

abdominal thrust	fracture	EMS
splints	symptoms	swath

_______________ **a.** Broken bone.

_______________ **b.** Forceful thrust on the abdomen, between the sternum and the navel, in an upward motion toward the head.

_______________ **c.** Emergency medical system.

_______________ **d.** Bandage.

_______________ **e.** Firm objects used to support an unstable body part.

_______________ **f.** Signs that indicate a condition, usually a disorder or disease.

2. Match each definition in column B with the correct vocabulary word in column A (8 points).

Column A	*Column B*
____ 1. Cardiopulmonary	a. Condition in which the skin is bruised, swollen, and painful but is not broken.
____ 2. Contusion	b. Especially sensitive, capable of being affected.
____ 3. Dressings	c. Having to do with the heart and lungs.
____ 4. Susceptible	d. Bandages, usually gauze pads that are used to cover a wound.
____ 5. Definitive	e. Wound or tear of the skin.
____ 6. Saturated	f. Clear, without question, exacting.
____ 7. Laceration	g. Forceful upward thrust on the abdomen, between the sternum and the navel.
____ 8. Heimlich maneuver	h. Soaked; filled to capacity.

3. Define the following vocabulary words (3 points).

a. Impending ______________________________

b. Priorities ______________________________

c. Spurts ______________________________

There are 17 possible points in this worksheet.

• WORKSHEET 2

1. What is first aid (1 point)? ______________________________

____

2. Write the six general principles of first aid, and explain why each is important (12 points).

a. ______________________________

____

b. ______________________________

____

c. ______________________________

____

d. ______________________________

____

e. ______________________________

____

f. ______________________________

____

3. List the life-threatening situations discussed in the text (7 points).

   a. ______________________________

   b. ______________________________

   c. ______________________________

   d. ______________________________

   e. ______________________________

   f. ______________________________

   g. ______________________________

4. Explain why these situations are life threatening (2 points). ______________________________

   ____

   ____

   ____

5. Oxygen is necessary for ____________ to live (1 point).

6. Permanent brain damage can occur if (a) ____________ is not present for (b) ____________ to (c) ____________ minutes (3 points).

There are 26 possible points in this worksheet.

• WORKSHEET 3

1. List each step in the procedure for mouth-to-mouth or mouth-to-nose breathing for a victim who has stopped breathing (5 points).

   a. ______________________________

   b. ______________________________

   c. ______________________________

   d. ______________________________

   e. ______________________________

2. Fill in the missing words to complete the following sentences (3 points).

   a. If air does not inflate the lungs when giving mouth-to-mouth breathing, you should ____________ to ensure an open airway.

   b. If, after ensuring an open airway, the lungs still do not inflate, the victim should be treated for an ____________.

   c. If the lungs do inflate during mouth-to-mouth breathing, give one breath every ____________ seconds for an adult.

There are 8 possible points in this worksheet.

• WORKSHEET 4

1. Fill in the missing words to complete the following sentences (4 points).
   a. Obstructed airway occurs when an ____________________ blocks the airway.
   b. The two types of obstructions discussed are ____________________ and ____________________.
   c. Do not ____________________ with the victim's attempt to cough the object out.
2. List the signs of poor air exchange (5 points).
   a. ____________________
   b. ____________________
   c. ____________________
   d. ____________________
   e. ____________________
3. ____________________ occurs when there is no air exchange or there is poor air exchange (1 point).
4. List the signs of a complete airway obstruction (3 points).
   a. ____________________
   b. ____________________
   c. ____________________
5. List each step in the procedure to correct an obstructed airway of a conscious victim (2 points).
   a. ____________________
   b. ____________________
6. Should you begin the Heimlich maneuver if the victim is coughing (1 point)? ____________________
7. List each step in the procedure for obstructed airway in an unconscious victim (6 points).
   a. ____________________
   b. ____________________
   c. ____________________
   d. ____________________
   e. ____________________
   f. ____________________

There are 22 possible points in this worksheet.

• WORKSHEET 5

1. The first two hours after the onset of a heart attack are the ______________ period (1 point).
2. List the early warning signs of a heart attack (3 points).
   a. ______________________________
   b. ______________________________
   c. ______________________________
3. If the bleeding is pulsating in a serious wound, the ______________ has been cut (1 point).
4. When an artery is cut, it is necessary to apply ______________ to stop the bleeding (1 point).
5. Covering a serious wound decreases the chance of ______________ (1 point).
6. When performing first aid for a serious wound, you may use a piece of (a) ______________ or (b) ______________ if gauze dressings are not available (2 points).
7. List the procedure for performing first aid on a serious wound (3 points).
   a. ______________________________
   b. ______________________________
   c. ______________________________
8. List the procedure for performing first aid on a serious wound when direct pressure does not control the bleeding (4 points).
   a. ______________________________
   b. ______________________________
   c. ______________________________
   d. ______________________________

There are 16 possible points in this worksheet.

• WORKSHEET 6

1. Fill in the missing words to complete the following sentences (4 points).
   a. Shock after a serious injury can be ______________.
   b. Shock ______________ body functions and keeps the ______________ from functioning normally.
   c. A victim can be treated correctly for a wound and still ______________ from shock.

2. List the procedure for preventing shock (7 points).

   a. ______________________

   b. ______________________

   c. ______________________

   d. ______________________

   e. ______________________

   f. ______________________

   g. ______________________

3. While following the procedure to prevent shock, you find an open fracture of the right leg. Should you elevate the right leg (1 point)?

   ____

4. How should you position a victim you are treating for shock if he or she is vomiting or bleeding from the mouth (1 point)? ______________________

   ____

5. Should victims with breathing problems, head injury, or neck injury have their feet elevated (1 point)? ______________________

There are 14 possible points in this worksheet.

• WORKSHEET 7

1. Poisoning often causes (a) ______________________, (b) ______________________, and (c) ______________________ (3 points).

2. List the first aid procedure for a conscious poison victim (5 points).

   a. ______________________

   b. ______________________

   c. ______________________

   d. ______________________

   e. ______________________

3. List the first aid procedure for an unconscious poison victim (6 points).

   a. ______________________

   b. ______________________

   c. ______________________

   d. ______________________

   e. ______________________

   f. ______________________

4. Fill in the missing words to complete the following sentences (8 points).

   a. Burns around the mouth or nose may indicate that the ________________ is burned.

   b. Always check a mild burn ________________ to ________________ hours after it occurs. ________________ and ________________ may not appear until then.

   c. When performing first aid on a burn victim, you strive to ________________, ________________, and ________________.

There are 22 possible points in this worksheet.

• WORKSHEET 8

1. What are the two main types of bone fractures (2 points)?

   a. ________________________________

   b. ________________________________

2. Bandages are necessary to prevent ________________ from entering a wound (1 point).

3. List the principles of bandaging (6 points).

   a. ________________________________

   b. ________________________________

   c. ________________________________

   d. ________________________________

   e. ________________________________

   f. ________________________________

There are 9 possible points in this worksheet.

Chapter 14 Employability and Leadership

UNIT 1

Job-Seeking Skills

• OBJECTIVES

When you have completed this unit, you will be able to do the following:

- List seven places to seek employment opportunities and explain the benefits of each.
- Explain four ways to contact an employer.
- Name three occasions when a cover letter is used.
- List eight items required on a résumé.
- Identify seven items generally requested on a job application form.
- Write a cover letter and a résumé.
- Complete a job application.
- List five do's and five don'ts of job interviewing.
- Compile a professional-looking vocational portfolio.

• DIRECTIONS

1. Read this unit.
2. Complete Worksheet 1.
3. Ask your instructor for directions to complete Worksheets/Activities 2 through 5.
4. Complete Worksheets/Activities 6 and 7.
5. Ask your instructor for directions to complete the Vocational Portfolio.
6. When you are confident that you can meet each objective listed above, ask your instructor for the unit evaluation.

• EVALUATION METHODS

- Worksheets/Activities
- Class participation
- Mock interview
- Vocational Portfolio

• WORKSHEET 1

1. Explain why a vocational portfolio is important (5 points). ______________

____

____

____

____

2. List seven places to seek employment opportunities, and explain the benefits of each (14 points).

 a. ____

 ____

 b. ____

 ____

 c. ____

 ____

 d. ____

 ____

 e. ____

 ____

 f. ____

 ____

 g. ____

 ____

3. List four ways to contact an employer (4 points).

 a. ____

 b. ____

 c. ____

 d. ____

4. Name three occasions when a cover letter is used (3 points).

 a. ____

 b. ____

 c. ____

5. List eight items required on a résumé (8 points).

a. ______________________________

b. ______________________________

c. ______________________________

d. ______________________________

e. ______________________________

f. ______________________________

g. ______________________________

h. ______________________________

6. Identify seven items generally requested on a job application form (7 points).

a. ______________________________

b. ______________________________

c. ______________________________

d. ______________________________

e. ______________________________

f. ______________________________

g. ______________________________

There are 41 possible points in this worksheet.

• WORKSHEET/ACTIVITY 2

Write a cover letter following the guidelines in your text in unit 1, "Ways to Contact an Employer." Figure 14–2 is an example of a block letter format. See the Vocational Portfolio for additional examples.

- Use 8.5-by-11-inch paper.
- Type, word-process, or write with ink on one side only.
- Use correct grammar and spell correctly.

There are 100 possible points in this worksheet/activity:

▪ Format	5
▪ Spelling	10
▪ Neatness	10
▪ Grammar	25
▪ Composition	25
▪ Content	25

• WORKSHEET/ACTIVITY 3

Write a résumé following the guidelines in your text in unit 1, "Ways to Contact an Employer." Figure 14–3 is an example résumé. See the Vocational Portfolio for additional samples.

- Use 8.5-by-11-inch paper.
- Type, word-process, or write with ink on one side only.
- Use correct grammar and spell correctly.

There are 100 possible points in this worksheet/activity:

- Format 5
- Spelling 10
- Neatness 10
- Grammar 25
- Composition 25
- Content 25

• WORKSHEET/ACTIVITY 4

Complete a job application provided by your instructor.

- Use a black pen.
- Fill in every line or answer every question.
- Spell correctly.
- Print neatly.

There are 75 possible points in this worksheet/activity:

- Spelling 25
- Neatness 25
- Completeness 25

• WORKSHEET/ACTIVITY 5

1. List five do's and five don'ts of job interviewing (10 points).

	Do's	**Don'ts**
a.	________________	________________
b.	________________	________________
c.	________________	________________
d.	________________	________________
e.	________________	________________

2. Participate in a mock interview. Be able to answer the following questions (10 points).
   a. What do you enjoy about working in health care?
   b. What are your strengths?
   c. What are your weaknesses?
   d. What would you do if the client started yelling at you and complaining about you?
   e. As a health care worker, what is the most important part of your job?
   f. Why do you want to work for [name of company]?
   g. Is there any reason why you cannot be here on a regular basis?
   h. The position requires lifting. Is there any reason why you cannot do it?
   i. If you had an opportunity to go to the beach but were scheduled for work, what would you do?
   j. This position requires weekend work. Is there any reason why you cannot work on weekends?

Class Critique of Mock Interview

Directions: Pretend you are interviewing a prospective employee for your own business. Answer the following questions, using your best judgment concerning the interviewee. Make a check next to *Yes* or *No* to indicate your answer.

1. Is the interviewee dressed appropriately? Yes No
2. Did the interviewee greet the interviewer by name? Yes No
3. Did the interviewee's handshake appear to be firm? Yes No
4. Did the interviewee wait for an invitation to be seated before sitting down? Yes No
5. Did the interviewee's answers leave a question in your mind about truthfulness and sincerity? Yes No

   Helpful comments: ____________________

   ____

   ____

6. Did the interviewee show enthusiasm? Yes No
7. Was the interviewee prepared with good answers to each question? Yes No

   If not, give examples. ____________________

   ____

   ____

   ____

8. What would you recommend the interviewee do differently for the next interview? ______________________________

There are 20 possible points in this worksheet/activity.

• WORKSHEET/ACTIVITY 6

Compile corrected, perfectly typed or word-processed, well-formatted, professional-looking documents from Vocational Portfolio worksheets.

Your instructor will explain how you will be graded.

• WORKSHEET/ACTIVITY 7

Work with your instructor and the whole class to create a bulletin board with classified advertising information.

Everyone in the class must bring in at least one ad from a classified newspaper, a Web site, the Yellow Pages, or another regional advertising source, such as a business journal.

Prepare a bulletin board with ad samples. Be sure to include employment agencies, area hospitals, nursing homes, and medical offices.

Keep the board updated as you find new listings.

Each listing brought in will earn a point and participation in the preparation of the board will earn points at the instructor's discretion.

UNIT 2 Keeping a Job

• OBJECTIVES

When you have completed this unit, you will be able to do the following:

- Define vocabulary words.
- List four employer responsibilities.
- List four responsibilities of a good employee.

• DIRECTIONS

1. Complete Worksheet 1 before beginning the reading.
2. Read this unit.
3. Ask your instructor for directions to complete Worksheet/Activity 2.
4. When you are confident that you can meet each objective listed above, ask your instructor for the unit evaluation.

• EVALUATION METHODS

- Worksheets/Activities
- Class participation
- Written evaluation

• WORKSHEET 1

1. Define the following vocabulary words (5 points).

a. Berating ______

b. Diligent ______

c. Productive ______

d. Initiative ______

e. Legitimate ______

2. List four employer responsibilities identified with the appropriate value (4 points).

a. Dignity ______

b. Excellence ______

c. Service ______

d. Fairness and Justice ______

3. List the responsibilities of a good employee identified with the appropriate value (11 points).

- Dignity

a. ______

b. ______

c. ______

- Excellence

a. ______

b. ______

c. ______

d. ______

- Service

a. ______

b. ______

- Fairness and Justice

a. ______

b. ______

There are 20 possible points in this worksheet.

• WORKSHEET 2

Write a one-or-two-page, double-spaced paper explaining what you consider your most important responsibility as an employee. Follow these guidelines when preparing your paper:

- Use 8.5-by-11-inch paper.
- Type, word-process, or write neatly in ink.
- Use correct spelling and grammar.

There are 100 possible points in this worksheet:

- Format 5
- Spelling 10
- Neatness 10
- Grammar 25
- Composition 25
- Content 25

UNIT 3

Becoming a Professional Leader

• OBJECTIVES

When you have completed this unit, you will be able to do the following:

- Define vocabulary words.
- Name the three main benefits of being a member of a student health vocational organization.
- Name six benefits of being a member of a professional organization.
- Identify ways to find a professional organization.
- Identify steps to become a leader.
- Define HOSA and VICA.
- Summarize why you plan to participate in a student and professional organization.

• DIRECTIONS

1. Read this unit.
2. Complete Worksheet 1.
3. Ask your instructor for directions to complete Worksheet/Activity 2.
4. Prepare responses to each item listed in the Chapter Review—Your Link to Success at the end of this chapter.
5. When you are confident that you can meet each objective for this unit, ask your instructor for the unit evaluation.

• EVALUATION METHODS

- Worksheets/Activities
- Class participation
- Written evaluation

• WORKSHEET 1

1. Define the following words (3 points).

a. Foster ______________________________

b. Prestige ______________________________

c. Extemporaneous ______________________________

2. Name the three main benefits of being a member of a student health vocational organization (3 points).

a. ______________________________

b. ______________________________

c. ______________________________

3. Name five benefits of being a member of a professional organization (5 points).

a. ______________________________

b. ______________________________

c. ______________________________

d. ______________________________

e. ______________________________

4. Identify six ways to find a professional organization (6 points).

a. ______________________________

b. ______________________________

c. ______________________________

d. ______________________________

e. ______________________________

f. ______________________________

5. Which of the following exhibit leadership qualities? Write an *X* in the appropriate spaces (5 points).

____ **a.** Coach	____ **f.** Clown	____**k.** Cop
____ **b.** Enthusiast	____ **g.** Naysayer	____**l.** Nurturer
____ **c.** Referee	____ **h.** Friend	____**m.** Cheerleader
____ **d.** Gossip	____ **i.** Facilitator	____**n.** Devil's advocate
____ **e.** Boss	____ **j.** Joiner	____**o.** Zealot

There are 22 possible points in this worksheet.

• WORKSHEET/ACTIVITY 2

Summarize in a one-page, double-spaced paper why you plan to participate in student and professional organizations.

- Use 8.5-by-11-inch paper.
- Type, word-process, or write neatly in ink.
- Spell correctly.
- Use proper grammar.

There are 75 possible points in this worksheet:

■ Spelling	10
■ Neatness	10
■ Grammar	28
■ Composition	27

Chapter 15 Nurse Assistant/ Patient Caregiver

UNIT 1

Basic Roles/Obra Care Skills/Long-Term Care

• OBJECTIVES

When you have completed this unit, you will be able to do the following:

- Complete all objectives in Part One of this text.
- Match vocabulary words with their correct meanings.
- Identify the following:
  - Responsibilities of the nurse assistant
  - Personal care equipment used by residents
  - Four skin conditions requiring special attention
  - Areas on the body where pressure sores usually develop
  - Antipressure aids
  - Occupied bed, closed bed, and open bed
  - Causes and symptoms of dehydration
  - Common types of specimens collected for analysis
  - Six common prosthetic devices
- List the following:
  - Four types of bathing
  - Two body areas requiring special attention during the bathing process
  - Four changes in the skin that may indicate the beginning of a pressure sore
  - Four techniques for positioning residents
  - Seven reasons why ambulation is important
  - Signs of diabetic coma and insulin shock
  - Nine steps to preparing a resident for a meal
  - Seven ways to prevent pressure sores
  - Causes and symptoms of edema
  - Ways to help residents who have a colostomy, ileostomy, or ureterostomy

    - Symptoms that indicate a resident is about to faint, and precautions that prevent injury
    - Five conditions that may develop when using postural supports
    - Five things you must do when using postural supports
- Explain the following:
    - Four important reasons to give mouth care
    - Six important reasons for routine bathing
    - Nine conditions poor body alignment causes
    - Why residents with diabetes must have their toenails cut by a podiatrist
    - Why a urinary drainage bag is not raised above the level of insertion
    - Six causes of incontinence
    - Procedures for bowel and/or bladder training
    - Important observations about urine
    - Important observations about stool
- Define the following terms:
    - AM and PM care
    - Good body alignment
    - Seizure
    - Syncope
    - Soft postural supports
    - Guarding technique and guarding belt from Chapter 19
- Match range-of-motion vocabulary words with their meanings.
- Calculate in cc and record fluid intake properly.
- Evaluate and determine appropriate action for a given situation.
- Demonstrate each procedure in this chapter.
- Demonstrate the following in Chapter 19:
    - Ambulating with a walking belt
    - Walking with crutches
    - Walking with a walker

• DIRECTIONS

1. Complete Worksheet 1 before beginning reading.
2. Read Unit 1.
3. Complete Worksheets/Activities 2 through 4 as directed by your instructor.
4. Complete Worksheets 5 through 7 as assigned.
5. Complete Worksheet/Activity 8 as directed by your instructor.
6. Complete Worksheets 9 and 10 as assigned.
7. Complete Worksheets/Activities 11 through 13 as directed by your instructor.
8. Complete Worksheets 14 through 17 as assigned.
9. Use the skills check-off sheets to practice and demonstrate all procedure in the chapter.
10. Prepare responses to each item listed in the Chapter Review—Your Link to Success at the end of this chapter.
11. When you are confident that you can meet each objective for this unit, ask your instructor for the unit evaluation.

• EVALUATION METHODS

- Worksheets/Activities
- Class participation
- Written evaluation
- Return demonstrations

• WORKSHEET 1

Fill in the crossword puzzle using the vocabulary words from Chapter 15 in your text (21 points).

Indicates a space between two words.

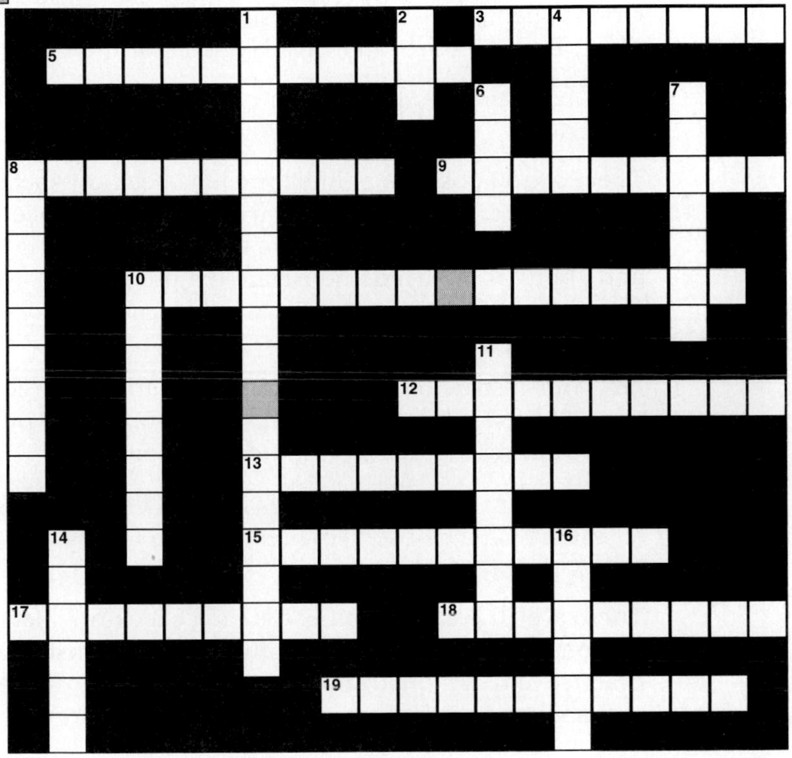

Clues

Across

3. Left over.
5. Severe loss of fluid from tissue and cells.
8. Walking.
9. Fecal material tightly wedged into the bowel.
10. Soft restraints used to protect residents.
12. Removal.
13. To get rid of something.
15. Unable to control the bowel or bladder.
17. Tubes inserted into a body opening or cavity.
18. Holding or keeping.
19. Ability to bend easily.

Down

1. Artificial parts made for the body.
2. Range of motion (abbreviation).
4. Opening.
6. Arm or leg.
7. Involuntary muscle contraction and relaxation.
8. Keeping a resident in proper position is called body __________.
10. Region between the vulva and anus in a female, or between the scrotum and anus in the male.
11. Liquid or pill that causes evacuation of the bowel.
14. Cold and wet.
16. Vomit.

There are 21 possible points in this worksheet.

• WORKSHEET/ACTIVITY 2

Find a partner and talk about how each of you likes to wake up in the morning and go to sleep at night. Be prepared to share your discussion with the class and think about the insights your own preferences give you into helping clients in your care with morning and nighttime routines.

There are 5 possible points in this worksheet/activity.

• WORKSHEET/ACTIVITY 3

1. Ask your instructor for directions. Bring a toothbrush to class for practice. In teams of three (a *resident, nurse assistant,* and *observer*), practice Self-Care Oral Hygiene, Brushing the Resident's Teeth, Oral Hygiene: Ambulatory Resident, Denture Care, and Oral Hygiene for the Unconscious Resident.

   The observer is responsible for checking that you carefully follow the procedure.

   There are 50 possible points for each check-off sheet you return and demonstrate. There are 200 points in this worksheet/activity. Points for practice and demonstration are assigned according to your participation and ability to return demonstrate the procedure to your instructor.

• WORKSHEET/ACTIVITY 4

1. Ask your instructor for directions. In teams of three (a *resident, nurse assistant,* and *observer*), use the skills check-off list to practice Offering the Bedpan, Offering the Urinal, and Bedside Commode.

   Each student will participate as (a) resident, (b) nurse assistant, and (c) observer. The observer is responsible for checking that you carefully follow the procedure.

   There are 50 possible points for each check-off sheet you return and demonstrate. There are 150 points in this worksheet/activity. Points for practice and demonstration are assigned according to your participation and ability to return demonstrate the procedure to your instructor.

• WORKSHEET 5

List seven reasons why ambulating the patient is important (7 points).

1. ______________________________
2. ______________________________
3. ______________________________
4. ______________________________
5. ______________________________
6. ______________________________
7. ______________________________

List eight complications of poor body alignment (8 points).

8. ______________________________
9. ______________________________

10. ______________________________

11. ______________________________

12. ______________________________

13. ______________________________

14. ______________________________

15. ______________________________

Match the following position names with their description (6 points).

_____ **16.** supine position	**a.** Facing down.
_____ **17.** semiprone	**b.** Sitting position.
_____ **18.** semisupine	**c.** Lying on side.
_____ **19.** prone position	**d.** Lying on side, front of body toward the mattress
_____ **20.** laterial	**e.** Lying on side with back of body leaning toward mattress.
_____ **21.** Fowler's position	**f.** Flat on back facing upward.

There are 21 possible points in this worksheet.

• WORKSHEET 6

Write the question for each of the following answers (15 points).

1. ______________________________

   Admit residents, provide AM and PM care, bathe residents, give good skin care, make beds, record intake and output, care for incontinent residents, perform range of motion.

2. ______________________________

   A list used when a new resident checks into a facility.

3. ______________________________

   A plastic bracelet with the resident's name on it.

4. ______________________________

   Residents use it to call for assistance.

5. ______________________________

   Special care given to residents in the morning and evening.

6. ______________________________

   Reduces odor, helps prevent tooth decay, is refreshing, relieves dry lips and mouth.

7. ______________________________

   Used to collect urine for a bedridden resident.

8. ______________________________

   To give baseline values for height and weight.

9. ______________________________

Used to collect fecal material.

10. ______________________________

Feces or stool.

11. ______________________________

Redness, heat, tenderness, or broken skin.

12. ______________________________

Shoulders, elbows, hips, sacrum, heels, ankles, ears, toes.

13. ______________________________

Change resident's position at least every two hours. Keep skin clean and dry. Massage reddened areas over sharp, bony areas. Provide backrubs to increase circulation and relax residents. Keep linen dry and free of wrinkles. Use foam padding or sheepskin.

14. ______________________________

Stimulates circulation, encourages flexibility, prevents contractures.

15. ______________________________

Pillow support at back, pillow support from the knee to ankle, trochanter support to prevent outward rotation, footboard and padded splints to prevent foot drop.

16. Mark on the diagram eight areas that are most sensitive to pressure sores (16 points).

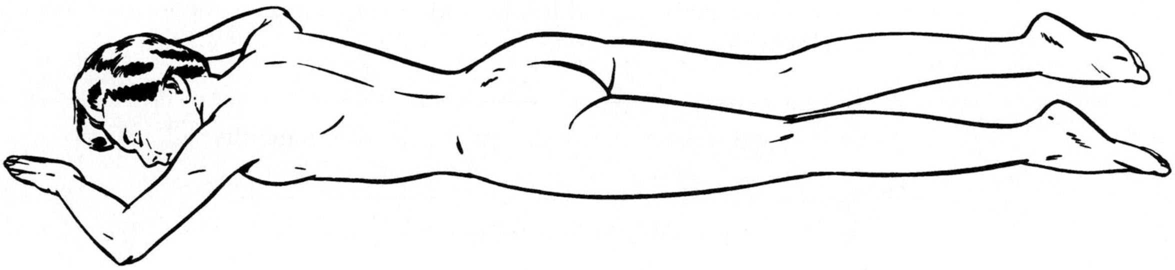

There are 31 possible points in this worksheet.

• WORKSHEET 7

Match each definition in column B with the correct vocabulary w
(13 points).

Column A	*Column B*
____ **1.** admit	**a.** Extending to ankle, toward the sole of
____ **2.** abduction	**b.** Between 12 midnight and 12 noon.
____ **3.** adduction	**c.** Moving an arm or leg toward the body.
____ **4.** extension	**d.** Between 12 noon and 12 midnight.
____ **5.** hyperextension	**e.** Moving an arm or leg away from the body.
____ **6.** flexion	**f.** Beyond the normal extension.
____ **7.** dorsiflexion	**g.** To figure out.
____ **8.** plantar flexion	**h.** To let someone in.
____ **9.** calculate	**i.** Flexing ankle, away from sole of foot.
____ **10.** syncope	**j.** False teeth.
____ **11.** denture	**k.** Straightening an arm or leg.
____ **12.** A.M.	**l.** Bending.
____ **13.** P.M.	**m.** Fainting.

Write the question for each of the following answers (5 points).

14. ____________________

Removes perspiration and dirt, removes odor, increases circulation, allows some exercise, provides an opportunity for skin to be observed, provides relaxation.

15. ____________________

Bed, tub, whirlpool, shower.

16. ____________________

Region between the vulva and anus in females and between the scrotum and anus in males.

17. ____________________

Observation and treatment for dryness, bruising, any unusual condition, and broken areas.

18. ____________________

To wheel residents into the shower.

There are 18 possible points in this worksheet.

• WORKSHEET/ACTIVITY 8

Use the skills check-off sheets provided in your book and by your teacher. Work with a partner to practice Measuring Weight on Standing Balance Scale, Measuring Weight on a Chair Scale, Measuring Weight on a Mechanical Lift and Measuring Height, Moving Resident and Belongings to Another Room, Discharging a Resident, AM and PM care, and Giving a Back Rub.

There are 50 possible points for each check-off sheet you return and demonstrate. There are 350 points in this worksheet/activity. Points for practice and demonstration are assigned according to your participation and ability to return demonstrate the procedure to your instructor.

WORKSHEET 9

1. List nine steps in preparing the patient for a meal (9 points).

   a. ____________________

   b. ____________________

   c. ____________________

   d. ____________________

   e. ____________________

   f. ____________________

   g. ____________________

   h. ____________________

   i. ____________________

2. Place the letter *E* next to causes of edema. Place the letter *D* next to causes of dehydration (12 points).

   _____ **a.** diarrhea
   _____ **b.** vomiting
   _____ **c.** high salt intake
   _____ **d.** bleeding
   _____ **e.** infections
   _____ **f.** excessive perspiration
   _____ **g.** injuries, burns
   _____ **h.** certain kidney diseases
   _____ **i.** certain heart diseases
   _____ **j.** poor fluid intake
   _____ **k.** infiltration of IV
   _____ **l.** sitting too long in one position

3. Place the letter *E* next to the symptoms of edema. Place the letter *D* next to symptoms of dehydration (8 points).

   _____ **a.** decrease in urine output
   _____ **b.** gain in weight
   _____ **c.** fever
   _____ **d.** sometimes shortness of breath
   _____ **e.** concentrated urine
   _____ **f.** weight loss
   _____ **g.** puffiness or swelling
   _____ **h.** increase in urine output

There are 29 possible points in this worksheet.

• WORKSHEET 10

1. From the following list, identify the nine items to be measured when the resident is on I & O. Circle the letter next to the appropriate items (9 points).

   a. water
   b. cereal
   c. gelatin
   d. egg salad sandwich
   e. juice
   f. fruit salad
   g. tea
   h. apple
   i. toast
   j. meat
   k. milk
   l. soup
   m. ice cream
   n. coffee
   o. custard

4. List oxygen safety rules (5 points).

   a. ______________________________

   b. ______________________________

   c. ______________________________

   d. ______________________________

   e. ______________________________

5. List four causes of seizures (4 points).

   a. ______________________________

   b. ______________________________

   c. ______________________________

   d. ______________________________

There are 35 possible points in this worksheet.

• WORKSHEET 16

1. List four symptoms that may indicate that a patient is about to faint (4 points).

   a. ______________________________

   b. ______________________________

   c. ______________________________

   d. ______________________________

2. List five things you must do when you use postural supports on a resident (5 points).

   a. ______________________________

   b. ______________________________

   c. ______________________________

   d. ______________________________

   e. ______________________________

3. Define soft postural supports (1 point).

   ____

   ____

4. Preparing a body after death is called ____________ (1 point).

There are 11 possible points in this worksheet.

• WORKSHEET 17

1. Mrs. Sherman is 96 years old. She experienced a stroke four months ago. She can walk with a walker and use her strong leg to push herself into a wheelchair. She is very independent and refuses help in washing and dressing herself. Every morning when you go in to see if she needs help, you find her sitting on her weak hand. She says she does not feel it, so it is OK. Explain what you will do to prevent Mrs. Sherman from sitting on her hand, and explain why it is important to protect the weak hand (20 points).

____

____

____

____

____

____

2. Mr. Cash calls for help to the bathroom. You know he has little control of his bladder. If you attend to him immediately, you will help him remain dry and clean. On your way to his room, you see a spilled urinal on the floor. Determine which situation requires attention first. Explain how you would handle both situations and what you expect the results to be (20 points).

____

____

____

____

____

____

3. Mrs. Collins is a resident with rheumatoid arthritis. She tries very hard to care for herself and becomes depressed when she is unable to do the activities of daily living. You deliver her lunch tray. As you are leaving, she says, "I hope I won't have trouble opening these containers." Explain what you think her concern and fear is. Determine how Mrs. Collins can be helped without her feeling helpless. Explain in detail what you will do and why (20 points).

____

____

____

____

____

____

4. Mr. Ramsey doesn't want to get out of bed or dress. He likes to stay in bed. He sometimes asks to have his breakfast tray brought to him. Then he asks to stay in bed and to read. You know that he wants to stay in bed all of the time. Explain how you can convince Mr. Ramsey how important it is to get up and attend activities (20 points).

5. When you are giving Mr. Gammons a back rub, you notice a reddened area on his shoulder and one on his hip. The reddened areas are both on his left side. Explain what steps you can take to be certain that he doesn't get a pressure sore. Write down the reasons why you give back rubs and explain why they are important (20 points).

6. Mr. Stevens is a new resident. When you ask him to get dressed, he refuses. You agree to allow him to rest an additional 20 minutes and ask him to get up again. He still refuses. Explain what you will do to encourage Mr. Stevens to get up and dress. Include in your explanation why it is important that he not be left in bed (20 points).

7. You are helping Ms. Hermans get out of bed. She has been in bed with the flu for three days. While she is sitting on the bedside, you notice that she is very pale and her face has beads of water on it. Her arm feels cool and wet. Explain what you will do for her (20 points).

8. Mr. White is short of breath after bathing and dressing. He still needs to shave and brush his teeth. He uses oxygen continuously and is afraid to have the oxygen turned off. He asks you to position his mirror and plug in his razor while his oxygen is on. Identify the problems in this situation. Explain what you will say to him and how you will assist him with shaving and brushing his teeth (20 points).

9. Mrs. Hughes experienced a stroke many years ago that left her paralyzed on the left side. She is usually out of bed in a wheelchair and in the recreation room. However, the last three days she has been sick to her stomach, so she stayed in bed. When rubbing her back, you notice a red area on her hip from lying on her side. You report it to the charge nurse and ask Mrs. Hughes to stay off her side. Later in the day you see her lying on the side where the red spot was. You also notice the sheets are wrinkled and half off the mattress. Think about the complications of the red hip after just three days in bed. Explain in detail the concerns you have about the red hip. Write the steps you will take to prevent further redness on the skin or other more serious complications (20 points).

10. Mrs. Allen has coarse hairs on her chin. She also has a slight mustache on her upper lip. She becomes irritated when she looks in the mirror. She tells you, "I was always such a pretty girl. Now I look old and ugly. Look at the awful hair on my face. I wish I could just die." Explain the steps you can take to help her. What can you do for her, and what can you say to raise her spirits (20 points)?

There are 200 possible points in this worksheet.

UNIT 2

Advanced Roles/Sub-Acute Care

• OBJECTIVES

When you have completed this unit, you will be able to do the following:

- List types of services in the sub-acute area.
- Explain transitional care.
- Describe the nurse assistant's role in the sub-acute area.
- List 12 observations for the postoperative patient.
- Explain why proper body alignment is important.
- List five devices used to align the body and explain how they work.

• DIRECTIONS

1. Complete vocabulary Worksheet 1.
2. Read this unit.
3. Complete Worksheet 2 as assigned.
4. Prepare responses to each item listed in the Chapter Review—Your Link to Success at the end of this chapter.
5. When you are confident that you can meet each objective for this unit, ask your instructor for the unit evaluation.

• EVALUATION METHOD

- Worksheets
- Class participation
- Oral quiz
- Written evaluation

• WORKSHEET 1

Directions: Using your text, or a medical dictionary, circle and number the words in the chart on the following page (horizontally, vertically, or diagonally) that match each of the following definitions. See example circled (18 points).

1. Abbreviation for intravenous
2. Unchangeable, cannot be changed
3. Collection of blood under the skin
4. Movement away from the midline of the body
5. Treatment
6. Fluid coming from the body
7. An unexpected occurence (diagonal answer)
8. Of vessels in the head (diagonal answer, from lower left to upper right)
9. Able to walk
10. Soaked through
11. A wound that reopens
12. Within a vein
13. A protrusion of a body organ through a wound
14. Abbreviation for a cerebrovascular accident
15. Inside the body
16. Placing a fluid into a vein
17. Outside of the body
18. Excessive bleeding

S	Q	W	D	V	S	E	R	O	S	A	N	G	U	I	N	E	O	U	S	V	K	U
A	Z	X	R	T	Y	J	K	H	L	P	T	Y	N	M	F	S	C	P	U	R	T	J
N	D	F	I	R	R	E	V	E	R	S	I	B	L	E	W	E	F	T	H	F	G	J
G	B	D	V	E	J	L	A	M	X	R	T	J	G	N	P	Z	A	H	F	E	H	B
U	Q	W	F	E	Y	R	J	A	B	D	U	C	T	I	O	N	K	E	B	N	M	H
I	P	U	R	U	L	E	N	T	E	W	Y	R	V	J	I	O	F	R	J	R	M	E
N	R	E	B	X	H	K	O	O	A	Q	E	T	D	R	A	I	N	A	G	E	M	M
E	R	E	G	B	V	C	Y	M	D	I	O	P	A	U	K	J	F	P	V	F	R	O
O	M	H	T	D	R	S	E	A	E	W	Q	L	H	C	J	K	L	Y	M	G	J	R
U	S	F	T	H	N	G	R	E	H	T	U	K	E	H	C	K	U	R	E	W	Z	R
S	M	A	J	K	L	O	I	O	I	C	Y	C	V	A	E	I	G	B	E	Y	I	H
K	Y	M	E	T	S	W	Q	Y	S	D	J	K	I	I	T	T	D	E	W	M	V	A
A	C	B	R	N	A	M	U	A	C	T	U	Q	S	R	G	R	C	E	D	G	S	G
W	F	U	S	H	T	K	V	L	E	B	I	E	C	I	N	T	E	R	N	A	L	E
Q	A	L	Z	X	U	O	S	W	N	E	D	C	E	V	F	R	B	G	T	T	N	H
Y	M	A	J	U	R	K	I	L	C	I	N	T	R	A	V	E	N	O	U	S	I	O
P	Z	T	A	B	A	Q	C	D	E	V	F	R	A	B	G	T	N	H	Y	M	J	U
K	I	O	E	L	T	O	P	Z	A	Q	C	X	T	W	C	D	E	V	F	R	B	G
T	N	R	N	H	E	T	Y	I	N	F	U	S	I	O	N	M	J	U	K	I	L	O
P	E	Y	B	V	D	C	X	Z	Q	W	E	R	O	F	D	S	A	L	K	J	H	Y
C	U	I	O	P	M	N	B	E	X	T	E	R	N	A	L	E	F	G	V	H	N	M

There are 18 possible points in this worksheet.

• WORKSHEET 2

Place an *X* next to each item that requires special attention by the sub-acute nurse assistant (21 possible points).

____ Labored respirations
____ Pink, warm, and dry skin
____ Loose dressings
____ Pail, clear drainage
____ Complaint of pain
____ Unusual odor
____ Slurred speech
____ Fresh blood on a bandage
____ Cyanosis of the skin or lips
____ Respiratory rate of 16 and regular
____ A moaning patient
____ Bubbles in a tracheostomy tube
____ Drainage from a wound
____ Client who is awake and alert
____ Smoothly flowing fluid in an IV
____ Stable blood pressure
____ Drainage tubes or catheters that are bent
____ Red, swollen skin color
____ Bradycardia
____ Client's discussing the daily news
____ Pulse rate of 80 and regular
____ Changing pupil size
____ Client suddenly not recognizing her family
____ Pulse rate of 100 and irregular
____ Blood in the IV tubing
____ Blood pressure of 120/80
____ IV site red and swollen
____ Nearly empty IV set
____ No urinary output in eight hours
____ Complaint of chest pain tube

There are 21 possible points in this worksheet.

Check-off Sheet:
15-1 Admitting a Resident

Name ______________________________ **Date** ______________

Directions: Practice this procedure, following each step. When you are ready to have your performance evaluated, give this sheet to your instructor. Review the detailed procedure in your textbook.

Procedure	Pass	Redo	Date Competency Met	Instructor Initials
Student must use Standard Precautions.	☐	☐	______	______
1. Wash hands.	☐	☐	______	______
2. Assemble equipment:				
a. Admission checklist				
b. Admission pack (may all be disposable depending on facility)				
1. Bedpan	☐	☐	______	______
2. Urinal	☐	☐	______	______
3. Emesis basin	☐	☐	______	______
4. Wash basin	☐	☐	______	______
5. Tissue	☐	☐	______	______
c. Gown or pajamas	☐	☐	______	______
d. Portable scale	☐	☐	______	______
e. Thermometer	☐	☐	______	______
f. Blood pressure cuff	☐	☐	______	______
g. Stethoscope	☐	☐	______	______
h. Clothing list	☐	☐	______	______
i. Envelope for valuables	☐	☐	______	______
3. Fan-fold bed covers to foot of bed. (See the check-off sheet "Making an Open Bed.")	☐	☐	______	______
4. Put resident's equipment away.	☐	☐	______	______
5. Put gown or pajamas on foot of bed.	☐	☐	______	______
6. Greet resident and introduce yourself.	☐	☐	______	______
7. Identify resident by looking at arm band and asking name.	☐	☐	______	______
8. Introduce resident to roommates.	☐	☐	______	______

Procedure	Pass	Redo	Date Competency Met	Instructor Initial
9. Explain				
a. How call signal works	☐	☐	______	______
b. How bed controls work	☐	☐	______	______
c. Hospital regulations	☐	☐	______	______
d. What you will be doing to admit him or her	☐	☐	______	______
10. Provide privacy by pulling privacy curtains.	☐	☐	______	______
11. Ask resident to put on gown or pajamas.	☐	☐	______	______
12. Check weight and height.	☐	☐	______	______
13. Help to bed, if ordered. (Check with nurse.)	☐	☐	______	______
14. Put side rails up, if required.	☐	☐	______	______
15. If resident has valuables:				
a. Make a list of jewelry, money, wallet, and so on	☐	☐	______	______
b. Have resident sign in	☐	☐	______	______
c. Have relative sign list	☐	☐	______	______
d. Either have relative take valuables home or send to cashier's office in valuables envelope.	☐	☐	______	______
16. Take and record the following:				
a. Temperature, pulse, respiration	☐	☐	______	______
b. Blood pressure	☐	☐	______	______
c. Urine specimen, if required	☐	☐	______	______
17. Complete admission checklist:				
a. Allergies	☐	☐	______	______
b. Medications being taken	☐	☐	______	______
c. Food preferences and dislikes	☐	☐	______	______
d. Any prosthesis	☐	☐	______	______
e. Skin condition	☐	☐	______	______
f. Handicaps (e.g., deafness, poor sight, lack of movement)	☐	☐	______	______
18. Orient resident to meal times, visiting hours, and so on.	☐	☐	______	______
19. Record information according to your facility's policy.	☐	☐	______	______
20. Wash hands.	☐	☐	______	______

Check-off Sheet:

15-2 Measuring Weight on Standing Balance Scale

Name ______________________________ **Date** ____________

Directions: Practice this procedure, following each step. When you are ready to have your performance evaluated, give this sheet to your instructor. Review the detailed procedure in your textbook.

Procedure	Pass	Redo	Date Competency Met	Instructor Initials
Student must use Standard Precautions.	☐	☐	______	______
1. Wash hands.	☐	☐	______	______
2. Assemble equipment:				
a. Portable balance scale	☐	☐	______	______
b. Paper towel	☐	☐	______	______
c. Paper and pencil/pen	☐	☐	______	______
3. Identify resident.	☐	☐	______	______
4. Explain what you are going to do.	☐	☐	______	______
5. Take resident to scale or bring scale to resident's room.	☐	☐	______	______
6. Place paper towel on platform of scale (with standing scale).	☐	☐	______	______
7. Put both weights to the very left on zero.	☐	☐	______	______
8. Balance beam pointer must stay steady in middle of balance area.				
9. Have resident remove shoes and stand on scale. (*Note:* the balance bar rises to top of bar guide when pointer is not centered.)	☐	☐	______	______
10. Move large weight to estimated weight of resident.	☐	☐	______	______
11. Move small weight to right until balance bar hangs free halfway between upper and lower bar guide.	☐	☐	______	______
12. Write weight down on a notepad.	☐	☐	______	______
13. Help resident with shoes and make him or her comfortable.	☐	☐	______	______
14. Replace scale.	☐	☐	______	______
15. Wash your hands.	☐	☐	______	______
16. Chart weight. Report any unusual increases or decreases in weight.	☐	☐	______	______

Check-off Sheet:

15-3 Measuring Weight on a Chair Scale

Name ______________________________ **Date** ______________

Directions: Practice this procedure, following each step. When you are ready to have your performance evaluated, give this sheet to your instructor. Review the detailed procedure in your textbook.

Procedure	Pass	Redo	Date Competency Met	Instructor Initials
Student must use Standard Precautions.	☐	☐	______	______
1. Place wheelchair on scale or transfer resident to chair on scale.	☐	☐	______	______
2. Follow the directions in the procedure "Measuring Weight on Standing Balance Scale."	☐	☐	______	______
3. Write down weight on notepad.	☐	☐	______	______
4. Make resident comfortable.	☐	☐	______	______
5. Wash hands.	☐	☐	______	______
6. Chart weight.	☐	☐	______	______

Check-off Sheet:

15-4 Measuring Weight on a Mechanical Lift

Name ______________________________ **Date** ______________

Directions: Practice this procedure, following each step. When you are ready to have your performance evaluated, give this sheet to your instructor. Review the detailed procedure in your textbook.

Procedure	Pass	Redo	Date Competency Met	Instructor Initials
Student must use Standard Precautions.	☐	☐	______	______
1. Wash hands.	☐	☐	______	______
2. Assemble equipment:				
a. Mechanical lift	☐	☐	______	______
b. Sling	☐	☐	______	______
c. Clean sheet	☐	☐	______	______
3. Identify resident.	☐	☐	______	______
4. Explain what you are going to do.	☐	☐	______	______
5. Pull privacy curtain.	☐	☐	______	______
6. Lower side rail on side you are working on.	☐	☐	______	______
7. Cover sling with clean sheet.	☐	☐	______	______
8. Help resident roll on side, and place sling with top at shoulders and bottom at knees.	☐	☐	______	______
9. Fan-fold remaining sling.	☐	☐	______	______
10. Help resident roll to other side onto half of sling, and pull other half of sling through.	☐	☐	______	______
11. Broaden base of lift.	☐	☐	______	______
12. Wheel lift to side of bed with base beneath bed.	☐	☐	______	______
13. Position lift over resident.	☐	☐	______	______
14. Attach sling using chains and hooks provided.	☐	☐	______	______
15. Use hand crank or pump handle to raise resident from bed. Make certain that buttocks are not touching bed.	☐	☐	______	______
16. Check to be certain that resident is in the center of sling and is safely suspended.	☐	☐	______	______

Procedure	Pass	Redo	Date Competency Met	Instructor Initials
17. To weigh resident:				
a. Swing feet and legs over edge of bed; move lift away from bed so that no body part contacts bed.	☐	☐	______	______
b. If bed is low enough, raise resident above bed so that no body part contacts bed.	☐	☐	______	______
18. Adjust weights until scale is balanced. (See the check-off sheet "Measuring Weight on Standing Balance Scale.")	☐	☐	______	______
19. Return resident to bed by reversing steps.	☐	☐	______	______
20. Replace mechanical lift.	☐	☐	______	______
21. Wash hands.	☐	☐	______	______
22. Note weight and write on pad.	☐	☐	______	______

Check-off Sheet:

15-5 Measuring Height

Name ______________________________ **Date** ______________

Directions: Practice this procedure, following each step. When you are ready to have your performance evaluated, give this sheet to your instructor. Review the detailed procedure in your textbook.

Procedure	Pass	Redo	Date Competency Met	Instructor Initials
Student must use Standard Precautions.	☐	☐	______	______
1. Wash hands.	☐	☐	______	______
2. Assemble equipment:				
a. Balance scale with height rod	☐	☐	______	______
b. Paper towels	☐	☐	______	______
3. Identify resident.	☐	☐	______	______
4. Explain what you are going to do.	☐	☐	______	______
5. Have resident remove shoes.	☐	☐	______	______
6. Raise measuring rod above head.	☐	☐	______	______
7. Have resident stand with back against measuring rod.	☐	☐	______	______
8. Instruct resident to stand straight, with heels touching measuring rod.	☐	☐	______	______
9. Lower measuring rod to rest on resident's head.	☐	☐	______	______
10. Check number of inches indicated on rod.	☐	☐	______	______
11. Record in inches, centimeters, or feet and inches according to facility policy.	☐	☐	______	______
12. Help resident with shoes.	☐	☐	______	______
13. Chart height.	☐	☐	______	______

Check-off Sheet:

15-6 Moving Resident and Belongings to Another Room

Name ______________________________ **Date** ______________

Directions: Practice this procedure, following each step. When you are ready to have your perfor mance evaluated, give this sheet to your instructor. Review the detailed procedure in your textbook.

Procedure	Pass	Redo	Date Competency Met	Instructor Initials
Student must use Standard Precautions.	☐	☐	______	______
1. Wash hands.	☐	☐	______	______
2. Assemble equipment:				
a. Resident's chart	☐	☐	______	______
b. Nursing care plan	☐	☐	______	______
c. Medications	☐	☐	______	______
d. Paper bag	☐	☐	______	______
3. Identify resident.	☐	☐	______	______
4. Explain what you are going to do.	☐	☐	______	______
5. Determine location to which resident is being transferred.	☐	☐	______	______
6. Gather resident's belongings. (Check admission list.)	☐	☐	______	______
7. Determine how resident is to be transported:				
a. Wheelchair	☐	☐	______	______
b. Stretcher	☐	☐	______	______
c. Entire bed	☐	☐	______	______
d. Ambulate	☐	☐	______	______
8. Transport resident to new unit.	☐	☐	______	______
9. Introduce to staff on new unit.	☐	☐	______	______
10. Introduce to new roommate.	☐	☐	______	______
11. Make resident comfortable.	☐	☐	______	______
12. Put away belongings.	☐	☐	______	______
13. Wash hands.	☐	☐	______	______
14. Give transferred medications, care plan, and chart to nurse.	☐	☐	______	______

Procedure	Pass	Redo	Date Competency Met	Instructor Initials
15. Before leaving unit, record the following:				
a. Date and time of transfer	☐	☐	______	______
b. How transported (e.g., wheelchair)	☐	☐	______	______
c. How transfer was tolerated by resident	☐	☐	______	______
16. Return to original unit and report completion of transfer.	☐	☐	______	______

Check-off Sheet:

15-7 Discharging a Resident

Name ______________________ **Date** ____________

Directions: Practice this procedure, following each step. When you are ready to have your performance evaluated, give this sheet to your instructor. Review the detailed procedure in your textbook.

Procedure	Pass	Redo	Date Competency Met	Instructor Initials
Student must use Standard Precautions.	☐	☐	______	______
1. Check chart for discharge order.	☐	☐	______	______
2. Wash hands.	☐	☐	______	______
3. Identify resident.	☐	☐	______	______
4. Explain what you are going to do.	☐	☐	______	______
5. Provide privacy by pulling the privacy curtain.	☐	☐	______	______
6. Help resident dress.	☐	☐	______	______
7. Collect resident's belongings.	☐	☐	______	______
8. Check belongings against admission list.	☐	☐	______	______
9. Secure and return valuables:				
a. Verify with resident that all valuables are present.	☐	☐	______	______
b. Have resident sign for them.	☐	☐	______	______
10. Check to see if resident has medications to take home.	☐	☐	______	______
11. Check to see if any equipment is to be taken home.	☐	☐	______	______
12. Help resident into wheelchair.	☐	☐	______	______
13. Help resident into car.	☐	☐	______	______
14. Return to unit:				
a. Remove all items left in unit.	☐	☐	______	______
b. Clean unit according to your facility's policy.	☐	☐	______	______
15. Wash hands.	☐	☐	______	______
16. Record discharge:				
a. Date and time	☐	☐	______	______
b. Method of transport	☐	☐	______	______
c. Whom resident left with	☐	☐	______	______

Check-off Sheet:

15-8 AM Care

Name ______________________________ **Date** ______________

Directions: Practice this procedure, following each step. When you are ready to have your performance evaluated, give this sheet to your instructor. Review the detailed procedure in your textbook.

Procedure	Pass	Redo	Date Competency Met	Instructor Initials
Student must use Standard Precautions.	☐	☐	______	______
1. Wash hands.	☐	☐	______	______
2. Gently awaken resident.	☐	☐	______	______
3. Assemble equipment:				
a. Washcloth and towel	☐	☐	______	______
b. Toothbrush and toothpaste	☐	☐	______	______
c. Emesis basin	☐	☐	______	______
d. Glass of water	☐	☐	______	______
e. Denture cup, if needed	☐	☐	______	______
f. Clean gown, if necessary	☐	☐	______	______
g. Clean linen, if necessary	☐	☐	______	______
h. Comb and brush	☐	☐	______	______
i. Disposable gloves (two pair)	☐	☐	______	______
4. Explain what you plan to do.	☐	☐	______	______
5. Provide privacy by pulling privacy curtain.	☐	☐	______	______
6. Elevate head of the bed, if allowed.	☐	☐	______	______
7. Put on disposable gloves.	☐	☐	______	______
8. Provide a bedpan or urinal, if needed, or escort resident to bathroom.	☐	☐	______	______
9. Empty bedpan or urinal, rinse it, and dispose of gloves.	☐	☐	______	______
10. Put bedpan or urinal out of sight.	☐	☐	______	______
11. Allow resident to wash hands and face.	☐	☐	______	______
12. Put on disposable gloves.	☐	☐	______	______
13. Provide oral hygiene.	☐	☐	______	______
14. Provide a clean gown, if necessary.	☐	☐	______	______

Procedure	Pass	Redo	Date Competency Met	Instructor Initials
15. Smooth sheets if resident remains in bed.	☐	☐	______	______
16. If resident is allowed out of bed, transfer to a chair.	☐	☐	______	______
17. Allow resident to comb hair; assist if necessary.	☐	☐	______	______
18. Prepare the overbed table:				
a. Clear tabletop.	☐	☐	______	______
b. Wipe off.	☐	☐	______	______
19. Position overbed table if resident is to remain in the room, or transport to dining room.	☐	☐	______	______
20. Remove and discard gloves.	☐	☐	______	______
21. Wash hands.	☐	☐	______	______

Check-off Sheet:

15-9 PM Care

Name ______________________________ Date ____________

Directions: Practice this procedure, following each step. When you are ready to have your performance evaluated, give this sheet to your instructor. Review the detailed procedure in your textbook.

Procedure	Pass	Redo	Date Competency Met	Instructor Initials
Student must use Standard Precautions.	☐	☐	______	______
1. Wash hands.	☐	☐	______	______
2. Tell resident what you are going to do.	☐	☐	______	______
3. Provide privacy.	☐	☐	______	______
4. Assemble equipment:				
a. Washcloth and towel	☐	☐	______	______
b. Toothbrush and toothpaste	☐	☐	______	______
c. Glass of water	☐	☐	______	______
d. Emesis basin	☐	☐	______	______
e. Denture cup, if necessary	☐	☐	______	______
f. Night clothes	☐	☐	______	______
g. Lotion	☐	☐	______	______
h. Linen as needed	☐	☐	______	______
i. Disposable gloves (two pair)	☐	☐	______	______
5. Encourage resident to do his or her own care if capable.	☐	☐	______	______
6. Assist if unable to do his or her own care.	☐	☐	______	______
7. Put on disposable gloves.	☐	☐	______	______
8. Provide bedpan or urinal, if necessary, or escort to bathroom.	☐	☐	______	______
9. Empty bedpan or urinal.	☐	☐	______	______
10. Rinse and place in a convenient place for nighttime use.	☐	☐	______	______
11. Remove and dispose of gloves.	☐	☐	______	______
12. Wash resident's hands and face.	☐	☐	______	______
13. Put on gloves.	☐	☐	______	______

Procedure	Pass	Redo	Date Competency Met	Instructor Initials
14. Provide for oral hygiene.	☐	☐	______	______
15. Change resident into night clothes.	☐	☐	______	______
16. Transfer resident from chair or wheelchair into bed, if out of bed.	☐	☐	______	______
17. Give back rub with lotion.	☐	☐	______	______
18. Observe skin for irritations or breakdown.	☐	☐	______	______
19. Smooth thc sheets.	☐	☐	______	______
20. Change draw sheets, if necessary.	☐	☐	______	______
21. Provide extra blankets, if necessary.	☐	☐	______	______
22. Position side rails as ordered after resident is in bed.	☐	☐	______	______
23. Remove and discard gloves.	☐	☐	______	______
24. Wash hands.	☐	☐	______	______
25. Provide fresh drinking water.	☐	☐	______	______
26. Place bedside table within resident's reach.	☐	☐	______	______
27. Secure call light within resident's reach.	☐	☐	______	______
28. Chart procedure.	☐	☐	______	______
29. Wash hands.	☐	☐	______	______

Check-off Sheet:

15-10 Skin-Care—Giving a Back Rub

Name ______________________________ **Date** ______________

Directions: Practice this procedure, following each step. When you are ready to have your performance evaluated, give this sheet to your instructor. Review the detailed procedure in your textbook.

Procedure	Pass	Redo	Date Competency Met	Instructor Initials
Student must use Standard Precautions.	☐	☐	______	______
1. Wash hands.	☐	☐	______	______
2. Assemble equipment:				
a. Lotion	☐	☐	______	______
b. Powder	☐	☐	______	______
c. Towel	☐	☐	______	______
d. Washcloth	☐	☐	______	______
e. Soap	☐	☐	______	______
f. Water (105°F)	☐	☐	______	______
g. Disposable gloves	☐	☐	______	______
3. Tell resident what you are going to do.	☐	☐	______	______
4. Provide privacy by pulling privacy curtains.	☐	☐	______	______
5. Place lotion container in warm water to help warm it.	☐	☐	______	______
6. Raise bed to a comfortable working height.	☐	☐	______	______
7. Lower side rail on the side you are working on.	☐	☐	______	______
8. Put on disposable gloves.	☐	☐	______	______
9. Position resident on side or in prone position.	☐	☐	______	______
10. Place a towel along the back to protect linen if resident is in a side-lying position.	☐	☐	______	______
11. Wash back thoroughly.	☐	☐	______	______
12. Rub a small amount of lotion into your hands.	☐	☐	______	______
13. Begin at base of spine and apply lotion over entire back.	☐	☐	______	______
14. Use firm, long strokes, beginning at buttocks and moving upward to neck and shoulders.	☐	☐	______	______

Procedure	Pass	Redo	Date Competency Met	Instructor Initials
15. Use firm pressure as you stroke upward, and light circular strokes returning to buttocks.	☐	☐	_______	_______
16. Use a circular motion over each area (shoulder blades, backbone). *Note:* Pay special attention to bony prominences.	☐	☐	_______	_______
17. Observe skin for irritation or breakdown. *Note:* Do not rub or apply lotion to any open area on the skin.	☐	☐	_______	_______
18. Repeat several times (3 to 5 minutes).	☐	☐	_______	_______
19. Dry back.	☐	☐	_______	_______
20. Adjust gown for comfort.	☐	☐	_______	_______
21. Remove towel.	☐	☐	_______	_______
22. Position resident comfortably.	☐	☐	_______	_______
23. Return bed to lowest height.	☐	☐	_______	_______
24. Put side rail up, if required.	☐	☐	_______	_______
25. Secure call light within reach of resident.	☐	☐	_______	_______
26. Remove and discard gloves.	☐	☐	_______	_______
27. Wash hands.	☐	☐	_______	_______
28. Record procedure and any observations (e.g., redness, broken areas, dry skin).	☐	☐	_______	_______

Check-off Sheet:

15-11 Oral Hygiene—Self-Care

Name ______________________________ **Date** ______________

Directions: Practice this procedure, following each step. When you are ready to have your performance evaluated, give this sheet to your instructor. Review the detailed procedure in your textbook.

Procedure	Pass	Redo	Date Competency Met	Instructor Initials
Student must use Standard Precautions.	☐	☐	______	______
1. Wash hands.	☐	☐	______	______
2. Assemble equipment:				
a. Toothbrush	☐	☐	______	______
b. Toothpaste	☐	☐	______	______
c. Mouthwash	☐	☐	______	______
d. Cup of water with straw, if needed	☐	☐	______	______
e. Emesis basin	☐	☐	______	______
f. Bath towel	☐	☐	______	______
g. Tissues	☐	☐	______	______
3. Identify resident and explain what you are going to do.	☐	☐	______	______
4. Screen resident by pulling privacy curtain around bed.	☐	☐	______	______
5. Raise head of the bed if resident is allowed to sit up.	☐	☐	______	______
6. Place towel over blanket and resident's gown.	☐	☐	______	______
7. Place toothbrush, toothpaste, mouthwash, emesis basin, and glass of water on overbed table.	☐	☐	______	______
8. Remove overbed table when resident has completed brushing.	☐	☐	______	______
9. Put towel away, and make resident comfortable.	☐	☐	______	______
10. Put side rails up if required.	☐	☐	______	______
11. Secure call bell within resident's reach.	☐	☐	______	______
12. Put all equipment away and tidy unit.	☐	☐	______	______
13. Wash hands.	☐	☐	______	______
14. Chart procedure.	☐	☐	______	______

Check-off Sheet:

15-12 Oral Hygiene—Brushing the Resident's Teeth

Name ______________________________ **Date** ______________

Directions: Practice this procedure, following each step. When you are ready to have your performance evaluated, give this sheet to your instructor. Review the detailed procedure in your textbook.

Procedure	Pass	Redo	Date Competency Met	Instructor Initials
Student must use Standard Precautions.	☐	☐	______	______
1. Wash hands.	☐	☐	______	______
2. Assemble equipment:				
a. Toothbrush	☐	☐	______	______
b. Toothpaste	☐	☐	______	______
c. Mouthwash	☐	☐	______	______
d. Cup of water with straw, if needed	☐	☐	______	______
e. Emesis basin	☐	☐	______	______
f. Bath towel	☐	☐	______	______
g. Tissues	☐	☐	______	______
h. Disposable nonsterile gloves	☐	☐	______	______
3. Identify resident and explain what you are going to do.	☐	☐	______	______
4. Screen resident by pulling privacy curtain around bed.	☐	☐	______	______
5. Raise head of bed if resident is allowed to sit up.	☐	☐	______	______
6. Place a towel over blanket and resident's gown.	☐	☐	______	______
7. Put on gloves.	☐	☐	______	______
8. Pour water over toothbrush; put toothpaste on brush.	☐	☐	______	______
9. Insert brush into the mouth carefully.	☐	☐	______	______
10. Starting at rear of mouth, place brush at an angle on upper teeth and brush in an up-and-down motion.	☐	☐	______	______
11. Repeat on lower teeth.	☐	☐	______	______

Procedure	Pass	Redo	Date Competency Met	Instructor Initials
12. Give resident water to rinse mouth. If necessary, use a straw.	☐	☐	______	______
13. Hold emesis basin under chin. Have resident expectorate (spit) water into the basin.	☐	☐	______	______
14. Offer tissues to resident to wipe mouth and chin. Discard tissues.	☐	☐	______	______
15. Provide mouthwash, if available. Use emesis basin and tissues as above.	☐	☐	______	______
16. Return all equipment.	☐	☐	______	______
17. Remove gloves and put in hazardous waste bin.	☐	☐	______	______
18. Wash hands.	☐	☐	______	______
19. Tidy up unit.	☐	☐	______	______
20. Put side rails up, if required.	☐	☐	______	______
21. Secure call bell within resident's reach.	☐	☐	______	______
22. Make resident comfortable before leaving the room.	☐	☐	______	______
23. Chart procedure and how resident tolerated it.	☐	☐	______	______

Check-off Sheet:

15-13 Oral Hygiene—Ambulatory Resident

Name ______________________________ **Date** ______________

Directions: Practice this procedure, following each step. When you are ready to have your performance evaluated, give this sheet to your instructor. Review the detailed procedure in your textbook.

Procedure	Pass	Redo	Date Competency Met	Instructor Initials
Student must use Standard Precautions.	☐	☐	______	______
1. Wash hands.	☐	☐	______	______
2. Tell resident what you are going to do.	☐	☐	______	______
3. Set up equipment at sink:				
a. Toothbrush	☐	☐	______	______
b. Toothpaste	☐	☐	______	______
c. Tablets or powder to soak dentures in	☐	☐	______	______
d. Towel	☐	☐	______	______
e. Glass	☐	☐	______	______
3. Rinse equipment and put away.	☐	☐	______	______
4. Wash hands.	☐	☐	______	______

Check-off Sheet:

15-14 Oral Hygiene—Denture Care

Name ______________________________ **Date** ______________

Directions: Practice this procedure, following each step. When you are ready to have your performance evaluated, give this sheet to your instructor. Review the detailed procedure in your textbook.

Procedure	Pass	Redo	Date Competency Met	Instructor Initials
Student must use Standard Precautions.	☐	☐	______	______
1. Wash hands.	☐	☐	______	______
2. Assemble equipment:				
a. Tissues	☐	☐	______	______
b. Paper towel or gauze squares	☐	☐	______	______
c. Mouthwash	☐	☐	______	______
d. Disposable denture cup	☐	☐	______	______
e. Toothbrush or denture brush	☐	☐	______	______
f. Denture paste or toothpowder	☐	☐	______	______
g. Towel	☐	☐	______	______
h. Disposable nonsterile gloves	☐	☐	______	______
3. Identify resident.	☐	☐	______	______
4. Explain what you are going to do.	☐	☐	______	______
5. Pull privacy curtain.	☐	☐	______	______
6. Lower side rails.	☐	☐	______	______
7. Raise head of bed, if allowed.	☐	☐	______	______
8. Place towel across resident's chest.	☐	☐	______	______
9. Prepare emesis basin by placing tissue or paper towel in bottom of basin.	☐	☐	______	______
10. Put on gloves.	☐	☐	______	______
11. Have resident remove his or her dentures.	☐	☐	______	______
12. Remove dentures if resident cannot.	☐	☐	______	______

Procedure	Pass	Redo	Date Competency Met	Instructor Initial
Upper Denture				
a. Explain what you are going to do.	☐	☐	______	______
b. Use a gauze square to grip upper denture.	☐	☐	______	______
c. Place your index finger between top ridge of denture and cheek.	☐	☐	______	______
d. Gently pull on denture to release suction.	☐	☐	______	______
e. Remove upper denture.	☐	☐	______	______
Lower Denture				
a. Use a gauze square to grip lower denture.	☐	☐	______	______
b. Place your index finger between lower ridge and cheek.	☐	☐	______	______
c. Gently pull on denture to release suction.	☐	☐	______	______
d. Remove lower denture.	☐	☐	______	______
13. Place dentures in lined emesis basin and take to sink or utility room.	☐	☐	______	______
14. Hold dentures firmly in palm of hand.	☐	☐	______	______
15. Put toothpowder or toothpaste on toothbrush.	☐	☐	______	______
16. Hold dentures under cold running water and brush dentures until clean.	☐	☐	______	______
17. Rinse dentures under cold running water.	☐	☐	______	______
18. Place in denture cup.	☐	☐	______	______
19. Place a solution of mouthwash and cool water in cup.	☐	☐	______	______
20. Help resident rinse mouth with mouthwash.	☐	☐	______	______
21. Have resident replace dentures.	☐	☐	______	______
22. Place dentures in labeled denture cup next to bed, if dentures are to be left out.	☐	☐	______	______
23. Rinse equipment and put away.	☐	☐	______	______
24. Remove gloves; dispose of in hazardous waste bin.	☐	☐	______	______
25. Wash hands.	☐	☐	______	______
26. Position resident.	☐	☐	______	______
27. Raise side rails, if required.	☐	☐	______	______
28. Secure call bell within resident's reach.	☐	☐	______	______
29. Chart procedure and how it was tolerated.	☐	☐	______	______

Check-off Sheet:

15-15 Oral Hygiene—for the Unconscious Resident

Name ______________________________ **Date** ______________

Directions: Practice this procedure, following each step. When you are ready to have your performance evaluated, give this sheet to your instructor. Review the detailed procedure in your textbook.

Procedure	Pass	Redo	Date Competency Met	Instructor Initials
Student must use Standard Precautions.	☐	☐	______	______
1. Wash hands.	☐	☐	______	______
2. Tell resident what you are going to do.	☐	☐	______	______
3. Provide privacy.	☐	☐	______	______
4. Assemble equipment:				
a. Emesis basin	☐	☐	______	______
b. Towel	☐	☐	______	______
c. Lemon glycerin swabs	☐	☐	______	______
d. Tongue blades	☐	☐	______	______
e. 4×4 gauze	☐	☐	______	______
f. Lip moisturizer	☐	☐	______	______
g. Disposable nonsterile gloves	☐	☐	______	______
5. Position bed at a comfortable working height.	☐	☐	______	______
6. Put on gloves.	☐	☐	______	______
7. Position resident's head to side and place towel on bed under resident's cheek and chin.	☐	☐	______	______
8. Secure emesis basin under resident's chin.	☐	☐	______	______
9. Wrap a tongue blade with 4×4 gauze and slightly moisten. Swab mouth, being certain to clean gums, teeth, tongue, and roof of mouth.	☐	☐	______	______
10. Apply lip moisturizer to lips and swab mouth with lemon glycerin, if available.	☐	☐	______	______
11. Remove towel and reposition resident.	☐	☐	______	______
12. Discard disposable equipment in hazardous waste bin.	☐	☐	______	______
13. Clean basin and put away.	☐	☐	______	______

Procedure	Pass	Redo	Date Competency Met	Instructor Initials
14. Remove gloves, put in hazardous waste bin.	☐	☐	________	________
15. Wash hands.	☐	☐	________	________
16. Report and document resident's tolerance of procedure.	☐	☐	________	________

Check-off Sheet:

15-16 Elimination—Offering the Bedpan

Name ______________________________ **Date** ____________

Directions: Practice this procedure, following each step. When you are ready to have your performance evaluated, give this sheet to your instructor. Review the detailed procedure in your textbook.

Procedure	Pass	Redo	Date Competency Met	Instructor Initials
Student must use Standard Precautions.	☐	☐	______	______
1. Wash hands.	☐	☐	______	______
2. Assemble equipment:				
a. Bedpan with cover	☐	☐	______	______
b. Toilet tissue	☐	☐	______	______
c. Soap and water	☐	☐	______	______
d. Towel	☐	☐	______	______
e. Disposable nonsterile gloves (two pair)	☐	☐	______	______
3. Ask visitors to wait outside room.	☐	☐	______	______
4. Provide privacy for resident.	☐	☐	______	______
5. Remove bedpan from storage space.	☐	☐	______	______
6. Warm metal bedpans by running warm water over them and drying.	☐	☐	______	______
7. Lower head of bed if it is elevated.	☐	☐	______	______
8. Put on gloves.	☐	☐	______	______
9. Fold top covers back enough to see where to place the pan. Do not expose resident.	☐	☐	______	______
10. Ask resident to raise hips off bed.	☐	☐	______	______
a. If the resident is unable to lift the hips, it will be necessary to roll the resident onto his or her side.	☐	☐	______	______
b. Place bedpan on buttocks.	☐	☐	______	______
c. Hold in place with one hand and help resident roll back onto bedpan.	☐	☐	______	______

Procedure	Pass	Redo	Date Competency Met	Instructor Initials
11. Slide bedpan into place.	☐	☐	______	______
12. Cover resident again.	☐	☐	______	______
13. Raise head of bed for comfort.	☐	☐	______	______
14. Remove gloves.	☐	☐	______	______
15. Leave call light with resident.	☐	☐	______	______
16. Wash your hands.	☐	☐	______	______
17. Leave room to provide privacy.	☐	☐	______	______
18. Watch for call light to signal resident's readiness to be removed from bedpan.	☐	☐	______	______
19. Put on gloves.				
20. Assist resident as necessary to ensure cleanliness.	☐	☐	______	______
21. Remove bedpan and empty.				
22. Measure urine if on I & O.	☐	☐	______	______
23. Remove gloves.				
24. Wash hands.	☐	☐	______	______
25. Provide washcloth, water, and soap for resident to wash hands.	☐	☐	______	______
26. Provide comfort measures for resident.	☐	☐	______	______
27. Secure call light within resident's reach.	☐	☐	______	______
28. Open privacy curtain.	☐	☐	______	______
29. Chart the following:				
a. Bowel movement amount, color, consistency	☐	☐	______	______
b. Amount voided if on I & O	☐	☐	______	______

Check-off Sheet:

15-17 Elimination—Offering the Urinal

Name ______________________ **Date** ____________

Directions: Practice this procedure, following each step. When you are ready to have your performance evaluated, give this sheet to your instructor. Review the detailed procedure in your textbook.

Procedure	Pass	Redo	Date Competency Met	Instructor Initials
Student must use Standard Precautions.	☐	☐	______	______
1. Wash hands.	☐	☐	______	______
2. Assemble equipment:				
a. Urinal with cover	☐	☐	______	______
b. Soap and water	☐	☐	______	______
c. Towel	☐	☐	______	______
d. Disposable nonsterile gloves	☐	☐	______	______
3. Ask visitors to wait outside room.	☐	☐	______	______
4. Provide privacy for resident.	☐	☐	______	______
5. Hand urinal to resident:	☐	☐	______	______
a. Place call light at resident's side.	☐	☐	______	______
b. Wash your hands.	☐	☐	______	______
c. Leave room until resident signals with the call light.	☐	☐	______	______
(If the resident is unable to place urinal, place penis in urinal. If necessary, stand and hold urinal until resident has finished voiding.) Wear gloves for this step.				
6. Return to room when resident has finished voiding.	☐	☐	______	______
7. Put on gloves.	☐	☐	______	______
8. Place cover over urinal and carry it into bathroom.	☐	☐	______	______
9. Check to see if resident is on I & O or if a urine specimen is needed.	☐	☐	______	______
10. Observe urine for:				
a. color	☐	☐	______	______
b. consistency	☐	☐	______	______
c. odor	☐	☐	______	______

Procedure	Pass	Redo	Date Competency Met	Instructor Initials
11. Empty into toilet.	☐	☐	______	______
12. Rinse urinal with cold water.	☐	☐	______	______
13. Cover and place in a convenient location for the resident.	☐	☐	______	______
14. Remove gloves.	☐	☐	______	______
15. Wash hands.	☐	☐	______	______
16. Secure call light within reach of resident.	☐	☐	______	______
17. Report and document unusual color, odor, or consistency of urine.	☐	☐	______	______
18. Record amount if on I & O.	☐	☐	______	______

Check-off Sheet:

15-18 Elimination—Bedside Commode

Name ______________________________ **Date** ______________

Directions: Practice this procedure, following each step. When you are ready to have your performance evaluated, give this sheet to your instructor. Review the detailed procedure in your textbook.

Procedure	Pass	Redo	Date Competency Met	Instructor Initials
Student must use Standard Precautions.	☐	☐	______	______
1. Wash hands.	☐	☐	______	______
2. Assemble equipment:				
a. Bedside commode	☐	☐	______	______
b. Toilet tissue	☐	☐	______	______
c. Washcloth	☐	☐	______	______
d. Warm water	☐	☐	______	______
e. Soap	☐	☐	______	______
f. Towel	☐	☐	______	______
g. Disposable nonsterile gloves (two pair)	☐	☐	______	______
3. Identify resident.	☐	☐	______	______
4. Explain what you are going to do.	☐	☐	______	______
5. Place commode chair next to bed, facing its head. *Lock wheels!*	☐	☐	______	______
6. Check to see if receptacle is in place under seat.	☐	☐	______	______
7. Provide privacy by pulling privacy curtains.	☐	☐	______	______
8. Lower bed to lowest position.	☐	☐	______	______
9. Lower side rail.	☐	☐	______	______
10. Help resident to sitting position.	☐	☐	______	______
11. Help resident swing legs over side of bed.	☐	☐	______	______
12. Put resident's slippers on and assist to stand.	☐	☐	______	______
13. Have resident place hands on your shoulders.	☐	☐	______	______
14. Support under resident's arm, pivot resident to right, and lower to commode.	☐	☐	______	______

Procedure	Pass	Redo	Date Competency Met	Instructor Initials
15. Place call bell within reach.	☐	☐	______	______
16. Place toilet tissue in reach.	☐	☐	______	______
17. Remain nearby if resident seems weak.	☐	☐	______	______
18. Return immediately when resident signals.	☐	☐	______	______
19. Put gloves on.	☐	☐	______	______
20. Assist resident to stand.	☐	☐	______	______
21. Clean anus or perineum if resident is unable to help self.	☐	☐	______	______
22. Remove gloves and put in hazardous waste bin.	☐	☐	______	______
23. Help resident wash hands.	☐	☐	______	______
24. Assist resident back to bed and position comfortably.	☐	☐	______	______
25. Put side rail up, if required.	☐	☐	______	______
26. Put gloves on.	☐	☐	______	______
27. Put cover on commode chair down and remove receptacle.	☐	☐	______	______
28. Empty contents, measuring if on I & O.	☐	☐	______	______
29. Empty and clean per hospital policy.	☐	☐	______	______
30. Remove gloves and put in hazardous waste bin.	☐	☐	______	______
31. Wash hands.	☐	☐	______	______
32. Replace equipment and tidy unit.	☐	☐	______	______
33. Record the following:				
a. Bowel movement	☐	☐	______	______
(1) Amount	☐	☐	______	______
(2) Consistency	☐	☐	______	______
(3) Color	☐	☐	______	______
b. Any unusual observations, such as				
(1) Weakness	☐	☐	______	______
(2) Discomfort	☐	☐	______	______

Check-off Sheet:

15-19 Transferring—Pivot Transfer from Bed to Wheelchair

Name ______________________________ **Date** ______________

Directions: Practice this procedure, following each step. When you are ready to have your performance evaluated, give this sheet to your instructor. Review the detailed procedure in your textbook.

Procedure	Pass	Redo	Date Competency Met	Instructor Initials
Student must use Standard Precautions.	☐	☐	______	______
1. Wash hands.	☐	☐	______	______
2. *Lock* wheels on chair and bed.	☐	☐	______	______
3. Lift foot rests or swing leg supports out of the way.	☐	☐	______	______
4. Position wheelchair alongside of bed.	☐	☐	______	______
5. Move resident to edge of bed, with legs over side.	☐	☐	______	______
6. Have resident dangle legs for a few minutes. Encourage some slow, deep breaths and observe for dizziness.	☐	☐	______	______
7. Support resident at midriff and ask resident to stand if resident is not dizzy.	☐	☐	______	______
8. Once standing, have resident pivot (turn) and hold onto armrest of wheelchair with both arms or one strong arm.	☐	☐	______	______
9. Gently ease resident into a sitting position.	☐	☐	______	______
10. Position yourself at back of wheelchair. Ask resident to push on the floor with feet as you lift gently under each arm to ease resident into a comfortable position against backrest.	☐	☐	______	______
11. Return foot rests to normal position and place feet and legs in a comfortable position on rests.	☐	☐	______	______
12. Do not leave a resident who requires a postural support until it is in place.	☐	☐	______	______
13. Reverse above procedure to return resident to bed.	☐	☐	______	______
14. Wash hands.	☐	☐	______	______

Check-off Sheet:

15-20 Transferring—Sliding from Bed to Wheelchair and Back

Name ______________________________ **Date** ______________

Directions: Practice this procedure, following each step. When you are ready to have your performance evaluated, give this sheet to your instructor. Review the detailed procedure in your textbook.

Procedure	Pass	Redo	Date Competency Met	Instructor Initials
Student must use Standard Precautions.	☐	☐	______	______
1. Wash hands.	☐	☐	______	______
2. Assemble equipment: wheelchair with removable arms.	☐	☐	______	______
3. Position wheelchair at bedside with back parallel to head of bed. *Lock* wheels.	☐	☐	______	______
4. Remove wheelchair arm nearest to bedside.	☐	☐	______	______
5. Place bed level to chair seat height if possible. *Lock* bed wheels.	☐	☐	______	______
6. Raise head of bed so that resident is in sitting position.	☐	☐	______	______
7. Position yourself beside wheelchair and carefully assist resident to slide from bed to wheelchair.	☐	☐	______	______
8. Position resident for comfort and apply postural supports PRN.	☐	☐	______	______
9. Wash hands.	☐	☐	______	______

Check-off Sheet:

15-21 Transferring—Two-Person Lift from Bed to Chair and Back

Name ______________________________ **Date** ______________

Directions: Practice this procedure, following each step. When you are ready to have your performance evaluated, give this sheet to your instructor. Review the detailed procedure in your textbook.

Procedure	Pass	Redo	Date Competency Met	Instructor Initials
Student must use Standard Precautions.	☐	☐	______	______
1. Wash hands.	☐	☐	______	______
2. Assemble equipment: chair.	☐	☐	______	______
3. Ask one other person to help.	☐	☐	______	______
4. Tell resident what you are going to do.	☐	☐	______	______
5. Position chair next to bed with back of chair parallel with head of bed. *Lock* wheels.	☐	☐	______	______
6. Position resident near edge of bed.	☐	☐	______	______
7. Position co-worker on side of bed near feet.	☐	☐	______	______
8. Position yourself behind chair at head of bed.	☐	☐	______	______
9. Place your arms under resident's axillae, and clasp your hands together at resident's midchest.	☐	☐	______	______
10. Co-worker places hands under resident's upper legs.	☐	☐	______	______
11. Count to three. On the count of three, lift resident into chair.	☐	☐	______	______
12. Position for comfort and secure postural supports PRN.	☐	☐	______	______
13. Wash hands.	☐	☐	______	______

Check-off Sheet:

15-22 Transferring—Sliding from Bed to Gurney and Back

Name ______________________________ Date ______________

Directions: Practice this procedure, following each step. When you are ready to have your performance evaluated, give this sheet to your instructor. Review the detailed procedure in your textbook.

Procedure	Pass	Redo	Date Competency Met	Instructor Initials
Student must use Standard Precautions.	☐	☐	______	______
1. Wash hands.	☐	☐	______	______
2. Assemble equipment:				
a. Gurney	☐	☐	______	______
b. Cover sheet	☐	☐	______	______
3. Ask a co-worker to help.	☐	☐	______	______
4. Explain what you are going to do, and *lock* wheels on bed.	☐	☐	______	______
5. Cover resident with sheet and remove bed covers.	☐	☐	______	______
6. Raise bed to gurney height: lower side rail, and move resident to side of bed.	☐	☐	______	______
7. Loosen draw sheet on both sides so it can be used as a pull sheet.	☐	☐	______	______
8. Position gurney next to bed, and *lock* wheels on gurney.	☐	☐	______	______
9. Position yourselves on outside of gurney—one at the head, the other at the hips. Co-worker is on other side of bed.	☐	☐	______	______
10. Reach across gurney and securely hold edge of draw sheet. Pull resident onto gurney and cover.	☐	☐	______	______
11. Position resident for comfort.	☐	☐	______	______
12. Secure with safety straps or raise side rails.	☐	☐	______	______
13. Wash hands.	☐	☐	______	______

Check-off Sheet:

15-23 Transferring—Lifting with a Mechanical Lift

Name ______________________________ Date ______________

Directions: Practice this procedure, following each step. When you are ready to have your performance evaluated, give this sheet to your instructor. Review the detailed procedure in your textbook.

Procedure	Pass	Redo	Date Competency Met	Instructor Initials
Student must use Standard Precautions.	☐	☐	______	______
1. Wash hands.	☐	☐	______	______
2. Gather equipment:				
a. Mechanical lift	☐	☐	______	______
b. Sheet or blanket for resident comfort	☐	☐	______	______
c. Sling	☐	☐	______	______
3. Check all equipment to be sure it is in good working order and that the sling is not damaged or torn.	☐	☐	______	______
4. Ask one other person to help.	☐	☐	______	______
5. Prepare resident's destination:				
a. Chair	☐	☐	______	______
b. Gurney	☐	☐	______	______
c. Bathtub	☐	☐	______	______
d. Shower	☐	☐	______	______
6. *Lock* wheels on bed, and explain what you are going to do.	☐	☐	______	______
7. Roll resident toward you.	☐	☐	______	______
8. Place sling on bed behind resident:	☐	☐	______	______
a. Position top of sling at shoulders.	☐	☐	______	______
b. Position bottom of sling under buttocks.	☐	☐	______	______
c. Leave enough of sling to support body when the body is rolled back. Fan-fold remaining sling next to body.	☐	☐	______	______
9. Roll resident to other side of bed and pull fan-folded portion of sling flat. Remove all wrinkles and allow resident to lie flat on back.	☐	☐	______	______

Procedure	Pass	Redo	Date Competency Met	Instructor Initials
10. Position lift over resident, being sure to broaden base of lift. This stabilizes the lift while raising the resident.	☐	☐	______	______
11. Raise head of bed to a semi–Fowler's position.	☐	☐	______	______
12. Attach straps on lift to sling loops. Shorter straps must be attached to shoulder loops. Longer straps are attached to loops at hips.	☐	☐	______	______
13. Reassure resident. Let resident know you will keep him or her from falling. Gently raise resident from bed with hand crank or pump handle.	☐	☐	______	______
14. Keep resident centered over base of lift as you move lift and resident to his or her destination.	☐	☐	______	______
15. Position resident over chair, commode, bathtub, shower chair, and so on. Ask a co-worker to steady chair.	☐	☐	______	______
16. Slowly lower resident into chair using foot pedal positioning, as the person's weight becomes more dependent on chair.	☐	☐	______	______
17. Unhook sling from lift straps, and carefully move lift away from resident.	☐	☐	______	______
18. Provide all comfort measures for resident.	☐	☐	______	______
19. Secure postural supports, if necessary.	☐	☐	______	______
20. Return lift to storage area.	☐	☐	______	______
21. Wash hands.	☐	☐	______	______
22. Reverse procedure when returning resident to bed.	☐	☐	______	______

Check-off Sheet:

15-24 Transferring—Moving a Resident on a Gurney

Name ______________________________ Date ______________

Directions: Practice this procedure, following each step. When you are ready to have your performance evaluated, give this sheet to your instructor. Review the detailed procedure in your textbook.

Procedure	Pass	Redo	Date Competency Met	Instructor Initials
Student must use Standard Precautions.	☐	☐	______	______
1. Position bed to gurney height.	☐	☐	______	______
2. *Lock* all the brakes on gurney and bed.	☐	☐	______	______
3. Follow the procedure for transferring to and from gurney.	☐	☐	______	______
4. Stand at the resident's head and push the gurney with resident's feet moving first down the hallway.	☐	☐	______	______
5. Slow down when turning a corner. Always check the intersection mirrors for traffic.	☐	☐	______	______
6. Enter an elevator by standing at resident's head and pulling gurney into elevator. The feet will be the last to enter elevator.	☐	☐	______	______
7. Leave elevator by carefully pushing the gurney out of elevator into corridor.	☐	☐	______	______
8. Position yourself at resident's feet, and back resident on a gurney down a hill.	☐	☐	______	______
9. Never leave a resident unattended on a gurney.	☐	☐	______	______
10. Raise side rails and secure a safety strap.	☐	☐	______	______

Check-off Sheet:

15-25 Transferring—Moving a Resident in a Wheelchair

Name ______________________________ **Date** ______________

Directions: Practice this procedure, following each step. When you are ready to have your performance evaluated, give this sheet to your instructor. Review the detailed procedure in your textbook.

Procedure	Pass	Redo	Date Competency Met	Instructor Initials
Student must use Standard Precautions.	☐	☐	______	______
1. Position wheelchair.	☐	☐	______	______
2. *Lock* all brakes on wheelchair and bed.	☐	☐	______	______
3. Follow procedure for transferring to and from a wheelchair.	☐	☐	______	______
4. Push wheelchair carefully into hallway, watching for others who may be near doorway.	☐	☐	______	______
5. Move cautiously down hallway, being especially careful at intersections.	☐	☐	______	______
6. Always back a resident in a wheelchair over bumps, doorways, and into or out of elevators.	☐	☐	______	______
7. Always back a resident in a wheelchair down a hill.	☐	☐	______	______
8. Check resident for comfort measures before leaving.	☐	☐	______	______
9. Always notify appropriate person when resident has arrived.	☐	☐	______	______

Check-off Sheet:

15-26 Moving—Helping the Helpless Resident to Move Up in Bed

Name ______________________________ **Date** ______________

Directions: Practice this procedure, following each step. When you are ready to have your performance evaluated, give this sheet to your instructor. Review the detailed procedure in your textbook.

Procedure	Pass	Redo	Date Competency Met	Instructor Initials
Student must use Standard Precautions.	☐	☐	______	______
1. Wash hands	☐	☐	______	______
2. Ask a co-worker to help move resident. (Co-worker will work on opposite side of bed.)	☐	☐	______	______
3. Identify resident and explain what you are going to do.	☐	☐	______	______
4. *Lock* wheels of bed. Raise bed to comfortable working position, and lower side rails.	☐	☐	______	______
5. Remove pillow and place it at head of bed or on a chair.	☐	☐	______	______
6. Loosen both sides of draw sheet.	☐	☐	______	______
7. Roll edges toward side of resident's body.	☐	☐	______	______
8. Face head of bed and grasp rolled sheet edge with hand closest to resident.	☐	☐	______	______
9. Place your feet 12 inches apart with foot farthest from the edge of bed in a forward position.	☐	☐	______	______
10. Place your free hand and arm under resident's neck and shoulders, supporting head.	☐	☐	______	______
11. Bend your hips slightly.	☐	☐	______	______
12. On the count of three, move resident smoothly to head of bed.	☐	☐	______	______
13. Replace pillow under resident's head and check for good body alignment.	☐	☐	______	______
14. Tighten and tuck in draw sheet and smooth bedding.	☐	☐	______	______
15. Raise side rails and lower bed.	☐	☐	______	______
16. Wash hands.	☐	☐	______	______

Check-off Sheet:

15-27 Moving—Assisting Resident to Sit Up in Bed

Name ______________________________ **Date** ______________

Directions: Practice this procedure, following each step. When you are ready to have your performance evaluated, give this sheet to your instructor. Review the detailed procedure in your textbook.

Procedure	Pass	Redo	Date Competency Met	Instructor Initials
Student must use Standard Precautions.	☐	☐	______	______
1. Wash hands.	☐	☐	______	______
2. Identify resident and explain what you are going to do.	☐	☐	______	______
3. *Lock* bed and lower all the way down.	☐	☐	______	______
4. Face head of bed, keeping your outer leg forward.	☐	☐	______	______
5. Turn your head away from resident's face.	☐	☐	______	______
6. Lock your arm nearest resident with resident's arm. Have resident hold back of your upper arm.	☐	☐	______	______
7. Support resident's head and shoulder with your other arm.	☐	☐	______	______
8. Raise resident to sitting position. Adjust head of bed and pillows.	☐	☐	______	______
9. Wash hands.	☐	☐	______	______

Check-off Sheet:

15-28 Moving—Logrolling

Name ______________________________ **Date** ______________

Directions: Practice this procedure, following each step. When you are ready to have your performance evaluated, give this sheet to your instructor. Review the detailed procedure in your textbook.

Procedure	Pass	Redo	Date Competency Met	Instructor Initials
Student must use Standard Precautions.	☐	☐	______	______
1. Wash hands.	☐	☐	______	______
2. Identify resident and explain what you are going to do.	☐	☐	______	______
3. Provide privacy by pulling privacy curtain.	☐	☐	______	______
4. *Lock* wheels of bed. Raise bed to a comfortable working position.	☐	☐	______	______
5. Lower side rail on side you are working on.	☐	☐	______	______
6. Be certain that side rail on opposite side of bed is in up position.	☐	☐	______	______
7. Leave pillow under head.	☐	☐	______	______
8. Place a pillow lengthwise between resident's legs.	☐	☐	______	______
9. Fold resident's arms across chest.	☐	☐	______	______
10. Roll resident onto his or her side like a log, turning body as a whole unit, without bending joints.	☐	☐	______	______
11. Check for good body alignment.	☐	☐	______	______
12. Tighten and tuck in draw sheet and smooth bedding.	☐	☐	______	______
13. Tuck pillow behind back for support.	☐	☐	______	______
14. Raise side rails and lower bed.	☐	☐	______	______
15. Secure call light within resident's reach.	☐	☐	______	______
16. Wash hands.	☐	☐	______	______
17. Chart position of resident and how procedure was tolerated.	☐	☐	______	______

Check-off Sheet:

15-29 Moving—Turning Resident Away from You

Name ______________________________ **Date** ______________

Directions: Practice this procedure, following each step. When you are ready to have your performance evaluated, give this sheet to your instructor. Review the detailed procedure in your textbook.

Procedure	Pass	Redo	Date Competency Met	Instructor Initials
Student must use Standard Precautions.	☐	☐	______	______
1. Wash hands.	☐	☐	______	______
2. Identify resident and explain what you are going to do.	☐	☐	______	______
3. *Lock* bed and elevate to a comfortable working height.	☐	☐	______	______
4. Lower side rail on side you are working from.	☐	☐	______	______
5. Have resident bend knees. Cross arms on chest.	☐	☐	______	______
6. Place arm nearest head of bed under resident's shoulders and head. Place other hand and forearm under small of the resident's back. Bend your body at hips and knees, keeping your back straight. Pull resident toward you.	☐	☐	______	______
7. Place forearms under resident's hips and pull resident toward you.	☐	☐	______	______
8. Place one hand under ankles and one hand under knees, and move ankles and knees toward you.	☐	☐	______	______
9. Cross resident's leg closest to you over other leg at ankles.	☐	☐	______	______
10. Roll resident away from you by placing one hand under hips and one hand under shoulders.	☐	☐	______	______
11. Place one hand under resident's shoulders and one hand under resident's head. Draw resident back toward center of bed.	☐	☐	______	______
12. Place both hands under resident's hips and move hips toward center of bed.	☐	☐	______	______
13. Put a pillow behind resident's back to give support and keep resident from falling onto his or her back.	☐	☐	______	______

Procedure	Pass	Redo	Date Competency Met	Instructor Initials
14. Be certain resident is in good alignment.	☐	☐	______	______
15. Place upper leg on a pillow for support.	☐	☐	______	______
16. Replace side rail on near side of bed and return bed to lowest height.	☐	☐	______	______
17. Place a turning sheet under a helpless or heavy resident to help with turning.	☐	☐	______	______
18. Wash hands.	☐	☐	______	______

Check-off Sheet:

15-30 Moving—Turning Resident Toward You

Name ______________________________ **Date** ______________

Directions: Practice this procedure, following each step. When you are ready to have your performance evaluated, give this sheet to your instructor. Review the detailed procedure in your textbook.

Procedure	Pass	Redo	Date Competency Met	Instructor Initials
Student must use Standard Precautions.	☐	☐	______	______
1. Wash hands.	☐	☐	______	______
2. Identify resident and explain what you are going to do.	☐	☐	______	______
3. *Lock* bed and elevate to a comfortable working height.	☐	☐	______	______
4. Lower side rail on side you are working from.	☐	☐	______	______
5. Cross resident's far leg over leg that is closest to you.	☐	☐	______	______
6. Place one hand on resident's far shoulder. Place your other hand on the hip.	☐	☐	______	______
7. Brace yourself against side of bed. Roll resident toward you in a slow, gentle, smooth movement.	☐	☐	______	______
8. Help resident bring upper leg toward you and bend comfortably (Sims position).	☐	☐	______	______
9. Put up side rail. Be certain it is secure.	☐	☐	______	______
10. Go to other side of bed and lower side rail.	☐	☐	______	______
11. Place hands under resident's shoulders and hips. Pull toward center of bed.	☐	☐	______	______
12. Be certain to align resident's body properly.	☐	☐	______	______
13. Use pillows to position and support legs if resident is unable to move self.	☐	☐	______	______
14. *Check tubing to make certain that it is not caught between legs or pulling in any way if resident has an indwelling catheter.*	☐	☐	______	______
15. Tuck a pillow behind resident's back.	☐	☐	______	______
16. Return bed to low position.	☐	☐	______	______
17. Secure call light within resident's reach.	☐	☐	______	______
18. Wash hands.	☐	☐	______	______

Check-off Sheet:

15-31 Moving—Range of Motion

Name ______________________________ **Date** ______________

Directions: Practice this procedure, following each step. When you are ready to have your performance evaluated, give this sheet to your instructor. Review the detailed procedure in your textbook.

Procedure	Pass	Redo	Date Competency Met	Instructor Initials
Student must use Standard Precautions.	☐	☐	______	______
1. Wash hands.	☐	☐	______	______
2. Assemble equipment:				
a. Sheet or bath blanket	☐	☐	______	______
b. Treatment table or bed	☐	☐	______	______
c. Good lighting	☐	☐	______	______
3. Identify resident.	☐	☐	______	______
4. Explain what you are going to do.	☐	☐	______	______
5. Ask visitor to wait outside, and provide privacy.	☐	☐	______	______
6. Place resident in a supine position on bed or treatment table, and cover with sheet or bath blanket. *Instruct resident to do the following movements at least five times each (or to tolerance for active ROM).*	☐	☐	______	______
7. Bend head until chin touches chest (flexion), then gently bend chin backward (extension).	☐	☐	______	______
8. Turn head to right (right rotation), then turn head to left (left rotation).	☐	☐	______	______
9. Move head so that right ear moves toward right shoulder (right lateral flexion), then move head to central position and continue moving head so that left ear moves toward left shoulder (left lateral flexion).	☐	☐	______	______
10. Raise one arm overhead, keeping elbow straight. Return to side position. Repeat with other arm.	☐	☐	______	______
11. Raise arm overhead, then lower. Keep arm out to side. Repeat with other arm.	☐	☐	______	______
12. Bend one hand and forearm toward shoulder (flexion) and straighten (extension). Repeat with other arm.	☐	☐	______	______

Procedure	Pass	Redo	Date Competency Met	Instructor Initials
13. Bend arm at elbow and rotate hand toward body (pronation), then rotate away from body (supination). Repeat with other arm.	☐	☐	_______	_______
14. Bend hand at wrist toward shoulder (flex), then gently force backward past a level position with arm (extension) to below arm level (hyperextension). Repeat with other hand.	☐	☐	_______	_______
15. Holding hand straight, move toward thumb (radial deviation), then move hand toward little finger (ulnar deviation). Repeat with other hand.	☐	☐	_______	_______
16. Bend thumb and fingers into hand, making a fist (flexion), then open hand by straightening fingers and thumb (extension). Repeat with other hand.	☐	☐	_______	_______
17. Move thumb away from hand (abduct), then toward hand (adduct). Repeat with other hand.	☐	☐	_______	_______
18. Move thumb toward little finger, touch tips. Touch tip of thumb to each finger. Open hand each time. Repeat with other hand.	☐	☐	_______	_______
19. Keeping fingers straight, separate them (abduction), then bring them together (adduction). Repeat with other hand.	☐	☐	_______	_______
20. Raise leg, bend knee, then return to bed, straightening knee. Repeat with other leg.	☐	☐	_______	_______
21. Keep knee straight. Slowly raise and lower leg. Repeat with other leg.	☐	☐	_______	_______
22. Separate legs (abduction), then bring back together (adduction). Then turn both legs so knees face outward. Turn legs so knees face inward.	☐	☐	_______	_______
23. Rotate one foot toward the other foot (internal rotation), then rotate away from other foot (external rotation). Repeat with other foot.	☐	☐	_______	_______
24. Move foot so that toes move toward knee (dorsal flexion), then move foot so that toes point away from head (plantar flexion). Repeat with other foot.	☐	☐	_______	_______

Procedure	Pass	Redo	Date Competency Met	Instructor Initials
25. Spread toes apart (abduction) on one foot, then bring toes together (adduction). Repeat on other foot.	☐	☐	______	______
26. Turn resident in a prone position.	☐	☐	______	______
27. Move arm toward ceiling; do not bend elbows (hyperextension), then return to bed. Repeat with other arm.	☐	☐	______	______
28. Bend leg so that foot moves toward resident's back (flexion), then straighten leg (extension). Repeat with other leg.	☐	☐	______	______
29. Position resident for comfort.	☐	☐	______	______
30. Place bath blanket or sheet in laundry basket.	☐	☐	______	______
31. Wash your hands.	☐	☐	______	______
32. Report and document resident's tolerance to procedure.	☐	☐	______	______

Check-off Sheet:

15-32 Giving a Bed Bath

Name ______________________________ **Date** ______________

Directions: Practice this procedure, following each step. When you are ready to have your performance evaluated, give this sheet to your instructor. Review the detailed procedure in your textbook.

Procedure	**Pass**	**Redo**	**Date Competency Met**	**Instructor Initials**
Student must use Standard Precautions.	☐	☐	______	______
1. Wash hands.	☐	☐	______	______
2. Assemble equipment:				
a. Soap and soap dish	☐	☐	______	______
b. Face towel	☐	☐	______	______
c. Bath towel	☐	☐	______	______
d. Washcloth	☐	☐	______	______
e. Hospital gown or resident's sleepwear	☐	☐	______	______
f. Lotion or powder	☐	☐	______	______
g. Nailbrush and emery board	☐	☐	______	______
h. Comb and brush	☐	☐	______	______
i. Bedpan or urinal and cover	☐	☐	______	______
j. Bed linen	☐	☐	______	______
k. Bath blanket	☐	☐	______	______
l. Bath basin, water at 105°F	☐	☐	______	______
m. Disposable nonsterile gloves	☐	☐	______	______
3. Place linens on chair in order of use, and place towels on overbed table.	☐	☐	______	______
4. Identify resident.	☐	☐	______	______
5. Explain what you are going to do.	☐	☐	______	______
6. Provide for privacy by pulling the privacy screen.	☐	☐	______	______
7. Raise bed to a comfortable working height.	☐	☐	______	______
8. Offer bedpan or urinal. *Empty and rinse* before starting bath. *Wash your hands.* (Remember to wear gloves when handling urine.)	☐	☐	______	______
9. Lower headrest and knee gatch (raised knee area of bed) so that bed is flat.	☐	☐	______	______

Procedure	Pass	Redo	Date Competency Met	Instructor Initials
10. Lower the side rail only on side where you are working.	☐	☐	_______	_______
11. Put on gloves.	☐	☐	_______	_______
12. Loosen top sheet, blanket, and bedspread. Remove and fold blanket and bedspread, and place over back of chair.	☐	☐	_______	_______
13. Cover resident with a bath blanket.	☐	☐	_______	_______
14. Ask resident to hold bath blanket in place. Remove top sheet by *sliding* it to foot of bed. *Do not expose resident*. (Place soiled linen in laundry container.)	☐	☐	_______	_______
15. Leave a pillow under resident's head for comfort.	☐	☐	_______	_______
16. Remove resident's gown and place in laundry container.	☐	☐	_______	_______
17. To remove gown when the resident has an IV:				
a. Loosen gown from neck.	☐	☐	_______	_______
b. Slip gown from free arm.	☐	☐	_______	_______
c. Be certain that resident is covered with a bath blanket.	☐	☐	_______	_______
d. Slip gown away from body toward arm with IV.	☐	☐	_______	_______
e. Gather gown at arm and slip downward over arm and tubing.	☐	☐	_______	_______
f. Gather material of gown in one hand and slowly draw gown over tip of resident's fingers.	☐	☐	_______	_______
g. Lift IV free of standard with free hand and slip gown over bag or bottle by raising gown.	☐	☐	_______	_______
h. *Do not lower bottle! Raise gown.*	☐	☐	_______	_______
18. Fill bath basin two-thirds full with warm water.	☐	☐	_______	_______
19. Help resident move to side of bed nearest you.	☐	☐	_______	_______
20. Fold face towel over upper edge of bath blanket. This will keep it dry.	☐	☐	_______	_______
21. Form a mitten by folding washcloth around your hand.	☐	☐	_______	_______

Procedure	Pass	Redo	Date Competency Met	Instructor Initials
22. Wash resident's eyes from nose to outside of face. Use different corners of washcloth.	☐	☐	______	______
23. Ask resident if he or she wants soap used on the face. Gently wash and rinse face, ears, and neck. Be careful not to get soap in eyes.	☐	☐	______	______
24. To wash resident's arms, shoulders, and axilla:				
a. Uncover resident's far arm (one farthest from you).	☐	☐	______	______
b. Protect bed from becoming wet with a bath towel placed under arm. Wash with long, firm, circular strokes, rinse, and dry.	☐	☐	______	______
c. Wash and dry armpits (axillae). Apply deodorant and powder.	☐	☐	______	______
25. To wash hand:				
a. Place basin of water on towel.	☐	☐	______	______
b. Put resident's hand into basin.	☐	☐	______	______
c. Wash, rinse, and dry and push back cuticle gently.	☐	☐	______	______
26. Repeat on other arm.	☐	☐	______	______
27. To wash chest:				
a. Place towel across resident's chest.	☐	☐	______	______
b. Fold bath blanket down to resident's abdomen.	☐	☐	______	______
c. Wash chest. Carefully dry skin under female breasts to prevent irritation.	☐	☐	______	______
28. To wash abdomen:				
a. Fold bath blanket down to pubic area.	☐	☐	______	______
b. Wash, rinse, and dry abdomen.	☐	☐	______	______
c. Pull bath blanket up to keep resident warm.	☐	☐	______	______
d. Slide towel out from under bath blanket.	☐	☐	______	______
29. To wash thigh, leg, and foot:				
a. Ask resident to flex knee, if possible.	☐	☐	______	______
b. Fold bath blanket to uncover thigh, leg, and foot of leg farthest from you.	☐	☐	______	______
c. Place bath towel under leg to keep bed from getting wet.	☐	☐	______	______

Procedure	Pass	Redo	Date Competency Met	Instructor Initials
d. Place basin on towel and put foot into basin.	☐	☐	______	______
e. Wash and rinse thigh, leg, and foot.	☐	☐	______	______
f. Dry well between toes. Be careful to support the leg when lifting it.	☐	☐	______	______
30. Follow same procedure for leg nearest you.	☐	☐	______	______
31. Change water. You may need to change water before this time if it is dirty or cold.	☐	☐	______	______
32. Raise side rail on opposite side if it is down.	☐	☐	______	______
33. To wash back and buttocks:				
a. Help resident turn on side away from you.	☐	☐	______	______
b. Have resident move toward center of bed.	☐	☐	______	______
c. Place a bath towel lengthwise on bed, under resident's back.	☐	☐	______	______
d. Wash, rinse, and dry neck, back, and buttocks.	☐	☐	______	______
e. Give resident a back rub. *Observe for reddened areas.* (See the check-off sheet "Giving a Back Rub.")	☐	☐	______	______
34. To wash genital area:				
a. Offer resident a clean, soapy washcloth to wash genital area.	☐	☐	______	______
b. Give the person a clean wet washcloth to rinse with and a dry towel to dry with.	☐	☐	______	______
35. Clean the genital area thoroughly if resident is unable to help. To clean the genital area:				
a. Put on a pair of disposable gloves and wash genitalia.	☐	☐	______	______
b. When washing a female resident, always wipe from front to back.	☐	☐	______	______
c. When washing a male resident, be sure to wash and dry penis, scrotum, and groin area carefully.	☐	☐	______	______
d. Remove gloves and put in hazardous waste bin.	☐	☐	______	______
36. If range of motion is ordered, complete at this time. (See the check-off sheet "Range of Motion.")	☐	☐	______	______
37. Put a clean gown on resident.	☐	☐	______	______

Procedure	Pass	Redo	Date Competency Met	Instructor Initials
38. If resident has an IV:				
a. Gather the sleeve on IV side in one hand.	☐	☐	______	______
b. Lift bag or bottle free of stand. *Do not lower bottle.*	☐	☐	______	______
c. Slip bag or bottle through sleeve from inside and rehang.	☐	☐	______	______
d. Guide gown along the IV tubing to bed.	☐	☐	______	______
e. Slip gown over the resident's hand. Be careful not to pull or crimp tubing.	☐	☐	______	______
f. Put gown on arm with IV, then on opposite arm.	☐	☐	______	______
39. Comb or brush hair.	☐	☐	______	______
40. Follow hospital policy for towels and washcloths.	☐	☐	______	______
41. Leave resident in a comfortable position and in good body alignment.	☐	☐	______	______
42. Place call bell within reach. Replace furniture and tidy unit.	☐	☐	______	______
43. Wash hands.	☐	☐	______	______
44. Chart procedure and how resident tolerated it. Note any unusual skin changes or resident complaints.	☐	☐	______	______

Check-off Sheet:

15-33 Giving a Partial Bath (Face, Hands, Axillae, Buttocks, and Genitals)

Name ______________________________ **Date** ______________

Directions: Practice this procedure, following each step. When you are ready to have your performance evaluated, give this sheet to your instructor. Review the detailed procedure in your textbook.

Procedure	Pass	Redo	Date Competency Met	Instructor Initials
Student must use Standard Precautions.	☐	☐	______	______
1. Wash hands.	☐	☐	______	______
2. Assemble equipment:				
a. Soap and soap dish	☐	☐	______	______
b. Face towel	☐	☐	______	______
c. Bath towel	☐	☐	______	______
d. Washcloth	☐	☐	______	______
e. Hospital gown or resident's sleepwear	☐	☐	______	______
f. Lotion or powder	☐	☐	______	______
g. Nailbrush and emery board	☐	☐	______	______
h. Comb and brush	☐	☐	______	______
i. Bedpan or urinal and cover	☐	☐	______	______
j. Bath blanket	☐	☐	______	______
k. Bath basin, water at 105°F	☐	☐	______	______
l. Clean linen, as needed	☐	☐	______	______
m. Disposable gloves (two pair)	☐	☐	______	______
3. Identify resident.	☐	☐	______	______
4. Explain what you are going to do.	☐	☐	______	______
5. Provide privacy by pulling privacy screen.	☐	☐	______	______
6. Offer bedpan or urinal. Empty and rinse before starting bath. (Wear gloves if handling body fluids.)	☐	☐	______	______
7. Raise headrest to a comfortable position, if permitted.	☐	☐	______	______
8. Lower side rails if permitted. If they are to remain up, only lower side rail on side where you are working.	☐	☐	______	______

Procedure	Pass	Redo	Date Competency Met	Instructor Initials
9. Put on gloves.	☐	☐	______	______
10. Loosen top sheet, blanket, and bedspread. Remove and fold blanket and bedspread and place over back of chair.	☐	☐	______	______
11. Cover resident with a bath blanket.	☐	☐	______	______
12. Ask resident to hold bath blanket in place. Remove top sheet by sliding it to the foot of bed. *Do not expose resident.* (Place soiled linen in laundry container.)	☐	☐	______	______
13. Leave a pillow under the resident's head for comfort.	☐	☐	______	______
14. Remove resident's gown and place in laundry container.	☐	☐	______	______
15. To remove gown if resident has an IV, see the check-off sheet "Giving a Bed Bath."	☐	☐	______	______
16. Fill bath basin two-thirds full with warm water and place on overbed table.	☐	☐	______	______
17. Put overbed table where resident can reach it comfortably.	☐	☐	______	______
18. Place towel, washcloth, and soap on overbed table.	☐	☐	______	______
19. Ask resident to wash as much as he or she is able to and tell the person that you will return to complete the bath.	☐	☐	______	______
20. Place call bell where resident can reach it easily. Ask resident to signal when ready.	☐	☐	______	______
21. Remove gloves, wash your hands, and leave unit.	☐	☐	______	______
22. When resident signals, return to unit, wash your hands, and put on gloves.	☐	☐	______	______
23. Change water. Complete bathing areas the resident was unable to reach.	☐	☐	______	______
24. Give a back rub. (See the check-off sheet "Giving a Back Rub.")	☐	☐	______	______
25. Put a clean gown on resident.	☐	☐	______	______

Procedure	Pass	Redo	Date Competency Met	Instructor Initials
26. If resident has an IV, see the check-off sheet "Giving a Bed Bath."	☐	☐	______	______
27. Assist resident in applying deodorant and putting on a clean gown.	☐	☐	______	______
28. Change bed according to hospital policy. Not all facilities change linen every day.	☐	☐	______	______
29. Put side rails up if required.	☐	☐	______	______
30. Leave resident in a comfortable position and in good body alignment.	☐	☐	______	______
31. Remove and discard gloves.	☐	☐	______	______
32. Wash hands.	☐	☐	______	______
33. Place call bell within reach. Replace furniture and tidy unit.	☐	☐	______	______
34. Chart procedure and how it was tolerated.	☐	☐	______	______

Check-off Sheet:

15-34 Tub/Shower Bath

Name ______________________ **Date** __________

Directions: Practice this procedure, following each step. When you are ready to have your performance evaluated, give this sheet to your instructor. Review the detailed procedure in your textbook.

Procedure	Pass	Redo	Date Competency Met	Instructor Initials
Student must use Standard Precautions.	☐	☐	______	______
1. Wash hands.	☐	☐	______	______
2. Assemble equipment on a chair near the tub (be certain the tub is clean):				
a. Bath towels	☐	☐	______	______
b. Washcloths	☐	☐	______	______
c. Soap	☐	☐	______	______
d. Bath thermometer	☐	☐	______	______
e. Wash basin	☐	☐	______	______
f. Clean gown	☐	☐	______	______
g. Bathmat	☐	☐	______	______
h. Disinfectant solution	☐	☐	______	______
i. Shower chair, if necessary	☐	☐	______	______
j. Disposable gloves (two pair)	☐	☐	______	______
3. Identify resident and explain what you are going to do.	☐	☐	______	______
4. Provide privacy by pulling privacy curtain.	☐	☐	______	______
5. Put on gloves.	☐	☐	______	______
6. Help resident out of bed.	☐	☐	______	______
7. Help with robe and slippers (if ambulatory).	☐	☐	______	______
8. Check with head nurse to see if the resident can ambulate or if a wheelchair or shower chair is needed. If a shower chair is used, always do the following:	☐	☐	______	______
a. Undress resident in room so that shower is not tied up for long periods of time while residents are dressing or undressing.	☐	☐	______	______

Procedure	Pass	Redo	Date Competency Met	Instructor Initials
b. Cover resident with a bath blanket or sheet so that resident is not exposed in any way.	☐	☐	_______	_______
c. Before leaving room with resident, step back and walk around resident to see if he or she is exposed from any view.	☐	☐	_______	_______
9. Take resident to shower or tub room.	☐	☐	_______	_______
10. For tub bath, place a towel in bottom of tub to help prevent falling.	☐	☐	_______	_______
11. Fill tub with water (95°–105°F) or adjust shower flow.	☐	☐	_______	_______
12. Help resident undress. Give a male resident a towel to wrap around his midriff.	☐	☐	_______	_______
13. Assist resident into tub or shower. If shower, leave weak resident in shower chair.	☐	☐	_______	_______
14. Wash resident's back. Observe carefully for reddened areas or breaks in skin.	☐	☐	_______	_______
15. Resident may be left alone to complete genitalia area if feeling strong enough.	☐	☐	_______	_______
16. If resident shows signs of weakness, remove plug from tub and drain water, or turn off shower. Allow resident to rest until feeling better.	☐	☐	_______	_______
17. Assist resident from tub or shower.	☐	☐	_______	_______
18. Wrap bath towel around resident to prevent chilling.	☐	☐	_______	_______
19. Assist in drying and dressing.	☐	☐	_______	_______
20. Remove and discard gloves.	☐	☐	_______	_______
21. Return to unit and make comfortable.	☐	☐	_______	_______
22. Put equipment away.	☐	☐	_______	_______
23. Put on gloves.	☐	☐	_______	_______
24. Clean bathtub with disinfectant solution.	☐	☐	_______	_______
25. Discard gloves.	☐	☐	_______	_______
26. Wash hands.	☐	☐	_______	_______
27. Chart procedure and how resident tolerated it.	☐	☐	_______	_______

Check-off Sheet:

15-35 Resident Gown Change

Name ______________________________ **Date** ______________

Directions: Practice this procedure, following each step. When you are ready to have your performance evaluated, give this sheet to your instructor. Review the detailed procedure in your textbook.

Procedure	Pass	Redo	Date Competency Met	Instructor Initials
Student must use Standard Precautions.	☐	☐	______	______
1. Wash hands.	☐	☐	______	______
2. Assemble equipment: clean resident gown.	☐	☐	______	______
3. Tell resident what you are going to do.	☐	☐	______	______
4. Provide privacy by pulling privacy curtain.	☐	☐	______	______
5. Untie strings of gown at neck and midback. (It may be necessary to assist resident onto side.)	☐	☐	______	______
6. Pull soiled gown out from sides of resident.	☐	☐	______	______
7. Unfold clean gown and position over resident.	☐	☐	______	______
8. Remove soiled gown one sleeve at a time.	☐	☐	______	______
9. Leave soiled gown laying over resident's chest; insert one arm into sleeve of clean gown.	☐	☐	______	______
10. Fold soiled gown to one side as clean gown is placed over resident's chest.	☐	☐	______	______
11. Insert other arm in empty sleeve of gown.	☐	☐	______	______
12. Tie neck string on side of neck.	☐	☐	______	______
13. Tie midback tie if resident desires.	☐	☐	______	______
14. Remove soiled gown; place in linen hamper.	☐	☐	______	______
15. Slip gown under covers, being careful not to expose resident.	☐	☐	______	______
16. Position resident for comfort.	☐	☐	______	______
17. Raise side rails when necessary.	☐	☐	______	______
18. Place bedside stand and call light within resident's reach.	☐	☐	______	______

Note: Use gloves if you are in contact with body fluids.

Check-off Sheet:

15-36 Perineal Care

Name ______________________________ **Date** ______________

Directions: Practice this procedure, following each step. When you are ready to have your performance evaluated, give this sheet to your instructor. Review the detailed procedure in your textbook.

Procedure	Pass	Redo	Date Competency Met	Instructor Initials
Student must use Standard Precautions.	☐	☐	______	______
1. Wash hands.	☐	☐	______	______
2. Assemble equipment:				
a. Bath blanket	☐	☐	______	______
b. Bedpan and cover	☐	☐	______	______
c. Graduate pitcher	☐	☐	______	______
d. Solution, water, or other, if ordered	☐	☐	______	______
e. Cotton balls	☐	☐	______	______
f. Waterproof protector for bed	☐	☐	______	______
g. Disposable gloves (two pair)	☐	☐	______	______
h. Perineal pad and belt, if needed	☐	☐	______	______
i. Bag to dispose of cotton balls	☐	☐	______	______
3. Identify resident.	☐	☐	______	______
4. Explain what you are going to do.	☐	☐	______	______
5. Provide privacy by pulling privacy curtain.	☐	☐	______	______
6. Put warm water in graduate pitcher (about 100°F).	☐	☐	______	______
7. Raise bed to a comfortable working height.	☐	☐	______	______
8. Lower side rail.	☐	☐	______	______
9. Put on disposable gloves.	☐	☐	______	______
10. Remove spread and blanket.	☐	☐	______	______
11. Cover resident with bath blanket.	☐	☐	______	______
12. Have resident hold top of bath blanket, and fold top sheet to bottom of bed.	☐	☐	______	______
13. Place waterproof protector under resident's buttocks.	☐	☐	______	______

Procedure	Pass	Redo	Date Competency Met	Instructor Initials
14. Pull bath blanket up to expose perineal area.	☐	☐	______	______
15. Provide male and female peri care:				
a. Circumcised male				
(1) Wipe away from urinary meatus as you wash with soap and water, rinse, and dry.	☐	☐	______	______
b. Uncircumsized male				
(1) Gently move foreskin back away from tip of penis.	☐	☐	______	______
(2) Wash as directed in step a.	☐	☐	______	______
(3) After drying, gently move foreskin back over tip of penis.	☐	☐	______	______
c. Female				
(1) Instruct resident to bend knees with feet flat on bed.	☐	☐	______	______
(2) Separate resident's knees.	☐	☐	______	______
(3) Separate the labia and wipe from front to back away from the urethra as you wash with soap and water, rinse, and dry.	☐	☐	______	______
16. Remove waterproof protector from bed, dispose of gloves, and wash hands.	☐	☐	______	______
17. Cover resident with sheet and remove bath blanket.	☐	☐	______	______
18. Return top covers.	☐	☐	______	______
19. Return bed to lowest position and put side rails up, if required.	☐	☐	______	______
20. Secure call bell within resident's reach.	☐	☐	______	______
21. Put on gloves.	☐	☐	______	______
22. Clean equipment; dispose of disposable material according to hospital policy.	☐	☐	______	______
23. Discard gloves and wash hands.	☐	☐	______	______

Check-off Sheet:

15-37 Vaginal Douche

Name ______________________________ **Date** ______________

Directions: Practice this procedure, following each step. When you are ready to have your performance evaluated, give this sheet to your instructor. Review the detailed procedure in your textbook.

Procedure	Pass	Redo	Date Competency Met	Instructor Initials
Student must use Standard Precautions.	☐	☐	______	______
1. Wash hands.	☐	☐	______	______
2. Assemble equipment:				
a. Disposable douche kit	☐	☐	______	______
(1) Tubing clamp	☐	☐	______	______
(2) Douche nozzle	☐	☐	______	______
(3) Irrigating container	☐	☐	______	______
b. Cleansing solution	☐	☐	______	______
c. Cotton balls	☐	☐	______	______
d. Bedpan and cover	☐	☐	______	______
e. Waterproof bed protector	☐	☐	______	______
f. Disposable gloves	☐	☐	______	______
3. Identify resident.	☐	☐	______	______
4. Explain what you are going to do.	☐	☐	______	______
5. Provide privacy by pulling privacy curtains.	☐	☐	______	______
6. Offer bedpan or urinal; empty if used. (Wear gloves if exposed to body fluid.)	☐	☐	______	______
7. Remove and discard gloves, if used; wash hands.	☐	☐	______	______
8. Raise bed to comfortable working height.	☐	☐	______	______
9. Place waterproof protector under resident's buttocks.	☐	☐	______	______
10. Open douche kit.	☐	☐	______	______
11. Clamp tubing and pour solution into douche container.	☐	☐	______	______
12. Put on gloves.	☐	☐	______	______
13. Place bedpan under resident.	☐	☐	______	______
14. Pour cleansing solution over cotton balls.	☐	☐	______	______

Procedure	Pass	Redo	Date Competency Met	Instructor Initials
15. Cleanse vulva with cotton balls by spreading lips (labia) and wiping one side from front to back.	☐	☐	______	______
16. Discard cotton balls into bedpan. Wipe other side and discard cotton ball.	☐	☐	______	______
17. Open clamp to expel air from tubing.	☐	☐	______	______
18. Allow solution to flow over vulva. Do not touch vulva with nozzle.	☐	☐	______	______
19. Insert douche nozzle into vagina as solution is flowing. Insert about 2 inches with an upward, then downward, and backward gentle movement.	☐	☐	______	______
20. Allow solution to flow into vagina while holding douche container no more than 18 inches above mattress.	☐	☐	______	______
21. Rotate nozzle until all solution has been used.	☐	☐	______	______
22. Clamp tubing and remove nozzle gently.	☐	☐	______	______
23. Place nozzle and tubing in douche container for disposal.	☐	☐	______	______
24. Assist resident to upright position on bedpan to help drain solution from vagina.	☐	☐	______	______
25. Help resident dry perineal area.	☐	☐	______	______
26. Remove bedpan.	☐	☐	______	______
27. Remove waterproof protector.	☐	☐	______	______
28. Empty bedpan; rinse, and put away.	☐	☐	______	______
29. Remove gloves and discard according to hospital policy.	☐	☐	______	______
30. Wash hands.	☐	☐	______	______
31. Lower bed to lowest position.	☐	☐	______	______
32. Position resident comfortably.	☐	☐	______	______
33. Put side rails up, if required.	☐	☐	______	______
34. Secure call bell within resident's reach.	☐	☐	______	______
35. Wash hands.	☐	☐	______	______
36. Record procedure.	☐	☐	______	______

Check-off Sheet:

15-38 Shampooing the Hair in Bed

Name ______________________________ **Date** ______________

Directions: Practice this procedure, following each step. When you are ready to have your performance evaluated, give this sheet to your instructor. Review the detailed procedure in your textbook.

Procedure	Pass	Redo	Date Competency Met	Instructor Initials
Student must use Standard Precautions.	☐	☐	______	______
1. Wash hands.	☐	☐	______	______
2. Assemble equipment:				
a. Chair	☐	☐	______	______
b. Basin of water (105°F)	☐	☐	______	______
c. Pitcher of water (115°F)	☐	☐	______	______
d. Paper or Styrofoam cup	☐	☐	______	______
e. Large basin	☐	☐	______	______
f. Shampoo tray or plastic sheet	☐	☐	______	______
g. Waterproof bed protector	☐	☐	______	______
h. Pillow with waterproof cover	☐	☐	______	______
i. Bath towels	☐	☐	______	______
j. Small towel	☐	☐	______	______
k. Cotton balls	☐	☐	______	______
3. Identify resident.	☐	☐	______	______
4. Explain what you are going to do.	☐	☐	______	______
5. Provide privacy by pulling privacy curtain.	☐	☐	______	______
6. Raise bed to a comfortable working position.	☐	☐	______	______
7. Place a chair at side of bed near resident's head.	☐	☐	______	______
8. Place small towel on chair.	☐	☐	______	______
9. Place large basin on chair to catch water.	☐	☐	______	______
10. Put cotton in resident's ears to keep water out of ears.	☐	☐	______	______
11. Have resident move to side of bed with head close to where you are standing.	☐	☐	______	______

Check-off Sheet:

15-41 Nail Care

Name ______________________________ **Date** ____________

Directions: Practice this procedure, following each step. When you are ready to have your performance evaluated, give this sheet to your instructor. Review the detailed procedure in your textbook.

Procedure	Pass	Redo	Date Competency Met	Instructor Initials
Student must use Standard Precautions.	☐	☐	______	______
1. Wash hands.	☐	☐	______	______
2. Identify resident.	☐	☐	______	______
3. Assemble equipment:				
a. Warm water	☐	☐	______	______
b. Orange sticks	☐	☐	______	______
c. Emery board	☐	☐	______	______
d. Nail clippers	☐	☐	______	______
Do not clip a diabetic resident's nails.				
4. Cleanse nails by soaking in water.	☐	☐	______	______
5. Use slanted edge of orange stick to clean dirt out from under nails.	☐	☐	______	______
6. File nails with emery board to shorten. (Clip if permitted by your facility.)	☐	☐	______	______
7. When nails are correct length, use smooth edge of emery board to smooth.	☐	☐	______	______
8. Apply lotion to help condition cuticle.	☐	☐	______	______
9. Massage hands and feet with lotion.	☐	☐	______	______
10. Make resident comfortable.	☐	☐	______	______
11. If bed resident, raise side rail, if required.	☐	☐	______	______
12. Return equipment.	☐	☐	______	______
13. Wash hands.	☐	☐	______	______
14. Record procedure and any unusual conditions (e.g., hangnails, broken nails).	☐	☐	______	______

Check-off Sheet:

15-42 Shaving the Resident

Name ______________________________ **Date** ______________

Directions: Practice this procedure, following each step. When you are ready to have your performance evaluated, give this sheet to your instructor. Review the detailed procedure in your textbook.

Procedure	Pass	Redo	Date Competency Met	Instructor Initials
Student must use Standard Precautions.	☐	☐	______	______
1. Wash hands.	☐	☐	______	______
2. Assemble equipment:				
a. Electric shaver or safety razor	☐	☐	______	______
b. Shaving lather or an electric preshave lotion	☐	☐	______	______
c. Basin of warm water	☐	☐	______	______
d. Face towel	☐	☐	______	______
e. Mirror	☐	☐	______	______
f. Aftershave	☐	☐	______	______
g. Disposable gloves	☐	☐	______	______
3. Identify resident and explain what you are going to do.	☐	☐	______	______
4. Provide privacy by pulling privacy curtains.	☐	☐	______	______
5. Raise head of bed, if permitted.	☐	☐	______	______
6. Place equipment on overbed table.	☐	☐	______	______
7. Place a towel over resident's chest.	☐	☐	______	______
8. Adjust light so that it shines on resident's face.	☐	☐	______	______
9. Shave resident:				
a. If you are using a safety razor				
(1) Put on gloves.	☐	☐	______	______
(2) Moisten face and apply lather.	☐	☐	______	______
(3) Start in front of ear; hold skin taut and bring razor down over cheek toward chin. Use short, firm strokes. Repeat until lather on cheek is removed and skin is smooth.	☐	☐	______	______

Procedure	Pass	Redo	Date Competency Met	Instructor Initials
(4) Repeat on other cheek.	☐	☐	______	______
(5) Wash face and neck. Dry thoroughly.	☐	☐	______	______
(6) Apply aftershave lotion or powder, if desired.	☐	☐	______	______
(7) Discard gloves according to facility policy.	☐	☐	______	______
b. If you are using an electric shaver				
(1) Put on gloves.	☐	☐	______	______
(2) Apply preshave lotion.	☐	☐	______	______
(3) Gently shave until beard is removed.	☐	☐	______	______
(4) Wash face and neck. Dry thoroughly.	☐	☐	______	______
(5) Apply aftershave lotion or powder, if desired.	☐	☐	______	______
(6) Remove gloves.	☐	☐	______	______
10. Wash hands.	☐	☐	______	______
11. Chart procedure and how procedure was tolerated.	☐	☐	______	______

Check-off Sheet:

15-43 Making a Closed Bed

Name ______________________ **Date** __________

Directions: Practice this procedure, following each step. When you are ready to have your performance evaluated, give this sheet to your instructor. Review the detailed procedure in your textbook.

Procedure	Pass	Redo	Date Competency Met	Instructor Initials
Student must use Standard Precautions.	☐	☐	______	______
1. Wash hands.	☐	☐	______	______
2. Assemble equipment:				
a. Mattress pad and cover	☐	☐	______	______
b. Plastic or rubber draw sheet (if used in your facility)	☐	☐	______	______
c. Two large sheets or fitted bottom sheet and one large sheet	☐	☐	______	______
d. Draw sheet or half-sheet	☐	☐	______	______
e. Blankets as needed	☐	☐	______	______
f. Spread	☐	☐	______	______
g. Pillow	☐	☐	______	______
h. Pillowcase	☐	☐	______	______
3. Raise bed to a comfortable working height. *Lock* wheels on bed.	☐	☐	______	______
4. Place a chair at the side of the bed.	☐	☐	______	______
5. Put linen on chair in the order in which you will use it. (First things you will use go on top.)	☐	☐	______	______
6. Position mattress at head of bed until it is against head board.	☐	☐	______	______
7. Place mattress cover even with top of mattress and smooth it out.	☐	☐	______	______
8. Work on one side of bed until that side is completed. Then go to other side of bed. This saves you time and energy.	☐	☐	______	______
9. Bottom sheet is folded lengthwise. Place it on bed with center fold in center of mattress from head to foot. Place large hem at head of bed and narrow hem even with foot of mattress.	☐	☐	______	______

Procedure	Pass	Redo	Date Competency Met	Instructor Initials
10. Open sheet. Check to see that it hangs the same distance over each side of bed.	☐	☐	______	______
11. Leave about 18 inches of sheet to tuck under head of mattress.	☐	☐	______	______
12. Make a mitered corner:				
a. Pick up edge of sheet at side of bed approximately 12 inches from head of bed.	☐	☐	______	______
b. Place folded corner (triangle) on top of mattress.	☐	☐	______	______
c. Tuck hanging portion of sheet under the mattress.	☐	☐	______	______
d. While you hold the fold at the edge of the mattress, bring folded section down over side of mattress.	☐	☐	______	______
e. Tuck sheet under mattress from head to foot. Start at head and pull toward foot of bed as you tuck.	☐	☐	______	______
13. Fold draw sheet in half and place about 14 inches down from top of mattress. Tuck it in.	☐	☐	______	______
14. Top sheet is folded lengthwise.	☐	☐	______	______
a. Place the center fold at center of bed from head to foot.	☐	☐	______	______
b. Put large hem at head of bed, even with top of mattress.	☐	☐	______	______
c. Open the sheet. Be certain rough edge of hem is facing up.	☐	☐	______	______
d. Tightly tuck the sheet under at foot of bed.	☐	☐	______	______
e. Following directions in step 12, make a mitered corner at foot of bed.	☐	☐	______	______
f. Do not tuck sheet in at side of bed.	☐	☐	______	______
15. Blanket is folded lengthwise. Place it on bed:	☐	☐	______	______
a. Place center fold of blanket on center of bed from head to foot.	☐	☐	______	______
b. Place upper hem 6 inches from top of mattress.	☐	☐	______	______
c. Open blanket and tuck it under foot tightly.	☐	☐	______	______
d. Make a mitered corner at foot of bed.	☐	☐	______	______
e. Do not tuck in at sides of bed.	☐	☐	______	______

Procedure	Pass	Redo	Date Competency Met	Instructor Initials
16. Bedspread is folded lengthwise. Place it on bed:	☐	☐	_______	_______
a. Place center fold in center of bed from head to foot.	☐	☐	_______	_______
b. Place upper hem even with upper edge of mattress.	☐	☐	_______	_______
c. Place rough edge down.	☐	☐	_______	_______
d. Open spread and tuck it under at foot of bed.	☐	☐	_______	_______
e. Make a mitered corner.	☐	☐	_______	_______
f. Do not tuck in at sides.	☐	☐	_______	_______
17. Go to other side of bed. Start with bottom sheet:				
a. Pull sheet tight and smooth out all wrinkles.	☐	☐	_______	_______
b. Make a mitered corner at top of bed.	☐	☐	_______	_______
c. Pull draw sheet tight and tuck it in.	☐	☐	_______	_______
d. Straighten out top sheet. Make a mitered corner at foot of bed.	☐	☐	_______	_______
e. Miter foot corners of blanket and bedspread.	☐	☐	_______	_______
18. Fold top hem of spread over top hem of blanket.	☐	☐	_______	_______
19. Fold top hem of sheet back over edge of spread and blanket to form cuff.	☐	☐	_______	_______
20. Put pillowcase on pillow:				
a. Hold pillowcase at center of end seam.	☐	☐	_______	_______
b. With your other hand, turn pillowcase back over hand holding end seam.	☐	☐	_______	_______
c. Grasp pillow through case at center of end of pillow.	☐	☐	_______	_______
d. Bring case down over pillow and fit pillow into corners of case.	☐	☐	_______	_______
e. Fold extra material over open end of pillow and place it on bed with open end away from door.	☐	☐	_______	_______
21. Put bed in lowest position.	☐	☐	_______	_______
22. Wash hands.	☐	☐	_______	_______

Check-off Sheet:

15-44 Making an Occupied Bed

Name ______________________________ **Date** ______________

Directions: Practice this procedure, following each step. When you are ready to have your performance evaluated, give this sheet to your instructor. Review the detailed procedure in your textbook.

Procedure	Pass	Redo	Date Competency Met	Instructor Initials
Student must use Standard Precautions.	☐	☐	______	______
1. Wash hands.	☐	☐	______	______
2. Assemble equipment:				
a. Draw sheet	☐	☐	______	______
b. Two large sheets or fitted bottom sheet and one large sheet	☐	☐	______	______
c. Two pillowcases	☐	☐	______	______
d. Blankets as needed	☐	☐	______	______
e. Bedspread (if clean one is needed)	☐	☐	______	______
f. Pillow	☐	☐	______	______
g. Disposable gloves (as needed)	☐	☐	______	______
3. Identify resident and explain what you are going to do.	☐	☐	______	______
4. Raise bed to comfortable working height. *Lock* wheels on bed.	☐	☐	______	______
5. Place chair at side of bed.	☐	☐	______	______
6. Put linen on chair in the order in which you will use it. (First things you will use go on top.)	☐	☐	______	______
7. Provide for privacy by pulling privacy curtain.	☐	☐	______	______
8. Lower headrest and kneerest until bed is flat, if allowed.	☐	☐	______	______
9. Loosen linens on all sides by lifting edge of mattress with one hand and pulling bedclothes out with the other.	☐	☐	______	______
10. Push mattress to top of bed. Ask for assistance if you need it.	☐	☐	______	______
11. Remove bedspread and blanket by folding them to the bottom, one at a time. Lift them from center and place over back of chair.	☐	☐	______	______

Procedure	Pass	Redo	Date Competency Met	Instructor Initials
12. Place bath blanket or plain sheet over top sheet. Ask resident to hold top edge of clean cover if he or she is able to do so. If resident cannot hold the sheet, tuck it under resident's shoulders.	☐	☐	______	______
13. Slide soiled sheet from top to bottom and put in dirty linen container. Be careful not to expose resident.	☐	☐	______	______
14. Ask resident to turn toward the opposite side of bed. Have resident hold onto the side rail.	☐	☐	______	______
15. Adjust pillow for resident to make him or her comfortable.	☐	☐	______	______
16. Fan-fold soiled draw sheet and bottom sheet close to resident and tuck against resident's back. This leaves mattress stripped of linen.	☐	☐	______	______
17. Work on one side of bed until that side is completed. Then go to other side of bed. This saves you time and energy.	☐	☐	______	______
18. Take large, clean sheet and fold it lengthwise. Be careful not to let it touch the floor.	☐	☐	______	______
19. Place sheet on bed, still folded, with fold on middle of mattress. Small hem should be even with foot of mattress.	☐	☐	______	______
20. Fold top half of sheet toward resident. Tuck folds against resident's back.	☐	☐	______	______
21. Miter corner at head of mattress. Tuck clean sheet on your side from head to foot of mattress.	☐	☐	______	______
22. Place clean bottom draw sheet that has been folded in half with fold along middle of mattress. Fold top half of sheet toward resident. Tuck folds against resident's back.	☐	☐	______	______
23. Raise side rail and lock in place.	☐	☐	______	______
24. Lower side rail on opposite side.	☐	☐	______	______
25. Ask resident to roll away from you to other side of bed and onto clean linen. Tell resident that there will be a bump in the middle. (Be careful not to let resident become wrapped up in bath blanket.)	☐	☐	______	______
26. Remove old bottom sheet and draw sheet from bed and put into laundry container.	☐	☐	______	______

Procedure	Pass	Redo	Date Competency Met	Instructor Initials
27. Pull fresh linen toward edge of mattress. Tuck it under mattress at head of bed and make mitered corner.	☐	☐	______	______
28. Tuck bottom sheet under mattress from head to foot of mattress. Pull firmly to remove wrinkles.	☐	☐	______	______
29. Pull draw sheet very tight and tuck under mattress.	☐	☐	______	______
30. Have resident roll on back, or turn resident yourself. Loosen bath blanket as resident turns.	☐	☐	______	______
31. Change pillowcase:				
a. Hold pillowcase at center of end seam.	☐	☐	______	______
b. With your other hand, turn pillowcase back over hand, holding end seam.	☐	☐	______	______
c. Grasp pillow through case at center of end of pillow.	☐	☐	______	______
d. Bring case down over pillow and fit pillow into corners of case.	☐	☐	______	______
e. Fold extra material over open end of pillow and place pillow under resident's head.	☐	☐	______	______
32. Spread clean top sheet over bath blanket with wide hem at the top. Middle of sheet should run along middle of bed with wide hem even with top edge of mattress. Ask resident to hold hem of clean sheet. Remove bath blanket by moving it toward foot of bed. (Be careful not to expose resident.)	☐	☐	______	______
33. Tuck clean top sheet under mattress at foot of bed. Make toepleat in top sheet so that resident's feet can move freely. Tuck in and miter corner.	☐	☐	______	______
34. Place blanket over resident, being sure that it covers the shoulders.	☐	☐	______	______
35. Place bedspread on bed in same way. Tuck blanket and bedspread under bottom of mattress and miter corners.	☐	☐	______	______
36. Make cuff:				
a. Fold top hem edge of spread over blanket.	☐	☐	______	______
b. Fold top hem of top sheet back over edge of bedspread and blanket, being certain that rough hem is turned down.	☐	☐	______	______

Procedure	Pass	Redo	Date Competency Met	Instructor Initials
37. Position resident and make comfortable.	☐	☐	______	______
38. Put bed in lowest position.	☐	☐	______	______
39. Open privacy curtains.	☐	☐	______	______
40. Raise side rails, if required.	☐	☐	______	______
41. Place call light where resident can reach it.	☐	☐	______	______
42. Tidy unit.	☐	☐	______	______
43. Wash hands.	☐	☐	______	______
44. Chart linen change and how the resident tolerated procedure.	☐	☐	______	______

Check-off Sheet:

15-45 Making an Open Bed

Name ______________________________ **Date** ______________

Directions: Practice this procedure, following each step. When you are ready to have your performance evaluated, give this sheet to your instructor. Review the detailed procedure in your textbook.

Procedure	Pass	Redo	Date Competency Met	Instructor Initials
Student must use Standard Precautions.	☐	☐	______	______
(Begin by following steps for making a closed bed. If you start with a closed bed, the steps will be the same.)				
1. Wash hands.	☐	☐	______	______
2. Grasp cuff of bedding in both hands and pull to foot of bed.	☐	☐	______	______
3. Fold bedding back on itself toward head of bed. The edge of cuff must meet fold. (This is called fan-folding.)	☐	☐	______	______
4. Smooth the hanging sheets on each side into folds.	☐	☐	______	______
5. Wash hands.	☐	☐	______	______

Check-off Sheet:

15-46 Preparing the Resident to Eat

Name ______________________ Date ____________

Directions: Practice this procedure, following each step. When you are ready to have your performance evaluated, give this sheet to your instructor. Review the detailed procedure in your textbook.

Procedure	Pass	Redo	Date Competency Met	Instructor Initials
Student must use Standard Precautions.	☐	☐	______	______
1. Wash hands.	☐	☐	______	______
2. Assemble equipment:				
a. Bedpan or urinal	☐	☐	______	______
b. Toilet tissue	☐	☐	______	______
c. Washcloth	☐	☐	______	______
d. Hand towel	☐	☐	______	______
3. Assist resident as needed to empty bladder and wash hands and face.	☐	☐	______	______
4. Explain that you are getting ready to give resident a meal.	☐	☐	______	______
5. Clear bedside table.	☐	☐	______	______
6. Position resident for comfort and a convenient eating position.	☐	☐	______	______
7. Wash your hands.	☐	☐	______	______
8. Identify resident and check name on food tray to ensure that you are delivering the correct diet to resident.	☐	☐	______	______
9. Place tray in a convenient position in front of resident.	☐	☐	______	______
10. Open containers if resident cannot.	☐	☐	______	______
11. If resident is unable to prepare food, do it for resident:				
a. Butter the bread.	☐	☐	______	______
b. Cut meat.	☐	☐	______	______
c. Season food, as necessary.	☐	☐	______	______
12. Follow the procedure for feeding a resident if resident needs to be fed.	☐	☐	______	______
13. Wash hands.	☐	☐	______	______

Check-off Sheet:

15-47 Preparing the Resident to Eat in the Dining Room

Name ______________________________ **Date** ____________

Directions: Practice this procedure, following each step. When you are ready to have your performance evaluated, give this sheet to your instructor. Review the detailed procedure in your textbook.

Procedure	Pass	Redo	Date Competency Met	Instructor Initials
Student must use Standard Precautions.	☐	☐	______	______
1. Wash hands.	☐	☐	______	______
2. Help resident take care of toileting needs.	☐	☐	______	______
3. Assist with handwashing.	☐	☐	______	______
4. Take resident to dining room.	☐	☐	______	______
5. Position resident in wheelchair at table that is proper height for wheelchair.	☐	☐	______	______
6. Be certain resident is sitting in a comfortable position in wheelchair.	☐	☐	______	______
7. Provide adaptive feeding equipment, if needed.	☐	☐	______	______
8. Bring resident tray.	☐	☐	______	______
9. Identify resident.	☐	☐	______	______
10. Serve tray and remove plate covers.	☐	☐	______	______
11. Provide assistance as needed (e.g., cut meat, butter bread, open containers).	☐	☐	______	______
12. Remove tray, when finished, noting what resident ate.	☐	☐	______	______
13. Assist with handwashing and take resident to area of choice.	☐	☐	______	______
14. Wash hands.	☐	☐	______	______
15. Record what resident ate.	☐	☐	______	______
16. Record I & O, if necessary.	☐	☐	______	______

Check-off Sheet:

15-48 Assisting the Resident with Meals

Name ______________________________ **Date** ______________

Directions: Practice this procedure, following each step. When you are ready to have your performance evaluated, give this sheet to your instructor. Review the detailed procedure in your textbook.

Procedure	Pass	Redo	Date Competency Met	Instructor Initials
Student must use Standard Precautions.	☐	☐	______	______
1. Wash hands.	☐	☐	______	______
2. Check resident's ID band with name on food tray.	☐	☐	______	______
3. Tell resident what food is being served.	☐	☐	______	______
4. Ask resident how he or she prefers food to be prepared.	☐	☐	______	______
5. Position resident in a sitting position, as allowed by physician. If ordered to lie flat, turn resident on side.	☐	☐	______	______
6. Position yourself in a comfortable manner so that you won't be rushing resident because you are uncomfortable. (Do not sit on bed.)	☐	☐	______	______
7. Cut food into small bite-size pieces.	☐	☐	______	______
8. Place a napkin or small hand towel under resident's chin.	☐	☐	______	______
9. Put a flex straw in cold drinks.	☐	☐	______	______
10. Use a spoon to feed resident small-to-average-size bites of food. (Encourage resident to help self as much as possible.)	☐	☐	______	______
11. Always feed resident at a slow pace.	☐	☐	______	______
12. Always be sure that one bite has been swallowed before you give another spoonful to resident.	☐	☐	______	______
13. Tell resident what is being served and ask which item he or she prefers first, if resident cannot see food.	☐	☐	______	______
14. Encourage resident to finish eating, but do not force.	☐	☐	______	______

Procedure	Pass	Redo	Date Competency Met	Instructor Initials
15. Assist resident in wiping face when resident is finished eating.	☐	☐	________	________
16. Observe amount of food eaten.	☐	☐	________	________
17. Remove tray from room.	☐	☐	________	________
18. Position resident for comfort and safety.	☐	☐	________	________
19. Place call light in a convenient place.	☐	☐	________	________
20. Wash hands.	☐	☐	________	________
21. Record amount of food eaten (half, three-fourths, one-fourth, and so on) on chart, and indicate if food was tolerated well or not well.	☐	☐	________	________

Check-off Sheet:

15-49 Serving Food to the Resident in Bed

Name ______________________________ **Date** ____________

Directions: Practice this procedure, following each step. When you are ready to have your performance evaluated, give this sheet to your instructor. Review the detailed procedure in your textbook.

Procedure	Pass	Redo	Date Competency Met	Instructor Initials
Student must use Standard Precautions.	☐	☐	______	______
1. Wash hands.	☐	☐	______	______
2. Assemble equipment:				
a. Food tray with diet card	☐	☐	______	______
b. Flex straws	☐	☐	______	______
c. Towel	☐	☐	______	______
3. Assist resident with bedpan or urinal.	☐	☐	______	______
4. Position in a sitting position, if possible.	☐	☐	______	______
5. Help resident wash hands and face.	☐	☐	______	______
6. Remove unsightly or odor-causing articles.	☐	☐	______	______
7. Clean overbed table.	☐	☐	______	______
8. Check tray with diet card for:				
a. Resident's name	☐	☐	______	______
b. Type of diet	☐	☐	______	______
c. Correct foods according to diet (e.g., diabetic, puréed, chopped, regular).	☐	☐	______	______
9. Set up tray and help with foods, if needed (e.g., cut meat, butter bread, open containers). *Do not add foods to the tray until you check on diet.*	☐	☐	______	______
10. Encourage resident to eat all foods on the tray.	☐	☐	______	______
11. Remove tray when finished and note what resident ate.	☐	☐	______	______
12. Help resident wash hands and face.	☐	☐	______	______
13. Position resident comfortably.	☐	☐	______	______

Procedure	Pass	Redo	Date Competency Met	Instructor Initials
14. Remove tray.	☐	☐	______	______
15. Be certain that water is within reach.	☐	☐	______	______
16. Wash hands.	☐	☐	______	______
17. Record I & O, if required.	☐	☐	______	______
18. Record amount eaten.	☐	☐	______	______

Check-off Sheet:

15-50 Feeding the Helpless Resident

Name ______________________________ **Date** ______________

Directions: Practice this procedure, following each step. When you are ready to have your performance evaluated, give this sheet to your instructor. Review the detailed procedure in your textbook.

Procedure	Pass	Redo	Date Competency Met	Instructor Initials
Student must use Standard Precautions.	☐	☐	______	______
1. Wash hands.	☐	☐	______	______
2. Bring resident's tray.	☐	☐	______	______
3. Check name on card with resident ID band.	☐	☐	______	______
4. Explain to resident what you are going to do.	☐	☐	______	______
5. Tuck a napkin under resident's chin.	☐	☐	______	______
6. Season food the way resident likes it.	☐	☐	______	______
7. Use a spoon and fill only half full.	☐	☐	______	______
8. Give food from tip, not side of spoon.	☐	☐	______	______
9. Name each food as you offer it if resident cannot see food.	☐	☐	______	______
10. Describe position of food on plate if resident cannot see but can feed self.	☐	☐	______	______
11. Tell resident if you are offering something that is hot or cold.	☐	☐	______	______
12. Use a straw for giving liquids.	☐	☐	______	______
13. Feed resident slowly, and allow time to chew and swallow.	☐	☐	______	______
14. Note amount eaten and remove tray when finished.	☐	☐	______	______
15. Help with washing hands and face.	☐	☐	______	______
16. Position resident comfortably.	☐	☐	______	______
17. Wash hands.	☐	☐	______	______
18. Record amount eaten and I & O, if required.	☐	☐	______	______

Check-off Sheet:

15-51 Serving Nourishments

Name ______________________________ **Date** ______________

Directions: Practice this procedure, following each step. When you are ready to have your performance evaluated, give this sheet to your instructor. Review the detailed procedure in your textbook.

Procedure	**Pass**	**Redo**	**Date Competency Met**	**Instructor Initials**
Student must use Standard Precautions.	☐	☐	______	______
1. Wash hands.	☐	☐	______	______
2. Assemble equipment:				
a. Nourishment	☐	☐	______	______
b. Cup, dish, straw, spoon	☐	☐	______	______
c. Napkin	☐	☐	______	______
3. Identify resident.	☐	☐	______	______
4. Take nourishment to resident.	☐	☐	______	______
5. Help, if needed.	☐	☐	______	______
6. After resident is finished, collect dirty utensils.	☐	☐	______	______
7. Return utensils to dietary cart or kitchen.	☐	☐	______	______
8. Record intake on I & O sheet, if required.	☐	☐	______	______
9. Wash hands.	☐	☐	______	______
10. Record nourishment taken.	☐	☐	______	______

Check-off Sheet:

15-52 Measuring Urinary Output

Name ______________________________ **Date** ____________

Directions: Practice this procedure, following each step. When you are ready to have your performance evaluated, give this sheet to your instructor. Review the detailed procedure in your textbook.

Procedure	Pass	Redo	Date Competency Met	Instructor Initials
Student must use Standard Precautions.	☐	☐	______	______
1. Wash hands.	☐	☐	______	______
2. Assemble equipment:				
a. Bedpan, urinal, or special container	☐	☐	______	______
b. Graduate or measuring cup	☐	☐	______	______
c. Disposable nonsterile gloves	☐	☐	______	______
3. Put on gloves.	☐	☐	______	______
4. Pour urine into measuring graduate.	☐	☐	______	______
5. Place graduate on flat surface and read amount of urine.	☐	☐	______	______
6. Observe urine for:				
a. Unusual color	☐	☐	______	______
b. Blood	☐	☐	______	______
c. Dark color	☐	☐	______	______
d. Large amounts of mucus	☐	☐	______	______
e. Sediment	☐	☐	______	______
7. If you notice any unusual appearance, save the specimen and report to nurse immediately.	☐	☐	______	______
8. Discard if urine is normal.	☐	☐	______	______
9. Rinse graduate or pitcher, and put away.	☐	☐	______	______
10. Remove gloves, and discard according to facility policy.	☐	☐	______	______
11. Wash hands.	☐	☐	______	______
12. Record amount of urine in cc on I & O sheet.	☐	☐	______	______

Check-off Sheet:

15-53 Oil Retention Enema

Name ______________________________ **Date** ______________

Directions: Practice this procedure, following each step. When you are ready to have your performance evaluated, give this sheet to your instructor. Review the detailed procedure in your textbook.

Procedure	Pass	Redo	Date Competency Met	Instructor Initials
Student must use Standard Precautions.	☐	☐	______	______
1. Wash hands.	☐	☐	______	______
2. Assemble equipment:				
a. Prepackaged oil retention enema	☐	☐	______	______
b. Bedpan and cover	☐	☐	______	______
c. Waterproof bed protector	☐	☐	______	______
d. Toilet tissue	☐	☐	______	______
e. Towel, basin of water, and soap	☐	☐	______	______
f. Disposable gloves (two pair)	☐	☐	______	______
3. Identify resident.	☐	☐	______	______
4. Ask visitors to leave the room. Pull privacy curtains.	☐	☐	______	______
5. Explain what you are going to do.	☐	☐	______	______
6. Put on gloves.	☐	☐	______	______
7. Cover resident with a bath blanket, and fan-fold linen to foot of bed.	☐	☐	______	______
8. Put bedpan on foot of bed.	☐	☐	______	______
9. Place bed protector under buttocks.	☐	☐	______	______
10. Help resident into the Sims position.	☐	☐	______	______
11. Tell resident to retain enema as long as possible.	☐	☐	______	______
12. Open a prepackaged oil retention enema.	☐	☐	______	______
13. Lift resident's upper buttock and expose anus.	☐	☐	______	______
14. Tell resident when you are going to insert prelubricated tip into anus. (Instruct resident to take deep breaths and try to relax.)	☐	☐	______	______

Procedure	Pass	Redo	Date Competency Met	Instructor Initials
15. Squeeze container until all solution has entered rectum.	☐	☐	______	______
16. Remove container, place in original package to be disposed of in contaminated waste according to facility policy and procedure.	☐	☐	______	______
17. Instruct resident to remain on side.	☐	☐	______	______
18. Remove gloves and discard according to facility policy.	☐	☐	______	______
19. Check resident every 5 minutes until fluid has been retained for at least 20 minutes.	☐	☐	______	______
20. Position resident on bedpan or assist to bathroom, if ambulatory. Instruct resident not to flush toilet.	☐	☐	______	______
21. If using a bedpan, raise head of bed, if permitted.	☐	☐	______	______
22. Place toilet tissue and call bell within easy reach.	☐	☐	______	______
23. If resident is in bathroom, stay nearby.	☐	☐	______	______
24. Put on gloves.	☐	☐	______	______
25. Remove bedpan or assist resident to return to bed. Observe contents of toilet or bedpan for:				
a. Color, consistency, unusual materials, odor	☐	☐	______	______
b. Amount of return	☐	☐	______	______
26. Cover bedpan and dispose of contents.	☐	☐	______	______
27. Remove gloves and discard.	☐	☐	______	______
28. Replace top sheet and remove bath blanket and plastic bed protector.	☐	☐	______	______
29. Give resident soap, water, and towel for hands and face.	☐	☐	______	______
30. Wash hands.	☐	☐	______	______
31. Chart the following:				
a. Type of enema given	☐	☐	______	______
b. Consistency and amount of bowel movement	☐	☐	______	______
c. How the procedure was tolerated	☐	☐	______	______

Check-off Sheet:

15-54 Prepackaged Enemas

Name ______________________________ **Date** ____________

Directions: Practice this procedure, following each step. When you are ready to have your performance evaluated, give this sheet to your instructor. Review the detailed procedure in your textbook.

Procedure	Pass	Redo	Date Competency Met	Instructor Initials
Student must use Standard Precautions.	☐	☐	______	______
1. Wash hands.	☐	☐	______	______
2. Assemble equipment:				
a. Prepackaged enema	☐	☐	______	______
b. Bedpan and cover	☐	☐	______	______
c. Waterproof bed protector	☐	☐	______	______
d. Toilet tissue	☐	☐	______	______
e. Towel, basin of water, and soap	☐	☐	______	______
f. Disposable gloves (two pair)	☐	☐	______	______
3. Identify resident.	☐	☐	______	______
4. Ask visitors to leave the room. Pull privacy curtains.	☐	☐	______	______
5. Explain what you are going to do.	☐	☐	______	______
6. Cover resident with a bath blanket, and fan-fold linen to foot of bed.	☐	☐	______	______
7. Put on gloves.	☐	☐	______	______
8. Place bed protector under buttocks.	☐	☐	______	______
9. Put bedpan on foot of bed.	☐	☐	______	______
10. Help resident into the Sims position.	☐	☐	______	______
11. Tell resident to retain enema as long as possible.	☐	☐	______	______
12. Open a prepackaged enema.	☐	☐	______	______
13. Lift resident's upper buttock and expose anus.	☐	☐	______	______
14. Tell resident when you are going to insert prelubricated tip into anus. (Have resident take deep breaths and try to relax.)	☐	☐	______	______

Procedure	Pass	Redo	Date Competency Met	Instructor Initials
15. Squeeze container until all solution has entered rectum.	☐	☐	______	______
16. Remove container; place in original package to be disposed of according to facility policy.	☐	☐	______	______
17. Remove gloves.	☐	☐	______	______
18. Instruct resident to remain on side and hold solution as long as possible.	☐	☐	______	______
19. Put on gloves.	☐	☐	______	______
20. Position resident on bedpan or assist to bathroom. Instruct resident not to flush toilet.	☐	☐	______	______
21. If resident is using a bedpan, raise head of bed, if permitted.	☐	☐	______	______
22. Place toilet tissue and call bell within easy reach.	☐	☐	______	______
23. If resident is in bathroom, stay nearby.	☐	☐	______	______
24. Remove bedpan or assist resident to return to bed.	☐	☐	______	______
25. Observe contents of toilet or bedpan for:				
a. Color, consistency, unusual materials, odor	☐	☐	______	______
b. Amount of return	☐	☐	______	______
26. Cover bedpan and dispose of contents.	☐	☐	______	______
27. Remove gloves and dispose of them according to facility policy.	☐	☐	______	______
28. Replace top sheet and remove bath blanket and plastic bed protector.	☐	☐	______	______
29. Give resident soap, water, and towel for hands and face.	☐	☐	______	______
30. Wash hands.	☐	☐	______	______
31. Chart the following:				
a. Type of enema given	☐	☐	______	______
b. Consistency and amount of bowel movement	☐	☐	______	______
c. How the procedure was tolerated	☐	☐	______	______

Check-off Sheet:

15-55 Tap Water, Soap Suds, Saline Enemas

Name ______________________________ **Date** ______________

Directions: Practice this procedure, following each step. When you are ready to have your performance evaluated, give this sheet to your instructor. Review the detailed procedure in your textbook.

Procedure	**Pass**	**Redo**	**Date Competency Met**	**Instructor Initials**
Student must use Standard Precautions.	☐	☐	______	______
1. Wash hands.	☐	☐	______	______
2. Assemble equipment:				
a. Disposable gloves	☐	☐	______	______
b. Disposable enema equipment	☐	☐	______	______
(1) Plastic container	☐	☐	______	______
(2) Tubing	☐	☐	______	______
(3) Clamp	☐	☐	______	______
(4) Lubricant	☐	☐	______	______
c. Enema solution as instructed by the head nurse. For example,				
(1) Tap water, 700–1,000cc (105°F)	☐	☐	______	______
(2) Soap suds, 700–1,000cc (105°F), one package enema soap	☐	☐	______	______
(3) Saline, 700–1,000cc (105°F), 2 teaspoons salt	☐	☐	______	______
d. Bedpan and cover	☐	☐	______	______
e. Urinal, if necessary	☐	☐	______	______
f. Toilet tissue	☐	☐	______	______
g. Waterproof disposable bed protector	☐	☐	______	______
h. Paper towel	☐	☐	______	______
i. Bath blanket	☐	☐	______	______
3. Identify resident.	☐	☐	______	______
4. Ask visitors to leave the room.	☐	☐	______	______
5. Tell resident what you are going to do.	☐	☐	______	______

Procedure	Pass	Redo	Date Competency Met	Instructor Initials
6. Attach tubing to irrigation container. Adjust clamp to a position where you can easily open and close it.	☐	☐	_______	_______
7. Fill container with warm water (105°F):				
a. For soap suds enema, add one package enema soap.	☐	☐	_______	_______
b. For saline enema, add 2 teaspoons of salt.	☐	☐	_______	_______
c. For tap water enema, do not add anything.	☐	☐	_______	_______
8. Provide privacy by pulling privacy curtain.	☐	☐	_______	_______
9. Cover resident with a bath blanket. Remove upper sheet by fan-folding to foot of bed.	☐	☐	_______	_______
10. Put on gloves.	☐	☐	_______	_______
11. Put waterproof protector under resident's buttocks.	☐	☐	_______	_______
12. Put bedpan on foot of bed.	☐	☐	_______	_______
13. Place resident in the Sims position.	☐	☐	_______	_______
14. Open clamp on enema tubing and let small amount of solution run into bedpan. (This eliminates air in tubing and warms tube.)	☐	☐	_______	_______
15. Put a small amount of lubricating jelly on tissue. Lubricate enema tip. Check to be certain that the opening is not plugged.	☐	☐	_______	_______
16. Expose buttocks by folding back bath blanket.	☐	☐	_______	_______
17. Lift the upper buttock to expose anus.	☐	☐	_______	_______
18. Tell resident when you are going to insert lubricated tip into anus.	☐	☐	_______	_______
19. Hold rectal tube about 5 inches from tip and insert slowly into rectum.	☐	☐	_______	_______
20. Tell resident to breathe deeply through mouth and to try to relax.	☐	☐	_______	_______
21. Raise container 12 to 18 inches above resident's hip.	☐	☐	_______	_______
22. Open clamp and let solution run in slowly. If resident complains of cramps, clamp tubing for a minute and lower container slightly.	☐	☐	_______	_______

Procedure	Pass	Redo	Date Competency Met	Instructor Initials
23. When most of solution has flowed into rectum, close clamp. Gently withdraw rectal tube. Wrap tubing with paper towel and place into enema container.	☐	☐	______	______
24. Ask resident to hold solution as long as possible.	☐	☐	______	______
25. Help resident onto bedpan and raise head of bed, if permitted.	☐	☐	______	______
26. If resident can go to bathroom, assist resident to bathroom and stay nearby.	☐	☐	______	______
27. Place call light within reach and check resident every few minutes.	☐	☐	______	______
28. Dispose of enema equipment while you are waiting for resident to expel enema. *Follow hospital policy.*	☐	☐	______	______
29. Remove bedpan or assist resident back to bed.	☐	☐	______	______
30. Observe contents for:				
a. Color, consistency, unusual materials, odor	☐	☐	______	______
b. Note amount of return (i.e., large or small)	☐	☐	______	______
31. Cover bedpan and remove bed protector.	☐	☐	______	______
32. Remove gloves and dispose of them according to facility policy. Wash hands.	☐	☐	______	______
33. Replace top sheet and remove bath blanket.	☐	☐	______	______
34. Give resident soap, water, and a towel to wash hands.	☐	☐	______	______
35. Secure call light within resident's reach.	☐	☐	______	______
36. Chart the following:				
a. Date and time	☐	☐	______	______
b. Type of enema given	☐	☐	______	______
c. Results (amount, color, consistency) of bowel movement	☐	☐	______	______
d. How the procedure was tolerated	☐	☐	______	______

Check-off Sheet:

15-56 Harris Flush

Name ______________________________ **Date** ____________

Directions: Practice this procedure, following each step. When you are ready to have your performance evaluated, give this sheet to your instructor. Review the detailed procedure in your textbook.

Procedure	Pass	Redo	Date Competency Met	Instructor Initials
Student must use Standard Precautions.	☐	☐	______	______
1. Wash hands.	☐	☐	______	______
2. Assemble equipment:				
a. Disposable gloves	☐	☐	______	______
b. Disposable enema equipment	☐	☐	______	______
(1) Plastic container	☐	☐	______	______
(2) Tubing	☐	☐	______	______
(3) Clamp	☐	☐	______	______
c. Lubricant	☐	☐	______	______
d. 500 mL of tap water (105°F)	☐	☐	______	______
e. Toilet tissue	☐	☐	______	______
f. Waterproof disposable bed protector	☐	☐	______	______
g. Bath blanket	☐	☐	______	______
3. Identify resident.	☐	☐	______	______
4. Ask visitors to leave the room.	☐	☐	______	______
5. Tell resident what you are going to do.	☐	☐	______	______
6. Attach tubing to irrigation container. Adjust clamp to a position where you can easily open and close it. Close clamp.	☐	☐	______	______
7. Fill container with warm water (105°F).	☐	☐	______	______
8. Provide privacy by pulling privacy curtain.	☐	☐	______	______
9. Cover resident with a bath blanket. Remove upper sheet by fan-folding to foot of bed. *Be careful not to expose resident.*	☐	☐	______	______
10. Put on gloves.	☐	☐	______	______

Procedure	Pass	Redo	Date Competency Met	Instructor Initials
11. Put waterproof protector under resident's buttocks.	☐	☐	_______	_______
12. Place resident in the Sims position.	☐	☐	_______	_______
13. Place bedpan on foot of bed.	☐	☐	_______	_______
14. Open clamp on enema tubing, and let a small amount of solution run into bedpan. (This eliminates air in tubing and warms tube.) Close clamp.	☐	☐	_______	_______
15. Put a small amount of lubricating jelly on tissue. Lubricate enema tubing tip. Check to make certain that opening is not plugged.	☐	☐	_______	_______
16. Expose buttocks by folding back bath blanket.	☐	☐	_______	_______
17. Lift upper buttock to expose anus.	☐	☐	_______	_______
18. Tell resident when you are going to insert lubricated tip into anus.	☐	☐	_______	_______
19. Hold rectal tube about 5 inches from tip and insert slowly into rectum.	☐	☐	_______	_______
20. Tell resident to breathe deeply through mouth and to try to relax.	☐	☐	_______	_______
21. Raise container 12 to 18 inches above resident's hip.	☐	☐	_______	_______
22. Open clamp and let 200 mL of solution run in slowly.	☐	☐	_______	_______
23. Lower irrigating container about 12 inches below level of bed; allow fluid to flow out of rectum into container.	☐	☐	_______	_______
24. Continue process until gas is expelled. When all fluid has returned, clamp tube, and gently withdraw rectal tube.	☐	☐	_______	_______
25. Position resident for comfort.	☐	☐	_______	_______
26. Dispose of equipment according to facility policy.	☐	☐	_______	_______
27. Remove gloves and dispose of them according to facility policy.	☐	☐	_______	_______
28. Replace top sheet and remove bath blanket and plastic protector. Straighten bed and make resident comfortable.	☐	☐	_______	_______

Procedure	Pass	Redo	Date Competency Met	Instructor Initials
29. Put up side rails, if required.	☐	☐	______	______
30. Secure call bell within resident's reach.	☐	☐	______	______
31. Wash hands.	☐	☐	______	______
32. Chart the following:				
a. Date and time	☐	☐	______	______
b. Type of procedure (Harris flush)	☐	☐	______	______
c. Amount of flatus expelled	☐	☐	______	______
d. How the procedure was tolerated	☐	☐	______	______

Check-off Sheet:

15-57 Inserting a Rectal Suppository

Name ______________________________ **Date** ______________

Directions: Practice this procedure, following each step. When you are ready to have your performance evaluated, give this sheet to your instructor. Review the detailed procedure in your textbook.

Procedure	Pass	Redo	Date Competency Met	Instructor Initials
Student must use Standard Precautions.	☐	☐	______	______
1. Wash hands.	☐	☐	______	______
2. Assemble equipment:				
a. Ordered suppository	☐	☐	______	______
b. Lubricant	☐	☐	______	______
c. Disposable gloves (three pair)	☐	☐	______	______
d. Toilet tissue	☐	☐	______	______
e. Bedpan with cover	☐	☐	______	______
3. Identify resident.	☐	☐	______	______
4. Ask visitors to leave the room.	☐	☐	______	______
5. Explain what you are going to do.	☐	☐	______	______
6. Provide privacy by pulling privacy curtain.	☐	☐	______	______
7. Raise bed to comfortable working position.	☐	☐	______	______
8. Position resident on left side with one knee bent toward chest (left Sims position).	☐	☐	______	______
9. Put on gloves.	☐	☐	______	______
10. Lift sheet and expose buttocks.	☐	☐	______	______
11. Apply lubricant to gloved finger.	☐	☐	______	______
12. Apply lubricant around anus.	☐	☐	______	______
13. Hold suppository between thumb and index finger. Insert as far as lubricated index finger will reach.	☐	☐	______	______
14. Remove finger and hold toilet tissue against anus for short time.	☐	☐	______	______

Procedure	Pass	Redo	Date Competency Met	Instructor Initials
15. Remove gloves by turning inside out, and discard in hazardous waste bin.	☐	☐	______	______
16. Reposition resident and ask him or her to hold suppository as long as possible.	☐	☐	______	______
17. When resident signals for assistance, lower bed and assist to bathroom, if ambulatory. Ask resident not to flush.	☐	☐	______	______
18. Put on gloves.	☐	☐	______	______
19. Provide privacy and assist resident onto bedpan.	☐	☐	______	______
20. Raise head of bed if permitted to a comfortable position.	☐	☐	______	______
21. Provide toilet paper and place call bell within resident's reach.	☐	☐	______	______
22. Remove gloves and discard according to facility policy.	☐	☐	______	______
23. Wash hands.	☐	☐	______	______
24. Return every few minutes until resident has expelled suppository or had a bowel movement.	☐	☐	______	______
25. Put gloves on to help resident clean self.	☐	☐	______	______
26. Dispose of waste.	☐	☐	______	______
27. Clean bedpan cover, and place in storage area.	☐	☐	______	______
28. Remove gloves and discard them; wash hands.	☐	☐	______	______
29. Reposition bed to lowest position (if bed resident).	☐	☐	______	______
30. Put side rail up, if required.	☐	☐	______	______
31. Secure call bell within resident's reach.	☐	☐	______	______
32. Wash hands.	☐	☐	______	______
33. Record time suppository was given and results.	☐	☐	______	______

Check-off Sheet:

15-58 Changing an Ostomy Bag

Name ________________________________ **Date** ______________

Directions: Practice this procedure, following each step. When you are ready to have your performance evaluated, give this sheet to your instructor. Review the detailed procedure in your textbook.

Procedure	Pass	Redo	Date Competency Met	Instructor Initials
Student must use Standard Precautions.	☐	☐	______	______
1. Wash hands.	☐	☐	______	______
2. Assemble equipment:				
a. Bedpan	☐	☐	______	______
b. Waterproof bed protector	☐	☐	______	______
c. Disposable gloves (two pair)	☐	☐	______	______
d. Basin of water and soap	☐	☐	______	______
e. Washcloth	☐	☐	______	______
f. Towel	☐	☐	______	______
g. Skin protector (ordered by doctor)	☐	☐	______	______
h. Biohazard waste bag	☐	☐	______	______
3. Identify resident.	☐	☐	______	______
4. Ask visitors to leave the room. Pull privacy curtains.	☐	☐	______	______
5. Explain what you are going to do.	☐	☐	______	______
6. Raise bed to comfortable working height.	☐	☐	______	______
7. Position resident on back with head elevated, if allowed.	☐	☐	______	______
8. Put waterproof protector on bed next to stoma (opening to ostomy).	☐	☐	______	______
9. Fill basin with water (105°F)	☐	☐	______	______
10. Put on gloves.	☐	☐	______	______
11. Place bedpan where you can reach it easily.	☐	☐	______	______
12. Expose abdomen; keep genital area covered.	☐	☐	______	______

Procedure	Pass	Redo	Date Competency Met	Instructor Initials
13. Carefully open ostomy belt.	☐	☐	______	______
14. Remove soiled or full ostomy bag by gently peeling away from skin. (Use toilet tissue to protect skin from feces.)	☐	☐	______	______
15. Put soiled ostomy bag in bedpan.	☐	☐	______	______
16. Check contents of ostomy bag for undigested food, blood, or any change in consistency of feces.	☐	☐	______	______
17. Remove belt if soiled.	☐	☐	______	______
18. Apply lubricant, skin protector, or skin cream around stoma.	☐	☐	______	______
19. Carefully observe surrounding area for redness, tenderness, or sores.	☐	☐	______	______
20. Place a clean ostomy bag over stoma.	☐	☐	______	______
21. Remove gloves and discard them according to facility policy.	☐	☐	______	______
22. Wash hands. Position patient comfortably.	☐	☐	______	______
23. Put a clean ostomy belt around resident.	☐	☐	______	______
24. Lower bed to lowest position.	☐	☐	______	______
25. Put side rail up, if required.	☐	☐	______	______
26. Secure call bell within resident's reach.	☐	☐	______	______
27. Put gloves on.	☐	☐	______	______
28. Dispose of bag according to your facility's policy.	☐	☐	______	______
29. Wash bedpan and return to storage.	☐	☐	______	______
30. Remove gloves and dispose of them according to facility procedure.	☐	☐	______	______
31. Wash hands.	☐	☐	______	______
32. Document procedure.	☐	☐	______	______
33. Report any unusual observations.	☐	☐	______	______

Check-off Sheet:

15-59 Disconnecting an Indwelling Catheter

Name ______________________________ **Date** ______________

Directions: Practice this procedure, following each step. When you are ready to have your performance evaluated, give this sheet to your instructor. Review the detailed procedure in your textbook.

Procedure	**Pass**	**Redo**	**Date Competency Met**	**Instructor Initials**
Student must use Standard Precautions.	☐	☐	______	______
1. Wash hands.	☐	☐	______	______
2. Assemble equipment:				
a. Disinfectant	☐	☐	______	______
b. Sterile gauze sponges	☐	☐	______	______
c. Sterile cap or plug	☐	☐	______	______
d. Disposable gloves	☐	☐	______	______
3. Identify resident.	☐	☐	______	______
4. Explain what you are going to do.	☐	☐	______	______
5. Put on gloves.	☐	☐	______	______
6. Disinfect connection between catheter and drainage tubing where it is to be disconnected by applying disinfectant with cotton or gauze.	☐	☐	______	______
7. Disconnect catheter and drainage tubing. *Do not allow catheter ends to touch anything!*	☐	☐	______	______
8. Insert a sterile plug in end of catheter. Place sterile cap over exposed end of drainage tube.	☐	☐	______	______
9. Carefully secure drainage tube to bed.	☐	☐	______	______
10. Remove gloves and discard them according to facility policy.	☐	☐	______	______
11. Wash hands.	☐	☐	______	______
12. Record procedure. *Reverse procedure to reconnect.*	☐	☐	______	______

Check-off Sheet:

15-60 Giving Indwelling Catheter Care

Name ______________________________ **Date** ______________

Directions: Practice this procedure, following each step. When you are ready to have your performance evaluated, give this sheet to your instructor. Review the detailed procedure in your textbook.

Procedure	Pass	Redo	Date Competency Met	Instructor Initials
Student must use Standard Precautions.	☐	☐	______	______
1. Wash hands.	☐	☐	______	______
2. Assemble equipment:				
a. Antiseptic solution	☐	☐	______	______
b. Waterproof bed protector	☐	☐	______	______
c. Disposable nonsterile gloves	☐	☐	______	______
3. Identify resident.	☐	☐	______	______
4. Explain what you are going to do.	☐	☐	______	______
5. Provide privacy by pulling the privacy curtains.	☐	☐	______	______
6. Put on gloves.	☐	☐	______	______
7. Put waterproof protector on bed.	☐	☐	______	______
8. Carefully clean perineum.	☐	☐	______	______
9. Observe around catheter for sores, leakages, bleeding, or crusting. Report any unusual observation to nurse.	☐	☐	______	______
10. For *female*, separate labia with forefinger and thumb. Apply antiseptic solution around area where catheter enters the urethra.	☐	☐	______	______
11. For *male*, pull back foreskin on uncircumcised resident and apply antiseptic ointment (if allowed in your facility).	☐	☐	______	______
12. Position resident so catheter does not have kinks and is not pulling. *Be sure the tubing is free of kinks and is draining.*	☐	☐	______	______
13. Remove waterproof protector.	☐	☐	______	______
14. Cover resident.	☐	☐	______	______

Procedure	Pass	Redo	Date Competency Met	Instructor Initials
15. Dispose of supplies according to facility policy.	☐	☐	______	______
16. Remove gloves.	☐	☐	______	______
17. Position resident comfortably.	☐	☐	______	______
18. Secure call light within resident's reach.	☐	☐	______	______
19. Wash hands.	☐	☐	______	______
20. Record procedure.	☐	☐	______	______

Check-off Sheet:

15-61 External Urinary Catheter

Name ______________________________ **Date** ______________

Directions: Practice this procedure, following each step. When you are ready to have your performance evaluated, give this sheet to your instructor. Review the detailed procedure in your textbook.

Procedure	Pass	Redo	Date Competency Met	Instructor Initials
Student must use Standard Precautions.	☐	☐	______	______
1. Wash hands.	☐	☐	______	______
2. Assemble equipment:				
a. Basin of warm water	☐	☐	______	______
b. Washcloth	☐	☐	______	______
c. Towel	☐	☐	______	______
d. Waterproof bed protector	☐	☐	______	______
e. Gloves	☐	☐	______	______
f. Plastic bag	☐	☐	______	______
g. Tincture of benzoin	☐	☐	______	______
h. Condom with drainage tip	☐	☐	______	______
i. Paper towels	☐	☐	______	______
3. Identify resident.	☐	☐	______	______
4. Explain what you are going to do.	☐	☐	______	______
5. Provide privacy by pulling privacy curtain.	☐	☐	______	______
6. Raise bed to comfortable working height.	☐	☐	______	______
7. Cover resident with bath blanket. Have resident hold top of blanket, and fold cover to bottom of bed.	☐	☐	______	______
8. Put on gloves.	☐	☐	______	______
9. Place waterproof protector under resident's buttocks.	☐	☐	______	______
10. Pull up bath blanket to expose genitals only.	☐	☐	______	______
11. Remove condom by rolling gently toward tip of penis.	☐	☐	______	______

Procedure	Pass	Redo	Date Competency Met	Instructor Initials
12. Wash and dry penis.	☐	☐	_______	_______
13. Observe for irritation, open areas, or bleeding.	☐	☐	_______	_______
14. Report any unusual observations.	☐	☐	_______	_______
15. Check condom for "ready stick" surface. If there is none, apply a thin spray of tincture of benzoin. *Do not spray on head of penis.*	☐	☐	_______	_______
16. Apply new condom and drainage tip to penis by rolling toward base of penis.	☐	☐	_______	_______
17. Reconnect drainage system.	☐	☐	_______	_______
18. Remove and dispose of gloves.	☐	☐	_______	_______
19. Pull up top bedding and remove bath blanket.	☐	☐	_______	_______
20. Replace equipment.	☐	☐	_______	_______
21. Lower bed to lowest position.	☐	☐	_______	_______
22. Put side rail up, if required.	☐	☐	_______	_______
23. Secure call light within resident's reach.	☐	☐	_______	_______
24. Tidy unit.	☐	☐	_______	_______
25. Wash hands.	☐	☐	_______	_______
26. Record procedure.	☐	☐	_______	_______

Check-off Sheet:

15-62 Emptying the Urinary Drainage Bag

Name ______________________________ **Date** ______________

Directions: Practice this procedure, following each step. When you are ready to have your performance evaluated, give this sheet to your instructor. Review the detailed procedure in your textbook.

Procedure	Pass	Redo	Date Competency Met	Instructor Initials
Student must use Standard Precautions.	☐	☐	______	______
1. Wash hands.	☐	☐	______	______
2. Assemble equipment:				
a. Graduate or measuring cup	☐	☐	______	______
b. Gloves	☐	☐	______	______
3. Put on disposable gloves.	☐	☐	______	______
4. Carefully open drain outlet on urinary bag. *Do not allow container outlet to touch floor!* This will introduce microorganisms into bag and can cause infection.	☐	☐	______	______
5. Drain bag into graduate, and reattach drainage outlet securely.	☐	☐	______	______
6. Observe urine for:				
a. Dark color	☐	☐	______	______
b. Blood	☐	☐	______	______
c. Unusual odor	☐	☐	______	______
d. Large amount of mucus	☐	☐	______	______
e. Sediment	☐	☐	______	______
7. Report any unusual observations to nurse immediately (do not discard urine).	☐	☐	______	______
8. Hold graduate at eye level and read amount of urine on measuring scale.	☐	☐	______	______
9. Discard urine if normal.	☐	☐	______	______
10. Rinse graduate and put away.	☐	☐	______	______
11. Remove gloves and discard in hazardous waste bin.	☐	☐	______	______
12. Wash hands.	☐	☐	______	______
13. Record amount of urine in cc on the I & O record.	☐	☐	______	______

Check-off Sheet:

15-63 Routine Urine Specimen

Name ______________________________ **Date** ____________

Directions: Practice this procedure, following each step. When you are ready to have your performance evaluated, give this sheet to your instructor. Review the detailed procedure in your textbook.

Procedure	Pass	Redo	Date Competency Met	Instructor Initials
Student must use Standard Precautions.	☐	☐	______	______
1. Wash hands.	☐	☐	______	______
2. Assemble equipment:				
a. Graduate (pitcher)	☐	☐	______	______
b. Bedpan or urinal	☐	☐	______	______
c. Urine specimen container	☐	☐	______	______
d. Label	☐	☐	______	______
e. Paper bag	☐	☐	______	______
f. Disposable nonsterile gloves	☐	☐	______	______
3. Identify resident.	☐	☐	______	______
4. Explain what you are going to do.	☐	☐	______	______
5. Label specimen carefully:				
a. Resident's name	☐	☐	______	______
b. Date	☐	☐	______	______
c. Time	☐	☐	______	______
d. Room number	☐	☐	______	______
6. Provide privacy by pulling privacy curtain.	☐	☐	______	______
7. Put on gloves.	☐	☐	______	______
8. Have resident void (urinate) into clean bedpan or urinal.	☐	☐	______	______
9. Ask resident to put toilet tissue into paper bag.	☐	☐	______	______
10. Pour specimen into graduate.	☐	☐	______	______
11. Pour from graduate into specimen container until about three-quarters full.	☐	☐	______	______
12. Place lid on container.	☐	☐	______	______

Procedure	Pass	Redo	Date Competency Met	Instructor Initials
13. Discard leftover urine.	☐	☐	______	______
14. Clean and rinse graduate, bedpan, or urinal, and put away.	☐	☐	______	______
15. Remove gloves.	☐	☐	______	______
16. Position resident comfortably.	☐	☐	______	______
17. Assist resident to wash hands.	☐	☐	______	______
18. Wash hands.	☐	☐	______	______
19. Store specimen according to directions for lab pickup.	☐	☐	______	______
20. Report and record procedure and observation of specimen.	☐	☐	______	______

Check-off Sheet:

15-64 Midstream Clean-Catch Urine, Female

Name ______________________________ **Date** ______________

Directions: Practice this procedure, following each step. When you are ready to have your performance evaluated, give this sheet to your instructor. Review the detailed procedure in your textbook.

Procedure	Pass	Redo	Date Competency Met	Instructor Initials
Student must use Standard Precautions.	☐	☐	______	______
1. Wash hands.	☐	☐	______	______
2. Assemble equipment:				
a. Antiseptic solution or soap and water or towelettes	☐	☐	______	______
b. Sterile specimen container	☐	☐	______	______
c. Tissues	☐	☐	______	______
d. Nonsterile gloves	☐	☐	______	______
3. Identify resident.	☐	☐	______	______
4. Explain what you are going to do.	☐	☐	______	______
5. Label specimen:				
a. Resident's name	☐	☐	______	______
b. Date	☐	☐	______	______
c. Time obtained	☐	☐	______	______
6. If resident is on bedrest:				
a. Put on gloves.	☐	☐	______	______
b. Lower side rail.	☐	☐	______	______
c. Position bedpan under resident.	☐	☐	______	______
7. Have resident carefully clean perineal area if able; if not, you will be responsible for cleaning perineum:				
a. Wipe with towelette or gauze with antiseptic solution from front to back.	☐	☐	______	______
b. Wipe one side and throw away wipe.	☐	☐	______	______
c. Use a clean wipe for other side.	☐	☐	______	______
d. Use another wipe down center.	☐	☐	______	______
e. Then proceed with collecting midstream urine.	☐	☐	______	______

Procedure	Pass	Redo	Date Competency Met	Instructor Initials
8. Explain procedure if resident is able to obtain own specimen.				
a. Have resident start to urinate into bedpan or toilet.	☐	☐	______	______
b. Allow stream to begin.	☐	☐	______	______
c. Stop stream, and place specimen container to collect midstream.	☐	☐	______	______
d. Remove container before bladder is empty.	☐	☐	______	______
9. Wipe perineum if on bedpan.	☐	☐	______	______
10. Remove bedpan.	☐	☐	______	______
11. Rinse bedpan and put away.	☐	☐	______	______
12. Remove gloves and discard according to facility policy and procedure.	☐	☐	______	______
13. Raise side rail.	☐	☐	______	______
14. Secure call light within resident's reach.	☐	☐	______	______
15. Dispose of equipment. Never handle contaminated equipment without gloves.	☐	☐	______	______
16. Wash hands.	☐	☐	______	______
17. Record specimen collection.	☐	☐	______	______
18. Report any unusual:				
a. Color	☐	☐	______	______
b. Odor	☐	☐	______	______
c. Consistency	☐	☐	______	______

Check-off Sheet:

15-65 Midstream Clean-Catch Urine, Male

Name ______________________________ Date ______________

Directions: Practice this procedure, following each step. When you are ready to have your performance evaluated, give this sheet to your instructor. Review the detailed procedure in your textbook.

Procedure	Pass	Redo	Date Competency Met	Instructor Initials
Student must use Standard Precautions.	☐	☐	______	______
1. Wash hands.	☐	☐	______	______
2. Assemble equipment:				
a. Antiseptic solution or soap and water or towelettes	☐	☐	______	______
b. Sterile specimen container	☐	☐	______	______
c. Tissues	☐	☐	______	______
d. Nonsterile gloves	☐	☐	______	______
3. Identify resident.	☐	☐	______	______
4. Label specimen:				
a. Resident's name	☐	☐	______	______
b. Date	☐	☐	______	______
c. Time obtained	☐	☐	______	______
5. Explain procedure (if possible allow resident to obtain his own specimen).				
a. Put on gloves.	☐	☐	______	______
b. Cleanse head of penis in a circular motion with towelette or gauze and antiseptic. (If resident is uncircumcised, have him pull back foreskin before cleaning.)	☐	☐	______	______
c. Have resident start to urinate into bedpan, urinal, or toilet. (If uncircumcised, have resident pull back foreskin before urinating.)	☐	☐	______	______
d. Allow stream to begin.	☐	☐	______	______
e. Stop stream, and place specimen container to collect midstream.	☐	☐	______	______
f. Remove container before bladder is empty.	☐	☐	______	______

Procedure	Pass	Redo	Date Competency Met	Instructor Initials
6. Dispose of equipment according to facility policy.	☐	☐	______	______
7. Remove and discard gloves according to facility policy and procedure.	☐	☐	______	______
8. Wash hands.	☐	☐	______	______
9. Record specimen collection.	☐	☐	______	______

Check-off Sheet:

15-66 HemaCombstix

Name ______________________________ **Date** ______________

Directions: Practice this procedure, following each step. When you are ready to have your performance evaluated, give this sheet to your instructor. Review the detailed procedure in your textbook.

Procedure	Pass	Redo	Date Competency Met	Instructor Initials
Student must use Standard Precautions.	☐	☐	______	______
1. Wash hands.	☐	☐	______	______
2. Assemble equipment:				
a. Bottle of HemaCombstix	☐	☐	______	______
b. Nonsterile gloves	☐	☐	______	______
3. Identify resident.	☐	☐	______	______
4. Explain what you are going to do.	☐	☐	______	______
5. Put gloves on.	☐	☐	______	______
6. Secure fresh urine sample from resident.	☐	☐	______	______
7. Take urine and reagent to bathroom.	☐	☐	______	______
8. Remove cap and place on flat surface. Be sure top side of cap is down.	☐	☐	______	______
9. Remove strip from bottle by shaking bottle gently. *Do not touch areas of strip with fingers.*	☐	☐	______	______
10. Dip reagent stick in urine. Remove immediately.	☐	☐	______	______
11. Tap edge of strip on container to remove excess urine.	☐	☐	______	______
12. Compare reagent side of test areas with color chart on bottle. Use time intervals that are given on bottle. *Note: Do not touch reagent strip to bottle.*	☐	☐	______	______
13. Remove gloves and discard according to facility policy and procedure.	☐	☐	______	______
14. Replace equipment.	☐	☐	______	______
15. Wash hands.	☐	☐	______	______

Procedure	Pass	Redo	Date Competency Met	Instructor Initials
16. Record results:				
a. Date and time	☐	☐	______	______
b. Name of procedure used	☐	☐	______	______
c. Results	☐	☐	______	______

Check-off Sheet:

15-67 Straining the Urine

Name ______________________________ **Date** ______________

Directions: Practice this procedure, following each step. When you are ready to have your performance evaluated, give this sheet to your instructor. Review the detailed procedure in your textbook.

Procedure	Pass	Redo	Date Competency Met	Instructor Initials
Student must use Standard Precautions.	☐	☐	______	______
1. Wash hands.	☐	☐	______	______
2. Assemble equipment:				
a. Paper strainers or gauze	☐	☐	______	______
b. Specimen container and label	☐	☐	______	______
c. Bedpan or urinal and cover	☐	☐	______	______
d. Laboratory request for analysis of specimen	☐	☐	______	______
e. Sign for resident's room or bathroom explaining that all urine must be strained	☐	☐	______	______
f. Nonsterile gloves	☐	☐	______	______
3. Identify resident.	☐	☐	______	______
4. Tell the resident to urinate into a urinal or bedpan and that the nurse assistant must be called to filter each specimen. Tell resident not to put paper in specimen.	☐	☐	______	______
5. Put on gloves.	☐	☐	______	______
6. Pour voided specimen through a paper strainer or gauze into a measuring container.	☐	☐	______	______
7. Place paper or gauze strainer into a dry specimen container if stones or particles are present after pouring urine through. *Note: Do not attempt to remove the particles from strainer.*	☐	☐	______	______
8. Measure the amount voided and record on the intake and output record.	☐	☐	______	______
9. Discard urine and container according to facility policy and procedure.	☐	☐	______	______
10. Clean urinal or bedpan and put away.	☐	☐	______	______

Procedure	Pass	Redo	Date Competency Met	Instructor Initials
11. Remove gloves and discard according to facility policy and procedure.	☐	☐	_______	_______
12. Wash hands.	☐	☐	_______	_______
13. Label specimen:				
a. Resident's name	☐	☐	_______	_______
b. Date	☐	☐	_______	_______
c. Room number	☐	☐	_______	_______
d. Time	☐	☐	_______	_______
14. Return resident to comfortable position.	☐	☐	_______	_______
15. Place call button within reach of resident.	☐	☐	_______	_______
16. Provide for resident safety by raising side rails when indicated or using postural supports as ordered.	☐	☐	_______	_______
17. Wash hands.	☐	☐	_______	_______
18. Report collection of specimen to supervisor immediately.	☐	☐	_______	_______
19. Record specimen collection.	☐	☐	_______	_______

Check-off Sheet:

15-68 Stool Specimen Collection

Name ______________________________ **Date** ______________

Directions: Practice this procedure, following each step. When you are ready to have your performance evaluated, give this sheet to your instructor. Review the detailed procedure in your textbook.

Procedure	Pass	Redo	Date Competency Met	Instructor Initials
Student must use Standard Precautions.	☐	☐	______	______
1. Wash hands.	☐	☐	______	______
2. Assemble equipment:				
a. Stool specimen container	☐	☐	______	______
b. Wooden tongue depressor	☐	☐	______	______
c. Disposable gloves	☐	☐	______	______
d. Bedpan and cover	☐	☐	______	______
3. Identify resident.	☐	☐	______	______
4. Explain what you are going to do.	☐	☐	______	______
5. Be certain container is properly labeled with:				
a. Resident's name	☐	☐	______	______
b. Date	☐	☐	______	______
c. Time	☐	☐	______	______
d. Room number	☐	☐	______	______
6. Provide privacy by pulling privacy curtains.	☐	☐	______	______
7. Put on gloves.	☐	☐	______	______
8. After resident has had bowel movement, take bedpan into bathroom.	☐	☐	______	______
9. Use tongue depressor to remove about 1 to 2 tablespoons of feces from bedpan.	☐	☐	______	______
10. Place specimen in specimen container.	☐	☐	______	______
11. Cover container immediately.	☐	☐	______	______
12. Wrap tongue depressor in paper towel and discard.	☐	☐	______	______
13. Remove gloves and dispose of them according to facility procedure.	☐	☐	______	______

Procedure	Pass	Redo	Date Competency Met	Instructor Initials
14. Wash hands.	☐	☐	______	______
15. Follow instruction for storage of specimen for collection by lab.	☐	☐	______	______
16. Position resident comfortably.	☐	☐	______	______
17. Report and record procedure.	☐	☐	______	______

Check-off Sheet:

15-69 Occult Blood Hematest

Name ______________________________ **Date** ______________

Directions: Practice this procedure, following each step. When you are ready to have your performance evaluated, give this sheet to your instructor. Review the detailed procedure in your textbook.

Procedure	Pass	Redo	Date Competency Met	Instructor Initials
Student must use Standard Precautions.	☐	☐	______	______
1. Wash hands.	☐	☐	______	______
2. Assemble equipment:				
a. Hematest reagent filter paper	☐	☐	______	______
b. Hematest reagent tablet	☐	☐	______	______
c. Distilled water	☐	☐	______	______
d. Tongue blade	☐	☐	______	______
e. Disposable gloves	☐	☐	______	______
3. Identify resident.	☐	☐	______	______
4. Explain what you are going to do.	☐	☐	______	______
5. Put on gloves.	☐	☐	______	______
6. Secure stool specimen from resident.	☐	☐	______	______
7. Place filter paper on glass or porcelain plate.	☐	☐	______	______
8. Use tongue blade to smear a thin streak of fecal material on filter paper.	☐	☐	______	______
9. Place Hematest reagent tablet on smear.	☐	☐	______	______
10. Place one drop of distilled water on tablet.	☐	☐	______	______
11. Allow 5 to 10 seconds for water to penetrate tablet.	☐	☐	______	______
12. Add second drop, allowing water to run down side of tablet onto filter paper and specimen.	☐	☐	______	______
13. Gently tap side of plate to knock water droplets from top of tablet.	☐	☐	______	______
14. Observe filter paper for color change (two minutes). Positive is indicated by blue halo on paper.	☐	☐	______	______

Procedure	Pass	Redo	Date Competency Met	Instructor Initials
15. Dispose of specimen and equipment according to your facility's policy.	☐	☐	______	______
16. Remove gloves and dispose of them according to your facility's policy.	☐	☐	______	______
17. Wash hands.	☐	☐	______	______
18. Report and record results (e.g., date, time, procedure, and results).	☐	☐	______	______

Check-off Sheet:

15-70 Sputum Specimen Collection

Name ______________________________ **Date** ______________

Directions: Practice this procedure, following each step. When you are ready to have your performance evaluated, give this sheet to your instructor. Review the detailed procedure in your textbook.

Procedure	Pass	Redo	Date Competency Met	Instructor Initials
Student must use Standard Precautions.	☐	☐	______	______
1. Wash hands.	☐	☐	______	______
2. Assemble equipment:				
a. Sputum container	☐	☐	______	______
b. Disposable nonsterile gloves	☐	☐	______	______
3. Identify resident.	☐	☐	______	______
4. Explain what you are going to do.	☐	☐	______	______
5. Label container:				
a. Resident's name	☐	☐	______	______
b. Date	☐	☐	______	______
c. Time taken	☐	☐	______	______
d. Room number	☐	☐	______	______
6. Put on gloves.	☐	☐	______	______
7. Help resident rinse mouth if he or she has just eaten.	☐	☐	______	______
8. Ask resident to take three deep breaths. On the third breath, tell resident to cough deep from lungs and try to bring up thick sputum. (Saliva is not adequate for this test.)	☐	☐	______	______
9. Have resident try several times until you get a good specimen. (You need 1 to 2 tablespoons.)	☐	☐	______	______
10. Cover container immediately.	☐	☐	______	______
11. Remove gloves and discard according to facility procedure.	☐	☐	______	______
12. Wash hands.	☐	☐	______	______
13. Report to nurse that specimen has been collected. (It needs to go to lab immediately.)	☐	☐	______	______
14. Record that specimen has been taken and record color, amount, odor, and consistency.	☐	☐	______	______

Check-off Sheet:

15-71 Seizure Precautions

Name ______________________ **Date** ____________

Directions: Practice this procedure, following each step. When you are ready to have your performance evaluated, give this sheet to your instructor. Review the detailed procedure in your textbook.

Procedure	Pass	Redo	Date Competency Met	Instructor Initials
Student must use Standard Precautions.	☐	☐	______	______
If you are with a resident who has a seizure:				
1. Use call signal or shout to get help. *Do not leave resident.*	☐	☐	______	______
2. Assist resident to lie down or prevent falling.	☐	☐	______	______
3. Protect head with pillow or soft cushion.	☐	☐	______	______
4. Move furniture to prevent limbs from bumping into it.	☐	☐	______	______
5. Turn resident on side to allow secretions to drain from mouth.	☐	☐	______	______
6. Observe seizure for:				
a. Length of time of seizure	☐	☐	______	______
b. Part of body where seizure began	☐	☐	______	______
c. Incontinence	☐	☐	______	______
d. Injury (where and severity)	☐	☐	______	______
e. Severity of convulsions	☐	☐	______	______
7. Help resident to bed when seizure is over.	☐	☐	______	______
8. Make resident comfortable.	☐	☐	______	______
9. Put side rails up.	☐	☐	______	______
10. Wrap side rails with blanket, sheet, or soft material to pad them.	☐	☐	______	______
11. Wash hands.	☐	☐	______	______
12. Chart seizure and observations.	☐	☐	______	______
13. Report seizure to charge nurse.	☐	☐	______	______

Check-off Sheet:

15-72 Elastic Hose (Antiembolism Hose)

Name ______________________________ **Date** ______________

Directions: Practice this procedure, following each step. When you are ready to have your performance evaluated, give this sheet to your instructor. Review the detailed procedure in your textbook.

Procedure	Pass	Redo	Date Competency Met	Instructor Initials
Student must use Standard Precautions.	☐	☐	______	______
1. Wash hands.	☐	☐	______	______
2. Select elastic hose. Check to be sure that they are the correct size and length.	☐	☐	______	______
3. Identify resident.	☐	☐	______	______
4. Have resident lie down; expose one leg at a time.	☐	☐	______	______
5. Hold the hose with both hands at top and roll toward toe end.	☐	☐	______	______
6. Place over toes, positioning opening at base of toes unless toes are to be covered. The raised seams should be on the outside.	☐	☐	______	______
7. Check to be sure that stocking is applied evenly and smoothly. There must be no wrinkles.	☐	☐	______	______
8. Repeat on opposite leg.	☐	☐	______	______
9. Record the following in the medical record:				
a. Date and time applied	☐	☐	______	______
b. Any skin changes, temperature change, or swelling	☐	☐	______	______
10. Remove and reapply at least once every eight hours, or more often if necessary.	☐	☐	______	______

Check-off Sheet:

15-73 How to Tie Postural Supports

Name ______________________________ **Date** ____________

Directions: Practice this procedure, following each step. When you are ready to have your performance evaluated, give this sheet to your instructor. Review the detailed procedure in your textbook.

Procedure	Pass	Redo	Date Competency Met	Instructor Initials
Student must use Standard Precautions.	☐	☐	______	______
1. Wash hands.	☐	☐	______	______
2. Assemble equipment: a postural support that has been ordered.	☐	☐	______	______
3. Tie a half-bow knot or quick-release knot.	☐	☐	______	______
4. Once bow is in place, grasp one loop and pull end of tie through knot.	☐	☐	______	______
5. Knot can be easily released by pulling end of loop.	☐	☐	______	______

Check-off Sheet:

15-74 Postural Supports: Limb

Name ______________________________ **Date** ______________

Directions: Practice this procedure, following each step. When you are ready to have your performance evaluated, give this sheet to your instructor. Review the detailed procedure in your textbook.

Procedure	Pass	Redo	Date Competency Met	Instructor Initials
Student must use Standard Precautions.	☐	☐	______	______
1. Wash hands.	☐	☐	______	______
2. Assemble equipment: a limb support.	☐	☐	______	______
3. Identify resident.	☐	☐	______	______
4. Explain what you are going to do.	☐	☐	______	______
5. Place soft side of limb support against skin.	☐	☐	______	______
6. Wrap around limb and put one tie through opening on other end of support.	☐	☐	______	______
7. Gently pull until it fits snugly around limb.	☐	☐	______	______
8. Buckle or tie in place so that support stays on limb.	☐	☐	______	______
9. Tie out of resident's reach (see the check-off sheet "How to Tie Postural Supports"):				
a. Tie to bed frame (*not side rails*).	☐	☐	______	______
b. Tie to wheelchair (*do not tie to stationary chair*).	☐	☐	______	______
10. Check for proper alignment and comfort of resident.	☐	☐	______	______
11. Check to be certain that knots or wrinkles are not causing pressure.	☐	☐	______	______
12. Check to be certain that support is snug but does not bind.	☐	☐	______	______
13. Place call light where it can be easily reached.	☐	☐	______	______
14. Check resident frequently and move at least every two hours.	☐	☐	______	______

Procedure	Pass	Redo	Date Competency Met	Instructor Initials
15. Chart the following:				
a. Reason for use of support	☐	☐	______	______
b. Type of support used	☐	☐	______	______
c. When it was applied	☐	☐	______	______
d. When it was released	☐	☐	______	______
e. Times of repositioning	☐	☐	______	______
f. How resident tolerated it	☐	☐	______	______

Check-off Sheet:

15-75 Postural Supports: Mitten

Name ______________________________ **Date** ______________

Directions: Practice this procedure, following each step. When you are ready to have your performance evaluated, give this sheet to your instructor. Review the detailed procedure in your textbook.

Procedure	Pass	Redo	Date Competency Met	Instructor Initials
Student must use Standard Precautions.	☐	☐	______	______
1. Wash hands.	☐	☐	______	______
2. Assemble equipment: a soft cloth.	☐	☐	______	______
3. Identify resident.	☐	☐	______	______
4. Explain what you are going to do.	☐	☐	______	______
5. Slip mitten on hand with padded side against palm and net on top of hand.	☐	☐	______	______
6. Lace mitten.	☐	☐	______	______
7. Gently pull until it fits snugly around wrist.	☐	☐	______	______
8. Tie with a double bow knot so that support stays on hand.	☐	☐	______	______
9. Check for proper alignment and comfort of resident.	☐	☐	______	______
10. Check to be certain that knots or wrinkles are not causing pressure.	☐	☐	______	______
11. Check to be certain that support is snug but does not bind.	☐	☐	______	______
12. Place call light where it can be easily reached.	☐	☐	______	______
13. Check resident frequently and move at least every two hours.	☐	☐	______	______
14. Chart the following:				
a. Reason for use of support	☐	☐	______	______
b. Type of support used	☐	☐	______	______
c. When it was applied	☐	☐	______	______
d. When it was released	☐	☐	______	______
e. Times of repositioning	☐	☐	______	______
f. How resident tolerated it	☐	☐	______	______

Check-off Sheet:

15-76 Postural Supports: Vest

Name ______________________________ **Date** ____________

Directions: Practice this procedure, following each step. When you are ready to have your performance evaluated, give this sheet to your instructor. Review the detailed procedure in your textbook.

Procedure	Pass	Redo	Date Competency Met	Instructor Initials
Student must use Standard Precautions.	☐	☐	______	______
1. Wash hands.	☐	☐	______	______
2. Assemble equipment: a vest support.	☐	☐	______	______
3. Identify resident.	☐	☐	______	______
4. Explain what you are going to do.	☐	☐	______	______
5. Put arms through armholes of vest with opening to back.	☐	☐	______	______
6. Cross back panels by bringing tie on left side over to right and right tie to left.	☐	☐	______	______
7. Carefully smooth material so that there are no wrinkles.	☐	☐	______	______
8. Tie where resident cannot reach (see the check-off sheet "How to Tie Postural Supports"):	☐	☐	______	______
a. Tie to bed frame (*not side rails*).	☐	☐	______	______
b. Tie to wheelchair (*not stationary chair*).	☐	☐	______	______
9. Check for proper alignment and comfort of resident.	☐	☐	______	______
10. Check to be certain that knots or wrinkles are not causing pressure.	☐	☐	______	______
11. Check to be certain that support is snug but does not bind.	☐	☐	______	______
12. Place call light where it can be easily reached.	☐	☐	______	______
13. Check resident frequently and move at least every two hours.	☐	☐	______	______

Procedure	Pass	Redo	Date Competency Met	Instructor Initials
14. Chart the following:				
a. Reason for use of support	☐	☐	______	______
b. Type of support used	☐	☐	______	______
c. When it was applied	☐	☐	______	______
d. When it was released	☐	☐	______	______
e. Times of repositioning	☐	☐	______	______
f. How resident tolerated it	☐	☐	______	______

Check-off Sheet:

15-77 Postmortem Care

Name ______________________ **Date** ____________

Directions: Practice this procedure, following each step. When you are ready to have your performance evaluated, give this sheet to your instructor. Review the detailed procedure in your textbook.

Procedure	Pass	Redo	Date Competency Met	Instructor Initials
Student must use Standard Precautions.	☐	☐	______	______
1. Wash hands.	☐	☐	______	______
2. Assemble equipment:				
a. Wash basin with warm water	☐	☐	______	______
b. Washcloth and towel	☐	☐	______	______
c. Shroud or postmortem set				
(1) Sheet or plastic container	☐	☐	______	______
(2) Strap to tie chin (to keep mouth closed)	☐	☐	______	______
(3) Identification tags	☐	☐	______	______
(4) Large container for personal belongings	☐	☐	______	______
(5) Plastic pad	☐	☐	______	______
d. Gurney or morgue cart	☐	☐	______	______
e. Nonsterile disposable gloves	☐	☐	______	______
3. Close privacy curtains.	☐	☐	______	______
4. Put on gloves.	☐	☐	______	______
5. Position body in good alignment in supine position.	☐	☐	______	______
6. Keep one pillow under head.	☐	☐	______	______
7. Straighten arms and legs.	☐	☐	______	______
8. Gently close each eye. Do not apply pressure to eyelids.	☐	☐	______	______
9. Put dentures in mouth or in a denture cup. If placed in a denture cup, put cup inside shroud so that mortician can find them.	☐	☐	______	______
10. Secure chin with a chin strap. Use pads under straps along side of face to prevent marking.	☐	☐	______	______

Procedure	Pass	Redo	Date Competency Met	Instructor Initials
11. Remove all soiled dressings or clothing.	☐	☐	______	______
12. Bathe body thoroughly.	☐	☐	______	______
13. Apply clean dressings where needed.	☐	☐	______	______
14. Tie wrists loosely together over abdomen. Use pads under ties to prevent marking.	☐	☐	______	______
15. Tie ankles loosely together. Use pads under ties to prevent marking.	☐	☐	______	______
16. Attach identification tags to wrists and ankles. Fill in tags with:				
a. Name	☐	☐	______	______
b. Sex	☐	☐	______	______
c. Facility ID number	☐	☐	______	______
d. Age	☐	☐	______	______
17. Place body in a shroud, sheet, or other appropriate container. Do this in the following way:				
a. Ask for assistance from a co-worker.	☐	☐	______	______
b. Logroll body to one side. Place shroud behind body, leaving enough material to support body when rolled back. Fan-fold remaining shroud next to body.	☐	☐	______	______
c. Place a plastic protection pad under buttocks.	☐	☐	______	______
d. Roll body on its back and then to the other side.	☐	☐	______	______
e. Pull fan-folded portion of shroud until flat.	☐	☐	______	______
f. Roll body on its back.	☐	☐	______	______
g. Cover entire body with shroud.	☐	☐	______	______
h. Tuck all loose edges of cover in.	☐	☐	______	______
i. Position a tie above elbows and below knees and secure around body.	☐	☐	______	______
j. Attach ID tag to tie just above elbows.	☐	☐	______	______
18. Remove gloves and discard according to facility policy and procedure.	☐	☐	______	______
19. Wash hands.	☐	☐	______	______

Procedure	Pass	Redo	Date Competency Met	Instructor Initials
20. Place all personal belongings in a large container. Label container with:				
a. Resident's name	☐	☐	______	______
b. Age	☐	☐	______	______
c. Room number	☐	☐	______	______
21. Place list of belongings in container and on resident's chart.	☐	☐	______	______
22. Follow your facility's procedure for transporting body and belongings through hallways.	☐	☐	______	______
23. Remove all linen and other supplies from room.	☐	☐	______	______
24. Wash hands.	☐	☐	______	______
25. Report procedure completed to charge nurse.	☐	☐	______	______

Chapter 16 Home Health Aide

• OBJECTIVES

When you have completed this unit, you will be able to do the following:

- Complete all objectives in Part One of this book.
- Complete all objectives in Chapter 15.
- Define vocabulary words.
- List the following:
  - Five causes of mental impairment
  - Items included when charting
  - Six rights to check when assisting a client with medication
  - Seven basic rules to follow when using household cleaners
  - Ten safety concerns specific to the client's home
  - Eight elements to remember when planning food and menus
- Explain the following:
  - Why correct charting is important
  - Proper care of a sterile and a nonsterile dressing
  - The basic guidelines to follow when storing medications
  - Why deep breathing is important for bedridden clients
  - The elements of an escape plan to use in case of fire
  - The basic guidelines for food storage
  - The definition of *sterile*
  - The home health aide's responsibilities when there are children in the home
- Develop an action plan to use when caring for:
  - Children
  - Aged
  - Dying

- Demonstrate all procedures in this chapter.
- Demonstrate all procedures in Chapter 15.
- Complete the following objectives in Chapter 20:
  - List three methods of packaging items
  - Demonstrate envelope wrap and square wrap
- Apply medical terminology when charting and discussing the client's condition.
- Demonstrate putting on a nonsterile dressing.

• DIRECTIONS

1. Complete Worksheet 1 before beginning the reading.
2. Read this chapter.
3. Complete Worksheet 2 as assigned.
4. Complete Worksheets/Activities 3 and 4 as assigned.
5. Complete Worksheets 5 and 6 as assigned.
6. Complete Worksheets/Activities 7, 8, and 9.
7. Use the skills check-off lists to practice and demonstrate all procedures in this chapter.
8. Prepare responses to each item listed in the Chapter Review—Your Link to Success at the end of this chapter.
9. When you are confident that you can meet each objective for this unit, ask your instructor for the unit evaluation.

• EVALUATION METHODS

- Worksheets/Activities
- Class participation
- Written evaluation
- Return demonstrations

• WORKSHEET 1

Write each word listed below in the space next to the statement that best defines it (10 points).

psychotherapy	heredity	geriatric
abrasive	implement	coping
autopsy	reimburse	specification
disoriented		

_______________ **a.** Medical procedure after death to determine cause of death.

_______________ **b.** To pay back for something given or spent.

_______________ **c.** Compound used to rub away or scrape away another substance.

_______________ **d.** Put into action.

_______________ **e.** Pertaining to aging people, usually over 65 years of age.

_______________ **f.** Being confused about time, place, and identity of person and objects.

_______________ **g.** Handling difficult situations.

_______________ **h.** Characteristics passed from parent to child.

_______________ **i.** Exact way something should be done.

_______________ **j.** Method of treatment using mental applications

There are 10 possible points in this worksheet.

• WORKSHEET 2

Circle the correct answer (3 points).

1. Children who are ill
  a. are interested in their care.
  b. prefer to be left alone.
  c. cannot understand about illness.

2. Mental impairments can be caused by several things. Four of these are:
  a. anger, frustration, heredity, and impaired circulation.
  b. impaired circulation, attitude, medication, and anger.
  c. high temperature, medication, impaired circulation, and heredity.

3. When the client is dying, it is best to
  a. listen to the person.
  b. keep your distance because the person is dying.
  c. pretend that everything is okay.

Respond to the following scenarios.

4. Mr. Dimas is very ill. He asks you to arrange for his priest to visit. You belong to a different religion and do not approve of his. You wonder if it is a good idea to call your minister to see him. What will you do, and why (5 points)?

____

____

____

____

5. Ms. De Mecilli has a hospital bed in her bedroom. She enjoys watching the birds at the feeder outside her window. Her grandchildren's fingerprints get all over the window, and the dirty windows really bother her. What will you do to relieve her anxiety (5 points)?

____

____

____

____

6. Mr. Vanderlong had a stroke six months ago. He is gradually recovering his speech and mobility. He is still very slow about moving from place to place. He prefers using his walker to the wheelchair. When you have a lot to do, it is easier to move him along in the wheelchair. What should you do, and why (5 points)?

____

____

____

____

7. Johnny is a four-year-old you have taken care of for about five months. He has leukemia, and it cannot be cured. You are very attached to him because he is such a loving child. Everyone around him feels very sad that he is going to die soon. What do you think you will feel when he dies, and how will you react to the situation (5 points)?

____

____

____

____

There are 23 possible points in this worksheet.

• WORKSHEET/ACTIVITY 3

Look up the policies and procedures on death and dying in the facility where you are assigned. Explain in writing why these steps are important. Be prepared to discuss the policies and procedures with other students. Are all of the facility policies and procedures the same?

There are 75 possible points in this worksheet/activity.

• WORKSHEET/ACTIVITY 4

Use the skills check-off sheets provided in your book and by your teacher. Work with a partner to practice Dressings: Clean Nonsterile, and Assisting with Medication in the Home.

There are 50 possible points in this worksheet/activity. Points for practice and demonstration are assigned according to your participation and ability to return demonstrate the procedure to your instructor.

• WORKSHEET 5

1. List nine items to include when charting (9 points).

a. ______________________________

b. ______________________________

c. ______________________________

d. ______________________________

e. ______________________________

f. ______________________________

g. ______________________________

h. ______________________________

i. ______________________________

2. Ms. Young has a wound that keeps draining. It is dressed with a sterile bandage. The bandage is soaked with drainage. What will you do, and why (2 points)?

____

____

3. You drop a sterile item on the floor. It is the last one, and you need it. Since you cannot see any dirt or germs on it, will you use it? Why (2 points)?

____

____

4. Explain the difference between moist heat and dry heat sterilization (1 point).

____

____

5. List the six rights to check when assisting a client with medication (6 points).

a. ____
b. ____
c. ____
d. ____
e. ____
f. ____

6. List the basic guidelines to follow when storing medications, and explain why each is important (8 points).

a. ____
____
b. ____
____
c. ____
____
d. ____
____

7. Deep breathing is very important for clients after surgery or when they are otherwise inactive. Explain why (2 points).

____

____

8. Why do you have your client sit on the bedside before getting up (1 point)?

____

There are 31 possible points in this worksheet.

• WORKSHEET 6

1. 1. List the seven basic rules to follow when using household cleaners (7 points).

a. ____
b. ____
c. ____
d. ____
e. ____
f. ____
g. ____

2. Safety is an important responsibility. Choose four safety rules, and explain why each is important (8 points).

a. ______________________________
____

b. ______________________________
____

c. ______________________________
____

d. ______________________________
____

3. Why is it important to have a disaster escape plan (2 points)?

____
____

4. List eight elements to remember when planning food and menus (8 points).

a. ______________________________

b. ______________________________

c. ______________________________

d. ______________________________

e. ______________________________

f. ______________________________

g. ______________________________

h. ______________________________

5. List 11 rules to follow for storing food to prevent spoilage or contamination (11 points).

a. ______________________________

b. ______________________________

c. ______________________________

d. ______________________________

e. ______________________________

f. ______________________________

g. ______________________________

h. ______________________________

i. ______________________________

j. ______________________________

k. ______________________________

There are 36 possible points in this worksheet.

• WORKSHEET/ACTIVITY 7

1. Read five food labels. What did you learn from the labels?

   ____

2. How does knowing the nutrients and calories in foods benefit your patient and you?

   ____

3. Ask your teacher to assign you to a group to plan menus. Plan a nutritionally balanced meal for a different culture than yours. What did you learn from this activity?

   ____

There are 15 points in this worksheet/activity.

• WORKSHEET/ACTIVITY 8

1. Discuss the importance of safety with your family. What are the things you and your family think are important for your home?

   ____

2. Walk through every area in your home and develop a safety plan. List below any hazardous areas you found and how you repaired them.

   ____

3. Why do you think that talking with your family about safety is important?

   ____

There are 25 points in this worksheet/activity.

• WORKSHEET/ACTIVITY 9

Develop an action plan to use when caring for children, the aged, and the dying. Identify the need. Determine how to meet the need. Include the health care team and the family in helping to meet the client's needs (50 points for each question).

1. Action plan for children:

____

____

____

____

____

____

2. Action plan for the aged:

____

____

____

____

____

____

3. Action plan for the dying:

____

____

____

____

____

____

There are 150 possible points in this worksheet/activity.

Check-off Sheet:

16-1 Dressings: Clean, Nonsterile

Name ______________________________ **Date** ____________

Directions: Practice this procedure, following each step. When you are ready to have your performance evaluated, give this sheet to your instructor. Review the detailed procedure in your textbook.

Procedure	Pass	Redo	Date Competency Met	Instructor Initials
Student must use Standard Precautions.	☐	☐	______	______
1. Wash hands.	☐	☐	______	______
2. Assemble equipment:				
a. Clean dressings	☐	☐	______	______
b. Tape	☐	☐	______	______
c. Cleansing solution	☐	☐	______	______
d. Paper or plastic bag	☐	☐	______	______
e. Medication to be applied by client	☐	☐	______	______
f. Disposable nonsterile gloves	☐	☐	______	______
3. Identify client.	☐	☐	______	______
4. Explain what you are going to do.	☐	☐	______	______
5. Position client comfortably.	☐	☐	______	______
6. Open paper bag.	☐	☐	______	______
7. Open clean dressings. *Do not touch center of bandage.*	☐	☐	______	______
8. Put on gloves.	☐	☐	______	______
9. Remove old dressings:				
a. Check amount of drainage.	☐	☐	______	______
b. Check color, consistency, odor.	☐	☐	______	______
c. Check skin around wound.	☐	☐	______	______
d. Note size of wound.	☐	☐	______	______
10. To cleanse wound:				
a. Use circular motions.	☐	☐	______	______
b. Clean from center of wound to skin.	☐	☐	______	______

Procedure	Pass	Redo	Date Competency Met	Instructor Initials
11. Assist client with application of medication, if ordered.	☐	☐	______	______
12. Apply clean dressing.				
a. Hold dressing by corner.	☐	☐	______	______
b. Tape bandage securely in place.	☐	☐	______	______
13. Discard bandages according to agency procedures.				
a. Close bag with soiled bandages inside.	☐	☐	______	______
b. Tape bag closed.	☐	☐	______	______
c. Discard in covered container.	☐	☐	______	______
14. Remove gloves and discard according to agency procedures.	☐	☐	______	______
15. Clean equipment and put away.	☐	☐	______	______
16. Wash hands.	☐	☐	______	______
17. Chart the following:				
a. Time and date	☐	☐	______	______
b. Any observation made:	☐	☐	______	______
(1) Drainage (amount, color, odor)	☐	☐	______	______
(2) Size of wound	☐	☐	______	______
(3) Surrounding skin condition	☐	☐	______	______
c. Type of bandage applied	☐	☐	______	______
d. How procedure was tolerated	☐	☐	______	______

Check-off Sheet:

16-2 Assisting with Medication in the Home

Name ______________________________ **Date** ______________

Directions: Practice this procedure, following each step. When you are ready to have your performance evaluated, give this sheet to your instructor. Review the detailed procedure in your textbook.

Procedure	Pass	Redo	Date Competency Met	Instructor Initials
Student must use Standard Precautions.	☐	☐	______	______
Always follow the six rights of medication.				
1. Wash hands.	☐	☐	______	______
2. Assemble supplies:				
a. Glass of water or juice	☐	☐	______	______
b. Appropriate medication	☐	☐	______	______
c. Spoon or measuring device, if needed	☐	☐	______	______
3. Remind client when it is time to take medication.	☐	☐	______	______
4. Read label on medication.	☐	☐	______	______
5. Read physician's order for medication.	☐	☐	______	______
6. Read label on medication again.	☐	☐	______	______
7. Steady or guide client's hand if necessary.	☐	☐	______	______
8. Assist with pouring correct amount of medication into a container. (Pills are to be counted and placed in a container; liquids are measured.)	☐	☐	______	______
9. Close medicine container and read label again.	☐	☐	______	______
10. Assist client in taking medication.	☐	☐	______	______
11. Record on client care notes: time, type, route, amount of medication taken.	☐	☐	______	______
12. Wipe up spills and replace soiled linen or client's clothing, if necessary.	☐	☐	______	______
13. Replace medication in proper storage place.	☐	☐	______	______
14. Wash hands.	☐	☐	______	______

Check-off Sheet:

16-3 Establishing a Work Plan

Name ______________________________ **Date** ______________

Directions: Practice this procedure, following each step. When you are ready to have your performance evaluated, give this sheet to your instructor. Review the detailed procedure in your textbook.

Procedure	Pass	Redo	Date Competency Met	Instructor Initials
Student must use Standard Precautions.	☐	☐	______	______
1. Evaluate the need for basic household duties to be performed.	☐	☐	______	______
2. Make a list of the duties you decide must be routinely completed.	☐	☐	______	______
3. Ask the family to make a list of duties they feel must be routinely completed.	☐	☐	______	______
4. Plan a meeting with family members to discuss routine duties to be completed.	☐	☐	______	______
5. Discuss and agree upon the basic duties that will be done by each member of the family.	☐	☐	______	______
6. See sample work plan and use it to develop your own.	☐	☐	______	______

Sample Work Plan

Day	***Duty***	***Responsible Person***
Monday		
Tuesday		
Wednesday		
Thursday		
Friday		
Saturday		
Sunday		

Procedure	Pass	Redo	Date Competency Met	Instructor Initials
12. Attach leads to snap-on electrode patches. Each lead is color coded to ensure proper placement:				
a. White lead to right arm	☐	☐	______	______
b. Black lead to left arm	☐	☐	______	______
c. Green lead to right leg	☐	☐	______	______
d. Red lead to left leg	☐	☐	______	______
e. Brown leads are chest leads—place each one as indicated:	☐	☐	______	______
(1) V1: fourth intercostal space just to the right of sternum	☐	☐	______	______
(2) V2: fourth intercostal space just to the left of sternum	☐	☐	______	______
(3) V3: midway between position of the fourth and fifth intercostal spaces	☐	☐	______	______
(4) V4: fifth intercostal space	☐	☐	______	______
(5) V5: same level as V4 and just anterior of midaxillary line	☐	☐	______	______
(6) V6: same level as V4 and V5 at midaxillary line	☐	☐	______	______
Setting Machine Controls				
13. Set machine controls.				
a. Set speed switch to run 25 mm per second. (If there is a severe tachycardia, it may be necessary to set at 50 mm per second.)	☐	☐	______	______
b. Position stylus in center of paper.	☐	☐	______	______
c. Set sensitivity at 1 for normal complexes. If complexes are too small to recognize each wave, set at 2. If complexes are so large that they will not fit on the graph paper, set the sensitivity at ½.	☐	☐	______	______
d. Standardize each lead as instructed by your instructor.	☐	☐	______	______
14. Turn on machine.	☐	☐	______	______
15. Press run button. (Most multichannel EKG machines automatically standardize and record each lead when the run button is pushed. See manufacturer's instructions to operate your machine properly.)	☐	☐	______	______

Procedure	Pass	Redo	Date Competency Met	Instructor Initials
16. Turn machine off when all leads are recorded.	☐	☐	______	______
17. Remove all leads and electrode patches.	☐	☐	______	______
18. Clean remaining gel or paste left from patches.	☐	☐	______	______
19. Assist patient in dressing if necessary.	☐	☐	______	______
20. Label EKG with patient's name and physician's name.	☐	☐	______	______
21. Clean machine so that it is ready for the next procedure.	☐	☐	______	______
22. Mount EKG and deliver as instructed for interpretation. (See the procedure "Mounting EKGs".)				

Chapter 17 Electrocardiogram Technician

• OBJECTIVES

When you have completed this chapter, you will be able to do the following:

- Complete all objectives in Part One of this book.
- Match vocabulary words with their correct meanings.
- List two reasons why the physician orders an EKG/ECG.
- List four conditions that are determined by an EKG/ECG.
- Label a diagram of an EKG/ECG machine and describe the function of each part.
- Label a normal EKG/ECG complex.
- List three waves recorded on the EKG/ECG cycle and relate them to the activity of the heart.
- List the 12 leads recorded on an EKG/ECG.
- Identify the leads according to color and correct placement.
- List three common sources of artifacts.
- Identify eight common causes of artifacts and their remedies.
- Perform an EKG/ECG.
- Mount EKG/ECG readings.
- Compare and contrast normal EKG/ECG readings with abnormal readings.
- Attach a Holter monitor to a client and give clear instructions to the client.
- Explain what a Holter monitor records and why it is used for diagnostic purposes.
- Demonstrate the following from Chapter 15:
  - Pivot transfer from bed to wheelchair and back.
  - Sliding from bed to gurney and back.
  - Moving a resident in a wheelchair.
  - Moving a resident on a gurney.

- Demonstrate the following from Chapter 22:
  - List five filing systems.
  - Demonstrate alpha and numeric filing.

• DIRECTIONS

1. Read this chapter.
2. Complete Worksheets 1 and 2 as assigned.
3. Complete Worksheet/Activity 3 as assigned.
4. Use the skills check-off sheets to practice and demonstrate all procedures in this chapter.
5. Prepare responses to each item listed in the Chapter Review—Your Link to Success at the end of this chapter.
6. When you are confident that you can meet each objective for this unit, ask your instructor for the unit evaluation.

• EVALUATION METHODS

- Worksheets/Activities
- Class participation
- Written evaluation
- Return demonstrations

• WORKSHEET 1

1. List two reasons why the doctor orders an EKG/ECG (2 points).
   a. ______________________________
   b. ______________________________
2. List four conditions that are determined by an EKG/ECG (4 points).
   a. ______________________________
   b. ______________________________
   c. ______________________________
   d. ______________________________

3. Label a normal EKG/ECG complex (5 points).

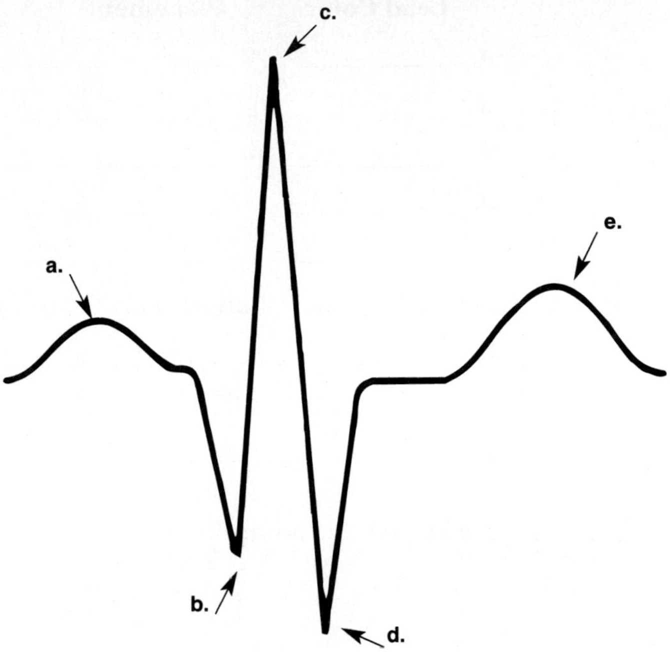

a. ______________________________

b. ______________________________

c. ______________________________

d. ______________________________

e. ______________________________

4. List 12 leads recorded on an EKG/ECG (12 points).

a. ______________________________

b. ______________________________

c. ______________________________

d. ______________________________

e. ______________________________

f. ______________________________

g. ______________________________

h. ______________________________

i. ______________________________

j. ______________________________

k. ______________________________

l. ______________________________

5. Identify the leads according to color and correct placement (10 points).

	Lead Color	Placement
a.	________	________________________
b.	________	________________________
c.	________	________________________
d.	________	________________________
e.	________	________________________

6. List three common sources of artifacts (3 points).

a. ________________________________

b. ________________________________

c. ________________________________

There are 36 possible points in this worksheet.

• WORKSHEET 2

Write the correct lead title under the appropriate graph (12 points).

Leads 1–3

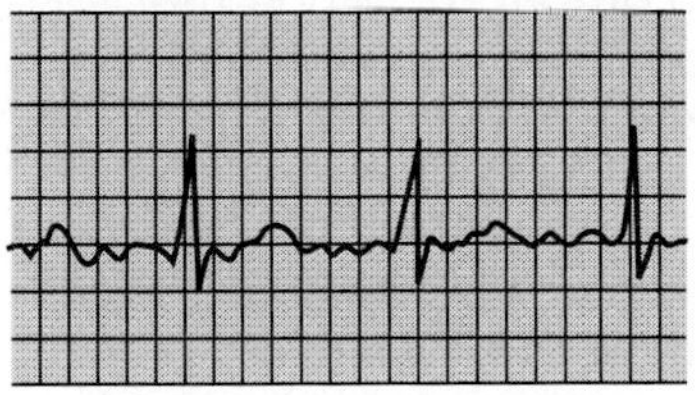

1. ____________________

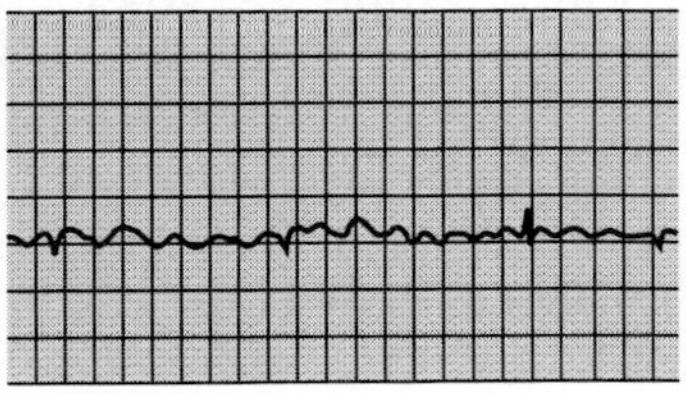

2. ____________________

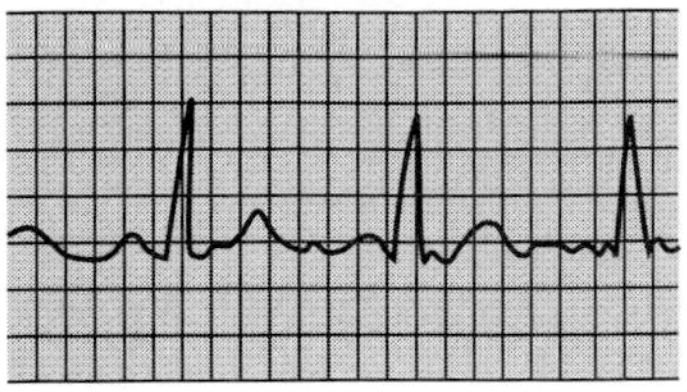

3. ____________________

Augmented Voltage Leads

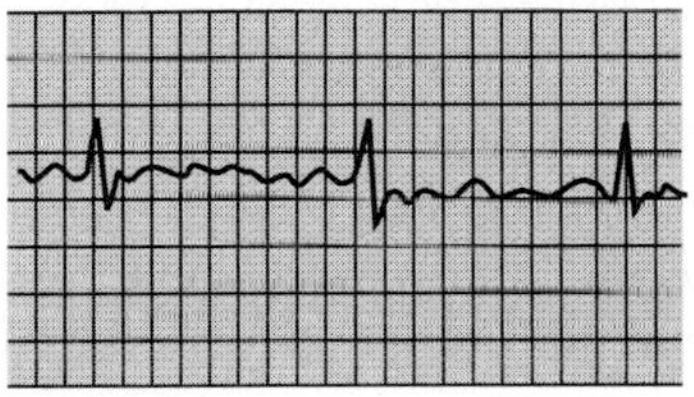

4. ____________________

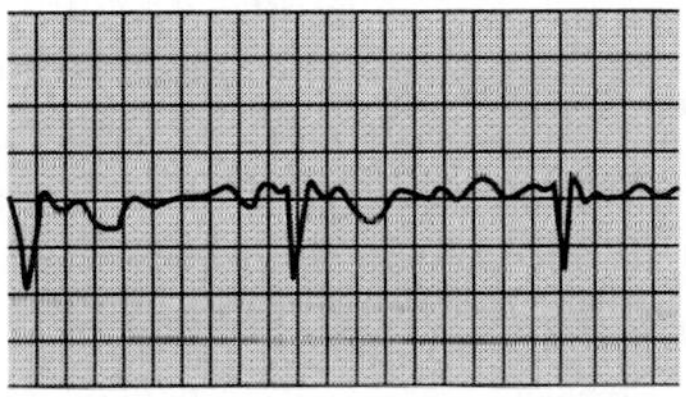

5. ____________________

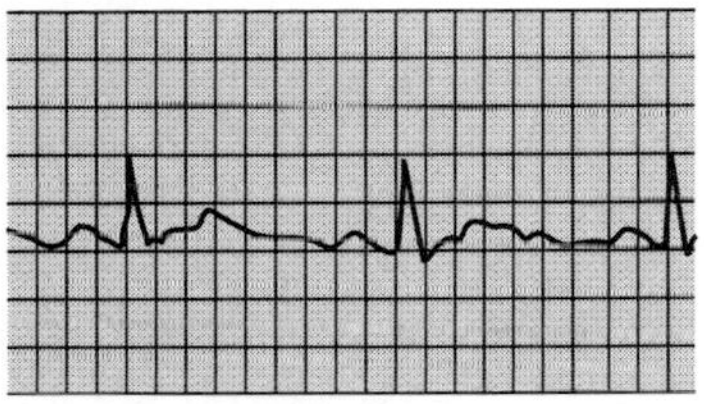

6. ____________________

V Leads

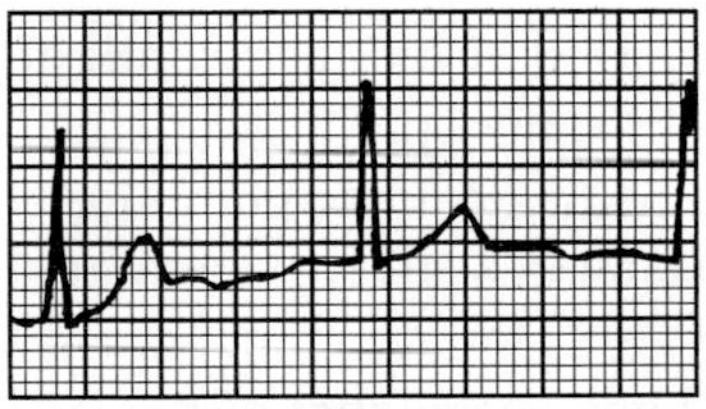

7. ____________________

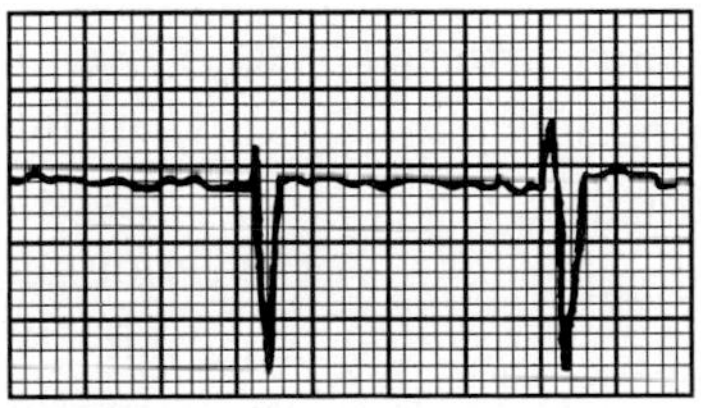

8. ____________________

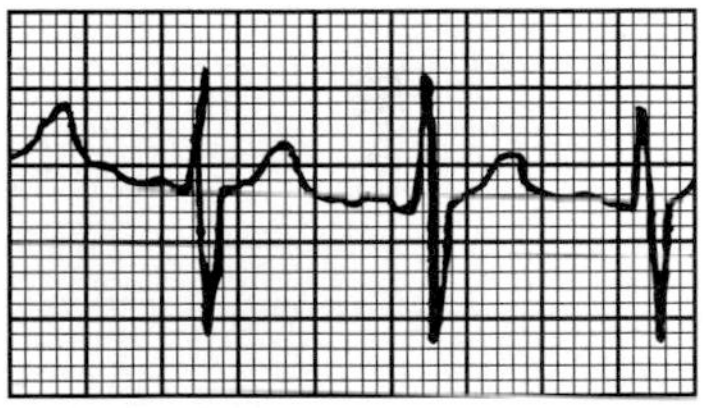

9. ____________________

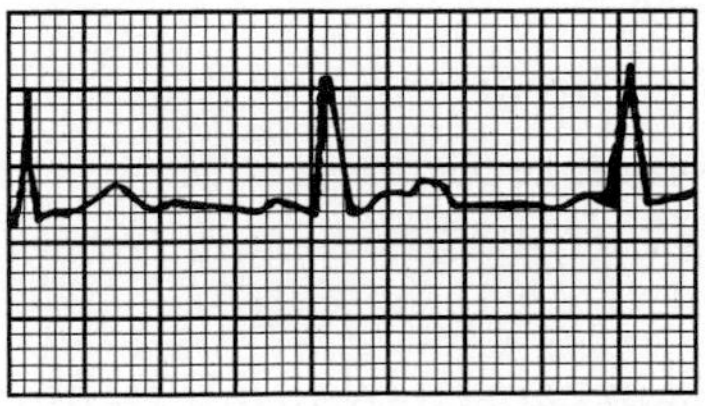

10. ____________________

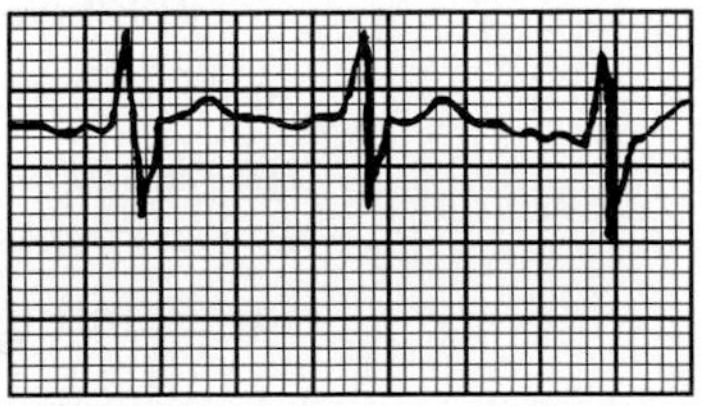

11. ____________________

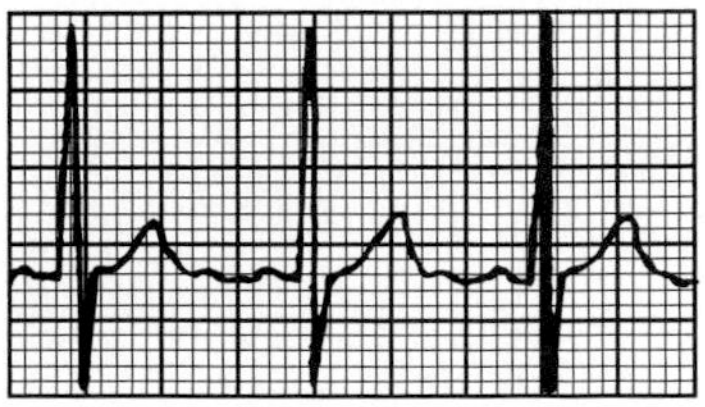

12. ____________________

Match each definition in column B with the correct vocabulary word in column A. Use a medical dictionary to find these terms (27 points).

Column A

____ **13.** electric cardiac pacemaker
____ **14.** electrocardiograph
____ **15.** embolism
____ **16.** heart block
____ **17.** hypertension
____ **18.** infarct
____ **19.** insufficiency
____ **20.** palpitation
____ **21.** paroxysmal tachycardia
____ **22.** pulse
____ **23.** stasis
____ **24.** syncope
____ **25.** tachycardia
____ **26.** thrombosis
____ **27.** angina pectoris
____ **28.** anoxia
____ **29.** arrhythmia
____ **30.** bradycardia
____ **31.** cardiac cycle
____ **32.** cardiac output
____ **33.** congestive heart failure
____ **34.** coronary arteries
____ **35.** cyanosis
____ **36.** defibrillator
____ **37.** dyspnea
____ **38.** edema
____ **39.** EKG/ECG

Column B

a. Abnormally high blood pressure.
b. Condition when the heart is unable to adequately pump out all the blood that returns to it, and there is a backing up of blood in the veins leading to the heart.
c. A graphic record of the electrical currents produced by the heart.
d. Abnormal rhythm of the heartbeat.
e. Two arteries, arising from the aorta, arching down over the top of the heart and conducting blood to the heart muscle.
f. One total heartbeat (i.e., one complete contraction and relaxation of the heart).
g. Any agent or procedure, such as an electrical shock, that stops incoordinate contraction of the heart muscle and restores normal rhythm.
h. An electric device that can control the beating of the heart by a rhythmic discharge of electrical impulses.
i. Blocking of a blood vessel by a clot or other substance carried in the blood stream.
j. Interference with the conduction of the electrical impulses of the heart, which is either partial or complete.
k. Tissue that is damaged or dies as a result of insufficient blood supply.
l. Condition when the heart is not pumping enough blood to supply a sufficient amount to parts of the body.
m. A period of rapid heartbeats that begins and ends suddenly.
n. Abnormally rapid heart rate; generally over 100 beats a minute.
o. Difficult or labored breathing.
p. An instrument which records electric currents produced by the heart.
q. Fainting.
r. Blueness of the skin caused by insufficient oxygen in the blood.
s. A stoppage or slackening of blood.
t. Pain in the chest due to coronary artery spasm.
u. Fluttering of the heart; abnormal rate or rhythm of the heart beat.

v. The formation or presence of a blood clot inside a blood vessel or cavity of the heart.

w. Without oxygen.

x. Slow heartbeat; generally below 60 beats per minute.

y. The amount of blood pumped by the heart per minute.

z. Swelling due to abnormally large amounts of fluid in the tissues of the body.

aa. The expansion and contraction of an artery, which may be felt by placing the fingers on the artery.

There are 39 possible points in this worksheet.

• WORKSHEET/ACTIVITY 3

Tour an EKG department, EEG department, and any associated area (END) to observe equipment and testing.

1. What do you find interesting about this department?

____

____

____

____

2. What did you learn that you didn't know about these diagnostic areas?

____

____

____

____

3. Does this department still interest you? Why?

There are 15 points in this worksheet/activity.

Check-off Sheet:

17-1 Using a Multilead Electrocardiograph (placing leads on the client, setting machine controls)

Name ______________________________ **Date** ______________

Directions: Practice this procedure, following each step. When you are ready to have your performance evaluated, give this sheet to your instructor. Review the detailed procedure in your textbook.

Procedure	Pass	Redo	Date Competency Met	Instructor Initials
Student must use Standard Precautions in placing leads on patient/client.	☐	☐	______	______
1. Wash hands.	☐	☐	______	______
2. Assemble equipment:				
a. EKG machine with electrodes	☐	☐	______	______
b. Electrode pads	☐	☐	______	______
c. Alcohol wipes or skin cleansing agent	☐	☐	______	______
d. Bath blanket or sheet	☐	☐	______	______
e. Patient gown	☐	☐	______	______
3. Identify patient/client.	☐	☐	______	______
4. Explain what you are doing, and reassure patient that this procedure is painless.	☐	☐	______	______
5. Help client change into a patient gown, if necessary.	☐	☐	______	______
6. Position patient on bed or treatment table in a supine position with arms relaxed beside body.	☐	☐	______	______
7. Cover patient with a blanket, leaving arms and legs exposed.	☐	☐	______	______
8. Position machine at the side of client.	☐	☐	______	______
9. Identify correct location for leg, arm, and chest leads. (Avoid bony areas.)	☐	☐	______	______
10. Wipe skin with a cleansing agent to remove oils, scaly skin, or perspiration.	☐	☐	______	______
11. Apply electrode patches.	☐	☐	______	______

Check-off Sheet:

17-2 Using a Single-Lead Electrocardiograph (placing leads on the client, setting machine controls, performing an EKG)

Name ______________________________ **Date** ______________

Directions: Practice this procedure, following each step. When you are ready to have your performance evaluated, give this sheet to your instructor. Review the detailed procedure in your textbook.

Procedure	Pass	Redo	Date Competency Met	Instructor Initials
Student must use Standard Precautions in placing leads on patient/client.	☐	☐	______	______
1. Wash hands.	☐	☐	______	______
2. Assemble equipment:				
a. EKG machine with electrodes	☐	☐	______	______
b. Conductive gel	☐	☐	______	______
c. Alcohol wipes or skin cleansing agent	☐	☐	______	______
d. Gauze	☐	☐	______	______
e. Rubber electrode straps	☐	☐	______	______
f. Bath blanket or sheet	☐	☐	______	______
g. Patient gown	☐	☐	______	______
3. Identify patient/client.	☐	☐	______	______
4. Explain what you are doing, and reassure client that this procedure is painless.	☐	☐	______	______
5. Help patient change into patient gown, if necessary.	☐	☐	______	______
6. Position patient on bed or treatment table in a supine position with arms relaxed beside the body.	☐	☐	______	______
7. Cover client with a blanket, leaving arms and legs exposed.	☐	☐	______	______
8. Position machine at the side of patient.	☐	☐	______	______
9. Identify correct location for leg, arm, and chest leads. (Avoid bony areas.)	☐	☐	______	______
10. Wipe skin with a cleansing agent to remove oils, scaly skin, or perspiration.	☐	☐	______	______
11. Apply conductive gel or paste and electrodes Secure with rubber straps.	☐	☐	______	______

Procedure	Pass	Redo	Date Competency Met	Instructor Initials
12. Connect leads to electrodes. Each lead is color coded to ensure proper placement:				
a. White lead to right arm	☐	☐	______	______
b. Black lead to left arm	☐	☐	______	______
c. Green lead to right leg	☐	☐	______	______
d. Red lead to left leg	☐	☐	______	______
e. Brown leads not attached at this time	☐	☐	______	______
Setting Machine Controls				
13. Set machine controls. Now that leads are in the proper place, it is important that you set each control on the machine in order to have a correct reading.				
a. Be certain to set speed switch to run 25 mm per second. (If there is a severe tachycardia, it may be necessary to set at 50 mm per second.)	☐	☐	______	______
b. Position stylus in center of paper.	☐	☐	______	______
c. Set sensitivity at 1 for normal complexes. If complexes are too small to recognize each wave, set at 2. If complexes are so large that they will not fit on the graph paper, set the sensitivity at ½.	☐	☐	______	______
d. Standardize each lead as instructed by your teacher.	☐	☐	______	______
14. Turn on machine. A light will come on if the machine is on.	☐	☐	______	______
15. Turn lead selector switch to standardization position and quickly press standardization button.	☐	☐	______	______
16. Turn lead selector to off position.	☐	☐	______	______
17. Check standardization mark on EKG paper. If machine is operating correctly, this mark will be 10 small blocks high, or two large blocks high. Press standardization button as you run each lead.	☐	☐	______	______
18. If the machine does not label each lead automatically, you will have to do so.	☐	☐	______	______
19. Turn lead selector to lead I and run an 8- to 10-inch strip.	☐	☐	______	______

Procedure	Pass	Redo	Date Competency Met	Instructor Initials
20. Repeat step 19 for leads II and III.	☐	☐	______	______
21. Repeat step 19 for AVL, AVR, AVF, but run only 4- to 6-inch strips.	☐	☐	______	______
22. Place brown chest leads in the following locations on the chest wall. After each placement, standardize and run a 4- to 6-inch strip.				
a. V1: fourth intercostal space just to the right of sternum	☐	☐	______	______
b. V2: fourth intercostal space just to the left of sternum	☐	☐	______	______
c. V3: midway between position of the fourth and fifth intercostal spaces	☐	☐	______	______
d. V4: fifth intercostal space	☐	☐	______	______
e. V5: same level as V4 and just anterior of midaxillary line	☐	☐	______	______
f. V6: same level as V4 and V5 at midaxillary line	☐	☐	______	______
23. Turn machine off.	☐	☐	______	______
24. Remove all leads and electrodes.	☐	☐	______	______
25. Clean remaining gel or paste from skin.	☐	☐	______	______
26. Assist client in dressing, if necessary.	☐	☐	______	______
27. Label EKG with patient's name and physician's name.	☐	☐	______	______
28. Clean electrodes thoroughly so that machine is ready for the next procedure.	☐	☐	______	______
29. Mount EKG and deliver as instructed for interpretation. (See the procedure "Mounting EKGs".)	☐	☐	______	______

Check-off Sheet:

17-3 Mounting EKGs

Name ______________________________ **Date** ______________

Directions: Practice this procedure, following each step. When you are ready to have your performance evaluated, give this sheet to your instructor. Review the detailed procedure in your textbook.

Procedure	Pass	Redo	Date Competency Met	Instructor Initials
Student must use Standard Precautions.	☐	☐	______	______
There are a variety of standard mount forms used in medicine. Mount the EKG records according to the physician's preference or the standard form used in your facility. Regardless of the form used, there are a few important steps you must follow in mounting every EKG.				
1. Neatly trim strips to fit in the space provided.	☐	☐	______	______
2. Include any unusual-looking complexes in the mounted strip.	☐	☐	______	______
3. Fill in the appropriate blanks on the form portion of mount.	☐	☐	______	______
4. Sign your name and deliver the completed EKG to the appropriate person for interpretation.	☐	☐	______	______

Check-off Sheet:

17-4 Using the Holter Monitor

Name ______________________________ **Date** ______________

Directions: Practice this procedure, following each step. When you are ready to have your performance evaluated, give this sheet to your instructor. Review the detailed procedure in your textbook.

Procedure	**Pass**	**Redo**	**Date Competency Met**	**Instructor Initials**
Student must use Standard Precautions.	☐	☐	______	______
1. Wash hands.	☐	☐	______	______
2. Assemble equipment:				
a. Prejelled adhesive electrodes	☐	☐	______	______
b. Holter monitor with lead wires	☐	☐	______	______
c. Alcohol wipes	☐	☐	______	______
d. Monitor belt	☐	☐	______	______
e. Razor and shaving cream	☐	☐	______	______
f. Cassette and batteries	☐	☐	______	______
g. Diary for patient records	☐	☐	______	______
h. Nonallergic tape to secure electrodes, if needed	☐	☐	______	______
i. Patient's medical record	☐	☐	______	______
j. Pen	☐	☐	______	______
k. Patient gown for women	☐	☐	______	______
3. Explain what you are going to do, and show monitor and leads to patient.	☐	☐	______	______
4. Ask client to remove clothes from the waist up. Provide a gown for women, instructing them to place the opening in front.	☐	☐	______	______
5. Test monitor for proper operation and insert new batteries each time you apply monitor.	☐	☐	______	______
6. Shave chest at electrode placement sites, if necessary.	☐	☐	______	______
7. Rub electrode sites with gauze to prepare skin for good contact.	☐	☐	______	______
8. Place electrode sites.	☐	☐	______	______

Procedure	Pass	Redo	Date Competency Met	Instructor Initials
9. Place monitor belt with monitor in place around patient's waist over the shoulder.	☐	☐	______	______
10. Instruct client in care of monitor according to manufacturer's instruction.	☐	☐	______	______
11. Give patient the diary and instruct him or her to follow a normal routine. If pain, discomfort, or any symptoms should occur, the patient is to				
a. Push the event button on monitor.	☐	☐	______	______
b. Document in diary time of event and length of time that symptoms last.	☐	☐	______	______
12. Assist client in dressing.	☐	☐	______	______
13. Wash hands.	☐	☐	______	______
14. Record the following in patient medical record:				
a. Date and time monitor was applied	☐	☐	______	______
b. What instructions were given to patient; your initials	☐	☐	______	______
15. Schedule client for a return visit.	☐	☐	______	______
To Remove Monitor:				
16. Wash hands.	☐	☐	______	______
17. Assist client in removing clothes from the waist up.	☐	☐	______	______
18. Remove monitor strap, electrodes, and wires.	☐	☐	______	______
19. Clean skin at electrode sites.	☐	☐	______	______
20. Assist patient in dressing, if necessary.	☐	☐	______	______
21. Collect diary from patient.	☐	☐	______	______
22. Instruct client according to physician's orders.	☐	☐	______	______
23. Wash hands.	☐	☐	______	______
24. Place diary in patient's medical record and record time monitor was returned; initial.	☐	☐	______	______
25. Place cassette in analyzer for reading.	☐	☐	______	______
26. When printout is received from analyzer, attach to medical record, initial, and send or give to physician.	☐	☐	______	______

Chapter 18 Laboratory Assistant/ Medical Assistant Laboratory Skills; Phlebotomist

UNIT 1 Laboratory Skills

• OBJECTIVES

When you have completed this unit, you will be able to do the following:

- Complete all objectives in Part One of this book.
- Match vocabulary words with their correct meanings.
- Follow 12 general laboratory guidelines.
- Practice laboratory safety.
- Practice the aseptic technique.
- Demonstrate loading and operating an autoclave.
- Dispose of hazardous materials according to facility policy.
- List six ways that laboratory tests help the physician.
- Identify information required on all laboratory slips.
- Discuss the importance of advance preparation for laboratory tests.
- List eight types of specimen studies.
- Identify general rules for testing specimens.
- List three methods for testing specimens.
- Discuss quality control in the laboratory.
- Label a diagram of a microscope.
- List five ways to prevent loss of your specimen in a centrifuge.
- Identify steps to acquire a midstream, clean-catch urine for male and female.
- Define *urinary sediment.*
- List three infectious diseases that can be diagnosed with a sputum test.

- Explain the reason for testing stool specimens for occult blood.
- Demonstrate:
  - Obtaining a throat culture
  - Preparing a direct smear
  - Streaking an agar plate
  - Preparing a slide from culture grown in an agar plate
  - Gram staining a slide
- Identify seven items learned from a complete blood test (CBC).
- Explain why a hematocrit and hemoglobin test is important.
- Explain the reason for blood glucose testing.
- Explain the importance of counting WBCs and RBCs.
- State reasons for doing a WBC differential.
- List the four blood types.
- Explain agglutination.
- Explain an erythrocyte sedimentation rate.
- Identify the tests done in blood chemistries.
- Demonstrate:
  - Finger stick
  - Hematocrit test
  - Blood glucose test with a glucose meter
  - Diluting blood cells with an Unopette
  - Preparing a blood smear slide
  - Completing a differential white cell count
  - Typing your blood
  - Determining the erythrocyte sedimentation rate

• DIRECTIONS

1. Complete Worksheet 1.
2. Complete Worksheets 2 through 7 and Worksheet/Activity 8 as assigned.
3. Read Unit 1 of Chapter 18.
4. Practice and demonstrate procedures P18-1 through P18-26 in this unit.
5. When you are confident that you can meet each objective listed above, ask your instructor for the unit evaluation.

• EVALUATION METHODS

- Worksheets
- Class participation
- Written evaluation
- Return demonstrations

• WORKSHEET 1

Define the following vocabulary words (12 points).

1. hazardous ____________________
2. contaminated ____________________
3. reagents ____________________
4. antigens ____________________
5. antibodies ____________________
6. parasite ____________________
7. heparinized ____________________
8. biconcave ____________________
9. plasma ____________________
10. NPO ____________________
11. diagnostic ____________________
12. uniformity ____________________

Match each definition in column B with the correct vocabulary word in column A (14 points).

Column A

____ 13. acids
____ 14. monocular
____ 15. biocular
____ 16. resistant
____ 17. agglutination
____ 18. polycythemia
____ 19. complex
____ 20. automated
____ 21. clumped
____ 22. classify
____ 23. consecutive
____ 24. invasive
____ 25. hematoma
____ 26. venipuncture

Column B

a. Having two eyepieces.
b. Condition of sticking together.
c. Having two or more related parts.
d. Substances that cause the urine to have an acid pH.
e. Having too much blood.
f. Put like items together.
g. Puncture of a vein.
h. Collection of blood beneath the skin.
i. Method of lab testing that uses equipment to perform a series of steps.
j. Having one eyepiece.
k. Following one after the other.
l. Penetrating the body.
m. Able to protect itself.
n. Stuck together.

There are 26 possible points in this worksheet.

• WORKSHEET 2

1. Define CLIA, and explain what it does (2 points). ____________________

____

____

2. List the 12 general laboratory guidelines (12 points).

   a. ____________________
   b. ____________________
   c. ____________________
   d. ____________________
   e. ____________________
   f. ____________________
   g. ____________________
   h. ____________________
   i. ____________________
   j. ____________________
   k. ____________________
   l. ____________________

3. Explain why laboratory standards are important (2 points). ____________

____

____

4. Personal safety in the laboratory is every health care worker's responsibility. Choose five safety guidelines from the text, and explain why they are important (10 points).

   a. ____________________

   ____

   b. ____________________

   ____

   c. ____________________

   ____

   d. ____________________

   ____

   e. ____________________

   ____

5. Define *aseptic technique* (in Chapter 12; 1 point). ____________________

6. Mark each of the following statements *T* for true or *F* for false (4 points).

   ____ **a.** All items that come in contact with body tissue or fluids must be sterilized.

   ____ **b.** Pack everything into the autoclave tightly to ensure that all items are sterilized.

   ____ **c.** Dispose of hazardous material according to facility policy.

   ____ **d.** Contaminated material that has contact with blood and body fluids can be placed in a regular container as long as there is only a small amount of blood.

There are 31 possible points in this worksheet.

• WORKSHEET 3

1. Put an *X* next to each piece of information required on all lab slips (10 points).

   ____ Time and date of collection
   ____ Client's name and address
   ____ Results of test
   ____ Spouse's name
   ____ Medications client is taking
   ____ Date of birth
   ____ Number of children
   ____ Client's age and sex
   ____ Physician's name and address
   ____ Marital status
   ____ Social Security number
   ____ Date entered facility
   ____ Method of collection
   ____ Name of test
   ____ Name of classification
   ____ Type and source of specimen
   ____ Possible diagnosis
   ____ Stat or routine

2. Explain why the patient's advance preparation for laboratory tests is important (1 point). ____

   ____

3. List eight types of studies commonly performed in a lab (8 points).

   a. ____

   b. ____

   c. ____

   d. ____

   e. ____

f. ______________________________

g. ______________________________

h. ______________________________

4. There are six basic steps to follow for testing all procedures. Put 1 next to the first step, 2 next to the second step, and so on (6 points).

___ a. Process the specimen correctly. For example, centrifuge, heat in a water bath, incubate, heat fix, and so on.
___ b. Combine the correct chemical reagent for the test with the specimen.
___ c. Measure the amount of specimen required for the test very carefully.
___ d. Calculate results by hand or machine.
___ e. Record all the information on lab report sheet.
___ f. Assess the sample by manual or automatic method.

5. Explain why quality control in the laboratory is important (1 point).

____

There are 26 possible points in this worksheet.

• WORKSHEET 4

1. Label the diagram of a microscope (7 points). Use the basic parts of a microscope in Chapter 18 of the text to label the diagram. Figure 18–2 is a newer type of microscope.

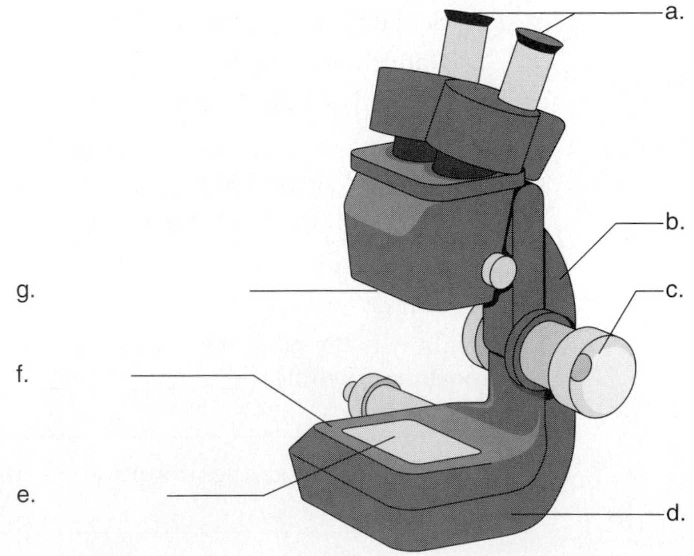

a. ____________________

b. ____________________

c. ____________________

d. ____________________

e. ____________________

f. ____________________

g. ____________________

2. List four ways to prevent loss of your specimen in a centrifuge (4 points).

a. ____________________

b. ____________________

c. ____________________

d. ____________________

3. Define *urinary sediment* (1 point). ____________________

____

See examples of urinary sediment on next page.

4. Explain a midstream, clean-catch urine (1 point). ____________________

____

5. List three infectious diseases that can be diagnosed with a sputum test (3 points).

a. ____________________

b. ____________________

c. ____________________

6. Explain the reason for testing stool specimens for occult blood (1 point).

____

There are 17 possible points in this worksheet.

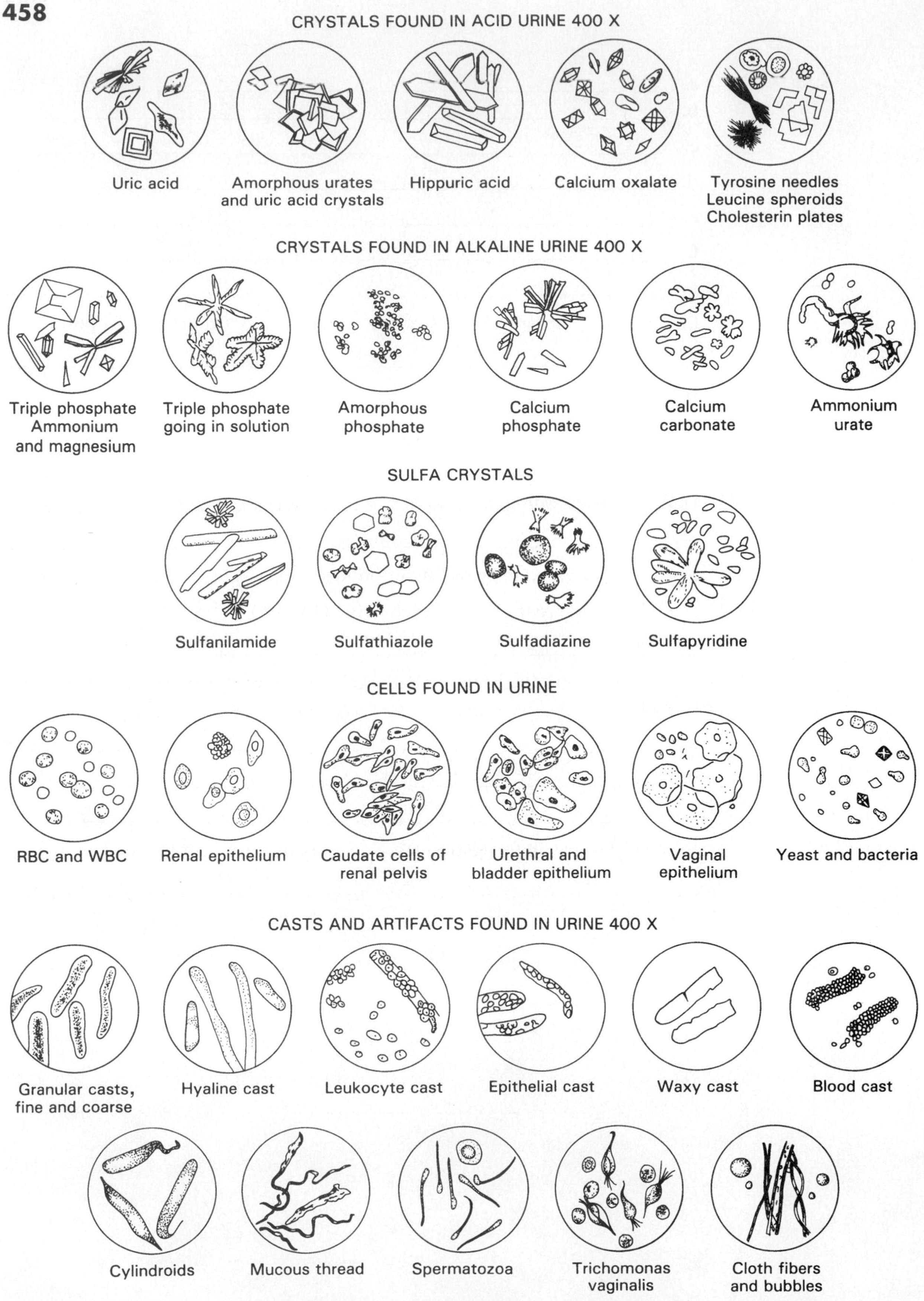
CRYSTALS FOUND IN ACID URINE 400 X
Uric acid
Amorphous urates and uric acid crystals
Hippuric acid
Calcium oxalate
Tyrosine needles
Leucine spheroids
Cholesterin plates
CRYSTALS FOUND IN ALKALINE URINE 400 X
Triple phosphate Ammonium and magnesium
Triple phosphate going in solution
Amorphous phosphate
Calcium phosphate
Calcium carbonate
Ammonium urate
SULFA CRYSTALS
Sulfanilamide
Sulfathiazole
Sulfadiazine
Sulfapyridine
CELLS FOUND IN URINE
RBC and WBC
Renal epithelium
Caudate cells of renal pelvis
Urethral and bladder epithelium
Vaginal epithelium
Yeast and bacteria
CASTS AND ARTIFACTS FOUND IN URINE 400 X
Granular casts, fine and coarse
Hyaline cast
Leukocyte cast
Epithelial cast
Waxy cast
Blood cast
Cylindroids
Mucous thread
Spermatozoa
Trichomonas vaginalis
Cloth fibers and bubbles

Examples of urinary sediment: crystals, cells, and casts found in urine sediment.

• WORKSHEET 5

1. Why is a culture ordered (1 point)?

    ____

2. List six places cultures are usually taken (6 points).

    a. ______________________________
    b. ______________________________
    c. ______________________________
    d. ______________________________
    e. ______________________________
    f. ______________________________

3. What is a direct smear (1 point)? ______________________________

    ____

4. What does an agar plate provide the microorganisms (1 point)? __________

    ____

5. A culture and sensitivity test is ordered. What will you learn from this test (2 points)? ______________________________

    ____

    ____

6. Why is a culture and sensitivity test important (1 point)? __________

    ____

7. Explain the term "fix the slide" (1 point). ______________________________

    ____

8. Why do you use gram stain on slides (1 point)? ______________________________

    ____

9. List the solutions used to gram stain slides (5 points).

    a. ______________________________
    b. ______________________________
    c. ______________________________
    d. ______________________________
    e. ______________________________

There are 19 possible points in this worksheet.

• WORKSHEET 6

1. Plasma makes up __________________ % of whole blood (1 point).
2. Formed elements make up __________________ % of the blood (1 point).
3. __________________ protect against infection and disease (1 point).
4. __________________ start the clotting process (1 point).
5. __________________ carry oxygen to the cells and carry away carbon dioxide (1 point).
6. Place an *X* next to the items that can be learned from a CBC (7 points).

___ **a.** amount of plasma	___ **g.** patient height
___ **b.** hemoglobin determination	___ **h.** stool color
___ **c.** number of RBCs	___ **i.** number of WBCs
___ **d.** types of bacteria	___ **j.** WBC differential
___ **e.** number of platelets	___ **k.** RBC size and shape
___ **f.** patient intelligence	___ **l.** hematocrit determination

7. Explain why a hematocrit is important (1 point). __________________

____

____

8. Explain why a hemoglobin test is important (1 point). __________________

____

____

9. Explain the reason for blood glucose testing (1 point). __________________

____

____

10. List four medical problems that too much glucose in the blood can cause (4 points).

a. __________________

b. __________________

c. __________________

d. __________________

11. Define a WBC differential (1 point). __________________

____

____

12. Name the two types of blood-diluting pipettes (2 point).

a. __________________

b. __________________

13. Identify each marking on the pipettes (12 points).

1. ______________________ 1. ______________________

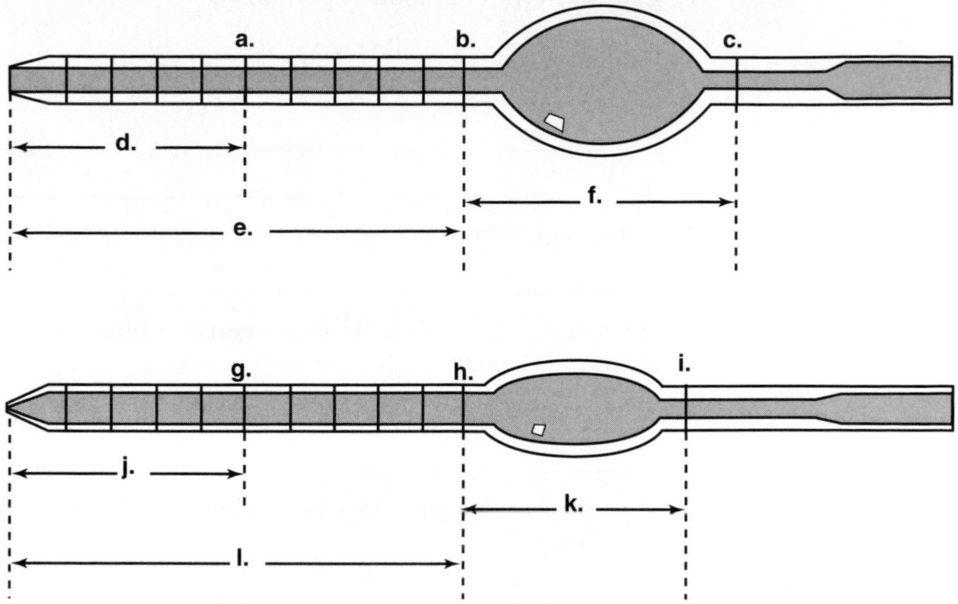

a. ______________________ g. ______________________

b. ______________________ h. ______________________

c. ______________________ i. ______________________

d. ______________________ j. ______________________

e. ______________________ k. ______________________

f. ______________________ l. ______________________

14. What steps do you use to calculate the red blood cell count after making a slide with one drop of diluted blood (3 points)?

a. ______________________

b. ______________________

c. ______________________

15. Determine the number of RBCs if your count has 88, 90, 75, 70, 68 (1 point). ______________________

There are 38 possible points in this worksheet.

• WORKSHEET 7

1. List four types of blood (4 points).

   a. ______________________________

   b. ______________________________

   c. ______________________________

   d. ______________________________

2. Define *agglutination* (1 point). ______________________________

   ____

3. What happens when a blood antigen combines with the same type of antibody (1 point)? ______________________________

4. What determines the type of blood that we have (1 point)? ______________________________

   ____

5. Why do you type and crossmatch blood before giving a transfusion (1 point)?

   ____

6. Define *erythrocyte sedimentation rate* (1 point). ______________________________

   ____

7. What are two things that an increased sedimentation rate might indicate (2 points)?

   a. ______________________________

   b. ______________________________

8. What are three problems a decreased sedimentation rate can indicate (3 points)?

   a. ______________________________

   b. ______________________________

   c. ______________________________

9. Define *blood chemistries* (1 point). ______________________________

   ____

There are 15 possible points in this worksheet.

• WORKSHEET/ACTIVITY 8

Working with your instructor as a class exercise, choose several scenarios to role-play (e.g., spilled materials or exposure to eyes and skin).

Divide into groups and act out the correct steps for each scenario.

There are 5 points for each participant in a correctly performed scenario in this worksheet/activity.

UNIT 2 Phlebotomist

• OBJECTIVES

When you have completed this unit, you will be able to do the following:

- Complete all objectives in Part One of this book.
- Define vocabulary words.
- List six things the physician can tell from blood samples.
- List three components of blood.
- Describe what changes occur in the blood after injury or infection.
- List four rules to follow when collecting blood samples.
- Match the blood collection tube stopper colors with their content and general use.
- Label a diagram of the arm, and identify the veins most often used in venipuncture.
- State three ways that blood samples are obtained.
- Give two reasons why a syringe and needle are used to draw a blood sample.
- Discuss why correct disposal of needles, syringes, and contaminated material is important.
- List two serious illnesses spread by contaminated needles and materials.
- Demonstrate how to use a Vacutainer correctly to withdraw blood.
- Demonstrate how to use a needle and syringe correctly to withdraw blood.
- Demonstrate how to complete a finger stick correctly.
- Apply all procedural techniques with confidence.

• DIRECTIONS

1. Read this unit.
2. Complete Worksheets 1 through 4 as assigned.
3. Practice and demonstrate procedures P18-27 and P18-28 in this unit.

4. Prepare responses to each item listed in the Chapter Review—Your Link to Success at the end of this chapter.
5. When you are confident that you can meet each objective listed above, ask your instructor for the unit evaluation.

• EVALUATION METHODS

- Worksheets
- Class participation
- Return demonstration
- Written test

• WORKSHEET 1

1. List six things the doctor can tell from blood samples (6 points).

   a. ____________________

   b. ____________________

   c. ____________________

   d. ____________________

   e. ____________________

   f. ____________________

2. List three components of blood (3 points).

   a. ____________________

   b. ____________________

   c. ____________________

3. Describe the changes that occur in the blood after injury or infection (1 point).

   ____

   ____

   ____

4. List four rules to follow when collecting blood samples (4 points).

   a. ____________________

   b. ____________________

   c. ____________________

   d. ____________________

5. List four reasons it may be difficult to find a vein (4 points).
   a. ______________________________
   b. ______________________________
   c. ______________________________
   d. ______________________________
6. Define the following words (4 points).
   a. venipuncture ______________________________
   b. plasma ______________________________
   c. invasive ______________________________
   d. hematoma ______________________________

There are 22 possible points in this worksheet.

• WORKSHEET 2

Divide into groups of four. Your teacher will give you a role-play. Work together to develop a skit demonstrating the correct way to meet the needs of your client and still obtain the specimens you need. Remember your communication skills, ethical behavior, and meeting people's needs.

• WORKSHEET 3

1. You have a long waiting list of clients who need their blood drawn. You know that your supervisor doesn't like to have clients waiting very long. You notice that when James draws blood during busy times, he doesn't change gloves. You could work much faster if you didn't change gloves. Identify four problems in this situation and explain how you will resolve them (5 points).

____

____

____

____

____

2. Mr. Jereman is a six-foot-tall muscular man. When he comes in to have his blood drawn, he jokes about being afraid of needles. As you prepare to draw his blood, you notice that he seems pale. What interventions will you take? Remember communication skills and syncope (5 points).

____

____

____

____

____

3. Ms. Tindell is obese. You've tried to get into a vein several times and are determined that this time you will be successful. But after sticking her three times, you are still unable to get into a vein. What will you do in order to obtain the specimen? Remember meeting the client's needs and proper procedure (5 points).

____

____

____

____

____

There are 15 possible points in this worksheet.

• WORKSHEET 4

Match the collection tube stopper colors with the correct explanation, using the colors more than once as needed (9 points).

a. red-brown **c.** violet **e.** gray
b. blue **d.** green

_____ **1.** Used for blood chemistry and other multipurpose tests
_____ **2.** Contains EDTA
_____ **3.** Used for glucose testing
_____ **4.** Contains citrate
_____ **5.** Contains heparin
_____ **6.** Tube is empty
_____ **7.** Used for coagulation tests
_____ **8.** Contains sodium fluoride
_____ **9.** Used for hematology testing

10. State three ways blood samples may be obtained (3 points).

a. ______________________________

b. ______________________________

c. ______________________________

11. State two reasons a syringe and needle may be used to draw a blood sample (2 points).

a. ______________________________

b. ______________________________

12. List two serious illnesses caused by contaminated needles and materials (2 points).

a. ______________________________

b. ______________________________

13. Label the following diagram of the veins in an arm (3 points).

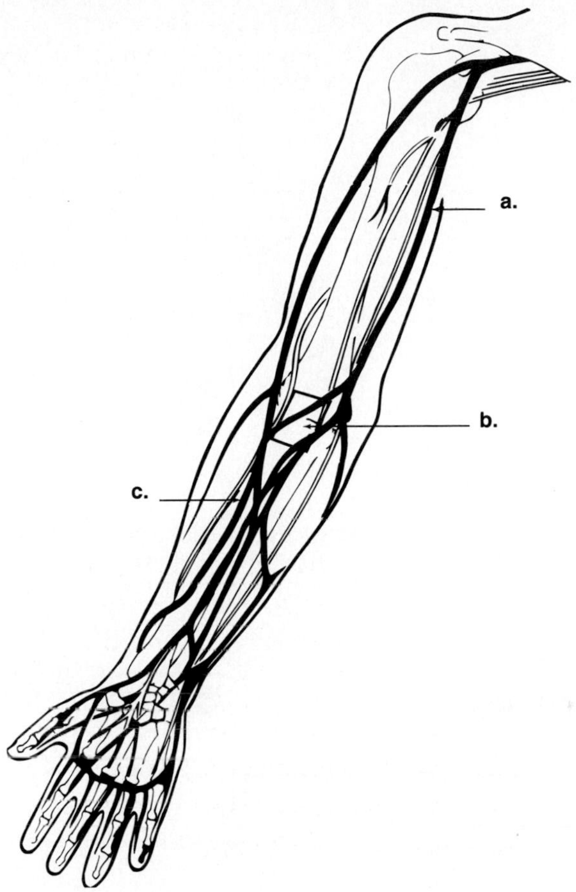

a. ______________________________

b. ______________________________

c. ______________________________

14. Explain why correct disposal of needles, syringes, and contaminated material is important (2 points).

____

____

____

There are 21 possible points in this worksheet.

Chapter 19 Physical Therapy Aide

• OBJECTIVES

When you have completed this unit, you will be able to do the following:

- Complete all objectives in Part One of this book.
- Describe the responsibilities of a physical therapy aide.
- Name four conditions treated with ultraviolet light.
- Describe four conditions treated with diathermy.
- Explain the physical therapy aide's main responsibility when setting up a patient for a diathermy treatment.
- List three conditions commonly treated by ultrasound.
- Document the most important question to ask a patient when preparing for an ultrasound treatment.
- Identify two kinds of thermotherapy and the conditions they treat.
- Identify two ways to give cryotherapy and the conditions they treat.
- Define *hydrotherapy* and list the three reasons hydrotherapy is used.
- Define *guarding technique* and *guarding belt.*
- Explain the purpose of range of motion (Chapter 15).
- List five commonly used ambulation devices.
- List two commonly used transporting devices (Chapter 15).
- Demonstrate each procedure in this chapter.
  - Demonstrate the following from Chapter 15:
    Pivot transfer from bed to wheelchair and back
    Sliding from bed to gurney and back
    Moving a resident on a gurney
    Lifting with a mechanical lift
    Moving a resident in a wheelchair
    Range of motion

- Demonstrate the following from Chapter 22: Customer service

• DIRECTIONS

1. Read this chapter.
2. Complete Worksheet 1.
3. Complete Worksheet/Activity 2 as assigned.
4. Demonstrate all procedures.
5. When you are confident that you can meet all of the objectives listed above, ask your instructor for the unit evaluation.

• EVALUATION METHODS

- Worksheets/Activities
- Class participation
- Written evaluation
- Return demonstrations

• WORKSHEET 1

1. Place an *X* next to the duties of a physical therapy aide (8 points).

_____ Suction the mouth	_____ Prepare equipment
_____ Feed the client	_____ Prepare hot packs
_____ Clean work area	_____ Give medication
_____ Position client	_____ Clean equipment
_____ Prepare paraffin baths	_____ Daily census
_____ Fold linen	_____ Assist client to dress and undress
_____ Take x-rays	_____ Prepare food

2. Describe the responsibilities of a physical therapy aide (5 points).

____

____

____

____

3. List four conditions for which ultraviolet light treatments are used (4 points).

   a. ____

   b. ____

   c. ____

   d. ____

4. List four conditions for which diathermy treatments are often used (4 points).

   a. ____________________

   b. ____________________

   c. ____________________

   d. ____________________

5. Describe in your own words what diathermy treatments do to the treated area (2 points).

   ____

   ____

   ____

6. Explain the physical therapy aide's main responsibility when setting up a client for a diathermy treatment (5 points).

   ____

   ____

   ____

7. List the three conditions commonly treated by ultrasound (3 points).

   a. ____________________

   b. ____________________

   c. ____________________

8. State the most important question a client must be asked when being prepared for an ultrasound treatment (1 point).

   ____

9. Define the following terms (3 points):

   a. hydrotherapy ____________________

   b. guarding technique ____________________

   c. guarding belt ____________________

10. Explain the purpose of range of motion (5 points). ____________________

    ____

    ____

11. Name two ways range of motion can be done (2 points).

    a. ____________________

    b. ____________________

12. Define adaptive devices (2 points). ____________________

    ____

    ____

There are 44 possible points in this worksheet.

• WORKSHEET/ACTIVITY 2

1. Locate the Policy and Procedure Book for your training site. What are your duties as a student physical therapy helper/aide?

____

____

____

____

____

2. Why are your duties written in a Policy and Procedure Book?

____

____

____

____

____

____

3. Does your understanding of what you are able to do protect the patient? How?

____

____

____

____

____

There are 30 points in this worksheet/activity.

Check-off Sheet:

19-5 Walking with a Cane

Name ______________________________ **Date** ______________

Directions: Practice this procedure, following each step. When you are ready to have your performance evaluated, give this sheet to your instructor. Review the detailed procedure in your textbook.

Procedure	Pass	Redo	Date Competency Met	Instructor Initials
Student must use Standard Precautions.	☐	☐	______	______
1. Wash hands.	☐	☐	______	______
2. Assemble equipment:				
a. Cane in good repair and with rubber tip	☐	☐	______	______
b. Client's footwear	☐	☐	______	______
c. Client's robe	☐	☐	______	______
3. Identify client.	☐	☐	______	______
4. Assist client with shoes and robe.	☐	☐	______	______
5. Explain what you are going to do.	☐	☐	______	______
6. Position client in a standing position (have a co-worker help you, if necessary).	☐	☐	______	______
7. Check height of cane. Top of cane should be at the client's hip joint.	☐	☐	______	______
8. Check arm position at side of body and holding top of cane. Arm should be bent at a 25° to 30° angle.	☐	☐	______	______
9. Have client hold cane in hand on stronger side of body (unaffected side).	☐	☐	______	______
10. Assist client as needed while ambulating:				
a. With cane in hand on stronger side, move cane and weaker foot forward.	☐	☐	______	______
b. Place the body weight forward on cane and move stronger foot forward.	☐	☐	______	______
11. When you have completed ordered ambulation, return client to the starting place.	☐	☐	______	______
12. Provide for client's comfort.	☐	☐	______	______

Procedure	Pass	Redo	Date Competency Met	Instructor Initials
13. Place cane in proper location. If client is capable and physician permits ambulation without assistance, leave cane in a convenient place for client.	☐	☐	______	______
14. Wash hands.	☐	☐	______	______
15. Report and document client's tolerance of procedure:				
a. Date	☐	☐	______	______
b. Time	☐	☐	______	______
c. Ambulated with cane (e.g., 15 minutes in hall)	☐	☐	______	______
d. How tolerated	☐	☐	______	______
e. Signature and classification	☐	☐	______	______

Check-off Sheet:
19-6 Walking with Crutches

Name ____ **Date** ______________

Directions: Practice this procedure, following each step. When you are ready to have your performance evaluated, give this sheet to your instructor. Review the detailed procedure in your textbook.

Procedure	Pass	Redo	Date Competency Met	Instructor Initials
Student must use Standard Precautions.	☐	☐	______	______
1. Wash hands.	☐	☐	______	______
2. Assemble equipment:				
a. Crutches in good repair with rubber tips	☐	☐	______	______
b. Client's footwear	☐	☐	______	______
c. Client's robe, if necessary	☐	☐	______	______
3. Identify client.	☐	☐	______	______
4. Explain what you are going to do.	☐	☐	______	______
5. Help client with shoes and robe.	☐	☐	______	______
6. Check fit of crutches to client.				
a. Have client stand with crutches in place.	☐	☐	______	______
b. Position foot of crutches about 4 inches to side of client's foot and slightly forward of foot.	☐	☐	______	______
c. Check distance between underarm and crutch underarm rest. It should be about 2 inches.	☐	☐	______	______
d. Check angle of client's arm. When hand is on hand rest bar and crutches are in walking position, arms should be at a 30° angle.	☐	☐	______	______
7. Remind client that the hands, not the underarms (axillae), support most of the body weight.	☐	☐	______	______
8. Assist client to ambulate following gait method ordered. There are a variety of crutch walking gaits:				
a. Three-point gait (beginners)				
(1) One leg is weight-bearing.	☐	☐	______	______

Procedure	Pass	Redo	Date Competency Met	Instructor Initials
(2) Place both crutches forward along with nonweight-bearing foot.	☐	☐	______	______
(3) Shift weight to *hands* on crutches and move weight-bearing foot forward.	☐	☐	______	______
b. Four-point gait (beginners)				
(1) Both legs are weight-bearing.	☐	☐	______	______
(2) Place one crutch forward.	☐	☐	______	______
(3) Move foot on opposite side of body forward, parallel with forward crutch.	☐	☐	______	______
(4) Place other crutch forward and parallel with first crutch.	☐	☐	______	______
(5) Move other foot forward so that it rests next to first foot.	☐	☐	______	______
c. Two-point gait (advanced)				
(1) Both legs are weight-bearing.	☐	☐	______	______
(2) Place one crutch forward and move opposite foot forward with it.	☐	☐	______	______
(3) Place other crutch forward and parallel with first crutch.	☐	☐	______	______
(4) Move opposite foot forward so that it is even with other foot.	☐	☐	______	______
d. Swing-to gait (arm and shoulder strength are needed)				
(1) One or both legs are weight-bearing.	☐	☐	______	______
(2) Balance weight on weight-bearing limb.	☐	☐	______	______
(3) Place both crutches forward.	☐	☐	______	______
(4) Shift weight to *hands* on crutches.	☐	☐	______	______
(5) Swing both feet forward until parallel with crutches.	☐	☐	______	______
e. Swing-through gait (advanced: arm and shoulder strength are needed)				
(1) One or both legs are weight-bearing.	☐	☐	______	______
(2) Balance weight on weight-bearing limb(s).	☐	☐	______	______
(3) Place both crutches forward.	☐	☐	___	___

Procedure	Pass	Redo	Date Competency Met	Instructor Initials
(4) Shift weight to *hands* on crutches.	☐	☐	______	______
(5) Swing both feet forward just ahead of crutches.	☐	☐	______	______
9. Return to room.	☐	☐	______	______
10. Ensure that client is comfortable.	☐	☐	______	______
11. Wash hands.	☐	☐	______	______
12. Record:				
a. Date	☐	☐	______	______
b. Time	☐	☐	______	______
c. Distance ambulated	☐	☐	______	______
d. How tolerated	☐	☐	______	______
e. Signature and classification	☐	☐	______	______

Check-off Sheet:

19-7 Walking with a Walker

Name ______________________________ Date ______________

Directions: Practice this procedure, following each step. When you are ready to have your performance evaluated, give this sheet to your instructor. Review the detailed procedure in your textbook.

Procedure	Pass	Redo	Date Competency Met	Instructor Initials
Student must use Standard Precautions.	☐	☐	______	______
1. Wash hands.	☐	☐	______	______
2. Assemble equipment:				
a. Walker in good condition	☐	☐	______	______
b. Client's footwear	☐	☐	______	______
c. Client's robe, if necessary	☐	☐	______	______
3. Identify client.	☐	☐	______	______
4. Tell client what you are going to do.	☐	☐	______	______
5. Stand client up with walker. (Ask a co-worker to help, if necessary.)	☐	☐	______	______
6. Check to see if walker fits client properly.				
a. Walker's handgrips should be at top of client's leg or bend of leg at hip joint.	☐	☐	______	______
b. Arm should be at a 25° to 30° angle.	☐	☐	______	______
7. Assist client to ambulate as ordered. Basic guidelines for walking with a walker are:				
a. Client begins by standing inside frame of walker.	☐	☐	______	______
b. Client lifts walker and places back legs of walker parallel with toes.	☐	☐	______	______
c. Client shifts weight onto hands and walker.	☐	☐	______	______
d. Client then walks into walker.	☐	☐	______	______
e. Place yourself just to the side and slightly behind client.	☐	☐	______	______
8. When you have completed the ordered ambulation, return client to his or her starting place.	☐	☐	______	______

Procedure	Pass	Redo	Date Competency Met	Instructor Initials
9. Provide for client's comfort.	☐	☐	______	______
10. Place walker in proper location.	☐	☐	______	______
11. Wash hands.				
12. Report and document client's tolerance of procedure:				
a. Date	☐	☐	______	______
b. Time	☐	☐	______	______
c. Distance and amount of time ambulated	☐	☐	______	______
d. How tolerated	☐	☐	______	______
e. Signature and classification	☐	☐	______	______

Chapter 20 Central Supply/Central Processing Worker

• OBJECTIVES

When you have completed this unit, you will be able to do the following:

- Complete all objectives in Part One of this book.
- Complete vocabulary words in the crossword puzzle.
- Describe the responsibilities of a central supply/central processing department worker.
- Describe the subdepartments of central supply/central processing.
- Identify six categories of cleaning agents with their specific functions.
- List items of appropriate clothing to be worn in decontamination, preparation, sterilization, and inventory areas.
- List three methods of packaging items.
- List two types of sterilization and explain two important things to remember about each.
- Select items that require special care during sterilization.
- Demonstrate proficiency in each procedure pertinent to central supply/central processing.

• DIRECTIONS

1. Complete Worksheet 1 before beginning reading.
2. Read this chapter.
3. Complete Worksheets 2 and 3 as assigned.
4. Complete Worksheet/Activity 4.
5. Complete Worksheet/Activity 5.
6. Use the skills check-off sheets to practice and demonstrate all procedures in this chapter.
7. Prepare responses to each item listed in the Chapter Review—Your Link to Success at the end of this chapter.
8. When you are confident that you can meet all of the objectives listed above, ask your instructor for the unit evaluation.

• EVALUATION METHODS

- Worksheets/Activities
- Class participation
- Written evaluation
- Return demonstrations

• WORKSHEET 1

Fill in the crossword puzzle using words from the glossary of your text and the clues on the following page (25 points).

Indicates space between two words

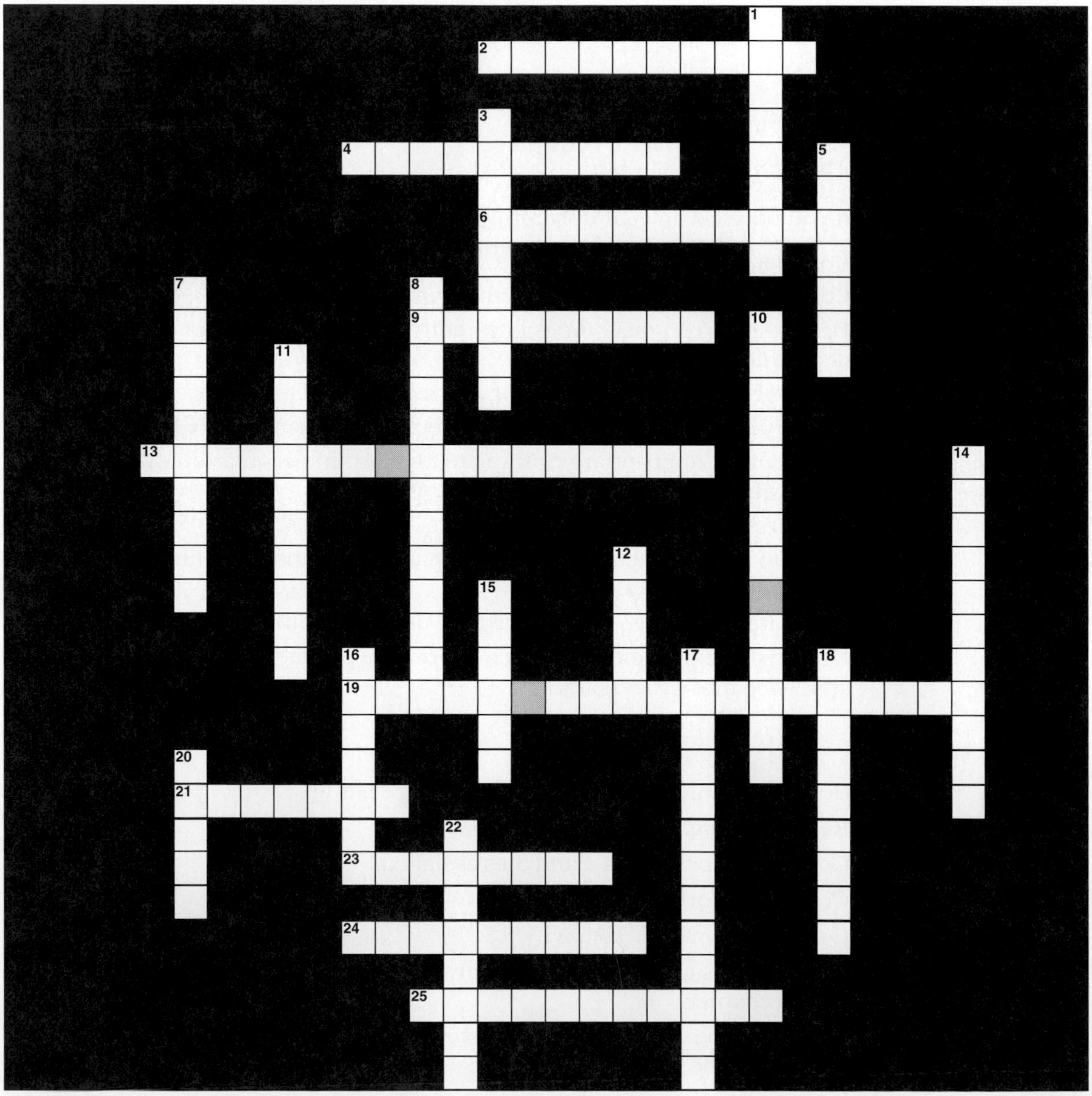

Clues

Across

2. Made a hole.
4. To put in various places.
6. To increase strength.
9. The special things needed for a task.
13. The method used to make the environment, the worker, and the patient as germ free as possible.
19. Use of steam at high pressure for a period of time so that microorganisms are killed.
21. A release of a substance through a vent or channel.
23. Mixture of substances.
24. Withstanding or being stronger than.
25. Movement from place to place.

Down

1. Describing the matter remaining after a process is complete.
3. The method used to accomplish a desired result.
5. Free of all living microorganisms.
7. Can be thrown away after use.
8. To rid of a harmful substance.
10. Gas that destroys microorganisms.
11. A tool used for delicate work.
12. Repeat process over a period of time.
14. What microorganisms do in contacting an area that is free of microorganisms.
15. Insects, bugs, or small animals.
16. State of being free from disease-producing microorganisms.
17. Living organism that can be seen only with the aid of a microscope.
18. Soaked through.
20. Abbreviation for *decontamination*.
22. Moisture.

There are 25 possible points to this worksheet.

• WORKSHEET 2

1. Place an *X* next to the correct duties of a central supply/central processing worker (9 points).

_____ Answer telephone calls
_____ Wash linen
_____ Type reports
_____ Clean instruments
_____ Maintain census sheet
_____ Operate autoclaves
_____ Maintain inventory
_____ Perform electrocardiograms
_____ Record charges and maintain files
_____ Clean floors
_____ Relay and record messages
_____ Maintain accurate files
_____ Assemble and wrap procedure trays
_____ Prepare medication
_____ Deliver supplies
_____ Admit clients
_____ Use antiseptic solutions
_____ Deliver kitchen supplies

2. Describe the responsibilities of the central supply/central processing worker (6 points).

____

____

____

There are 15 possible points in this worksheet.

• WORKSHEET 3

1. Describe the decontamination, preparation, sterilization, and inventory and distribution areas of central supply/central processing (8 points).

   a. Decontamination area _______________________

   ____

   b. Preparation area _______________________

   ____

   c. Sterilization area _______________________

   ____

   d. Inventory and distribution area _______________________

   ____

2. List six categories of cleaning agents and their specific functions (12 points).

Categories	Function
a. ______________	______________
b. ______________	______________
c. ______________	______________
d. ______________	______________
e. ______________	______________
f. ______________	______________

3. List items of appropriate clothing to be worn in the preparation area (3 points).

   a. ____

   b. ____

   c. ____

4. List three methods of packaging items (3 points).

   a. ____

   b. ____

   c. ____

5. List types of autoclaving and explain two important things to remember about each (6 points).

   a. ____
   ____
   ____

   b. ____
   ____
   ____

6. List items that require special care during sterilization (3 points).

   a. ____

   b. ____

   c. ____

There are 35 possible points in this worksheet.

• WORKSHEET/ACTIVITY 4

1. Set up a decontamination area and a preparation area.
2. Use a barrier and a window (cardboard covered with contact paper with an opening 2 feet by 2 1/2 feet works well).
3. Wear decontamination PPE.
4. Select the proper cleaning agent (empty bottle with cleaning agent labels).
5. Clean the instruments.
6. Pass the decontaminated items through the "window" to the clean area.
7. Change PPE when moving from the decontaminated area into the preparation area.

There are 100 possible points in this worksheet/activity.

• WORKSHEET/ACTIVITY 5

1. Ask your teacher for two 3-by-5-inch index cards, two square napkins, and one long strip of sterilizer tape.
2. Wrap a card in the napkin in an envelope wrap, then in a square wrap, following the procedure in your book.

There are 50 possible points in this worksheet/activity.

Chapter 21 Environmental Services Technician/ Housekeeper

• OBJECTIVES

When you have completed this unit, you will be able to do the following:

- Complete all objectives in Part One of this book.
- Define vocabulary words.
- Describe the responsibilities of an EVS/housekeeper.
- Match department names with their abbreviations.
- List seven supplies and types of equipment found on a service cart.
- Give two reasons why a service cart is important.
- Define *germicidal solution.*
- List 14 general guidelines to use in the EVS/housekeeping department.
- List five areas to check that are not usually found in your home.
- Describe HAI and explain how to prevent it.
- List seven general rules to follow when you clean a client's room.
- Explain the cleaning process for preparing a room for a new client.
- List seven specialized departments in the hospital.
- Identify the area within a specialized department that requires aseptic cleaning.
- Explain why it is important to keep all public areas clean and attractive.
- List duties required in the linen area.
- Differentiate between general cleaning, cleaning special areas, and cleaning sterile areas.
- Demonstrate each procedure pertinent to an EVS/housekeeper.

• DIRECTIONS

1. Read this chapter.
2. Complete Worksheets 1 through 3.
3. Complete Worksheets/Activities 4 through 6.
4. Practice all procedures in this chapter until you are proficient.
5. When you are confident that you can meet all of the objectives listed above, ask your instructor for the unit evaluation.

• EVALUATION METHODS

- Worksheets/Activities
- Class participation
- Demonstrated competency of procedures
- Written evaluation
- Written report

• WORKSHEET 1

Place an *X* next to the duties of an EVS/housekeeper (11 points).

_____ Type
_____ Answer telephones
_____ Disinfect
_____ Hang draperies
_____ Wash dishes
_____ Load service cart
_____ Replenish soap, towels
_____ Sweep, mop
_____ Prepare food
_____ Wash ceilings
_____ Empty trash
_____ Clean
_____ Wash windows
_____ Vacuum
_____ Polish floor

There are 11 possible points in this worksheet.

• WORKSHEET 2

Match the correct department name or definition in Column B with the abbreviation or word in column A (18 points).

Column A

____ **1.** Kick bucket
____ **2.** IV pole
____ **3.** Mayo stand
____ **4.** ER
____ **5.** EKG/ECG
____ **6.** EVS
____ **7.** Lab
____ **8.** X-ray
____ **9.** Ortho
____ **10.** OB
____ **11.** Med-Surg
____ **12.** Dietary

Column B

a. Neurology.
b. Emergency room.
c. Radiology.
d. Gynecology.
e. Food service.
f. Occupational therapy.
g. Bucket on wheels.
h. Rehabilitation.
i. Pole to hang intravenous fluid on.
j. Electrocardiology.
k. Laboratory.
l. Stand used to hold instruments; the tray is removable and wheels make it easy to move.

____ **13.** PT	**m.** Obstetric.
____ **14.** OT	**n.** Medical-surgical.
____ **15.** CS	**o.** Orthopedics.
____ **16.** Neuro	**p.** Physical therapy.
____ **17.** Rehab	**q.** Central supply.
____ **18.** GYN	**r.** Environmental services.

19. List seven supplies and/or types of equipment that should be on your service cart (7 points).

a. ____________________

b. ____________________

c. ____________________

d. ____________________

e. ____________________

f. ____________________

g. ____________________

20. Give two reasons why a service cart is important (2 points).

a. ____________________

b. ____________________

21. List 14 general guidelines used in the EVS/housekeeping department (14 points).

a. ____________________

b. ____________________

c. ____________________

d. ____________________

e. ____________________

f. ____________________

g. ____________________

h. ____________________

i. ____________________

j. ____________________

k. ____________________

l. ____________________

m. ____________________

n. ____________________

22. Define *germicidal solution* (1 point). ____________________

____

23. Name five areas in medical facilities that you do not have in your home that need cleaning every day (5 points).

a. ____________________

b. ______________________________

c. ______________________________

d. ______________________________

e. ______________________________

24. Explain why it is important to keep all public areas clean and attractive (1 point).

____

____

____

There are 48 possible points in this worksheet.

• WORKSHEET 3

1. What does HAI stand for (1 point)?

____

2. List seven general rules to follow when you clean a patient's room (7 points).

a. ______________________________

____

b. ______________________________

____

c. ______________________________

____

d. ______________________________

____

e. ______________________________

____

f. ______________________________

____

g. ______________________________

____

3. Explain the cleaning process when preparing a room for a new client (3 points).

a. ______________________________

____

b. ______________________________

____

c. ____

____

4. List seven specialized departments (7 points).

a. ____

b. ____

c. ____

d. ____

e. ____

f. ____

g. ____

5. Circle the areas that require aseptic cleaning (3 points).

labor and delivery	lobby	cath lab
nurses' station	pharmacy	front lobby
linen room	surgery suite	restrooms

6. List the duties required in the linen room (7 points).

a. ____

b. ____

c. ____

d. ____

e. ____

f. ____

g. ____

7. Differentiate between general cleaning, cleaning special areas, and cleaning sterile areas (11 points).

____

____

____

____

____

8. Mrs. Jones in room 6 asks you to go to the gift shop and buy her some candy. What will you do, and why (5 points)?

____

____

____

9. There is a large liquid spill in one of the supply rooms. When you go to clean it up, you notice very strong fumes. No one seems to know what spilled. What will you do, and why (5 points)?

____

____

____

10. The nearest area for you to get supplies is about five minutes away. As you check the stock on your service cart, you realize there are missing supplies. You are running behind schedule. What will you do, and why (5 points)?

____

____

____

11. There is a page for you to come immediately to the labor and delivery area to clean up a spill. You just started to wet mop the hallway. What will you do, and why (5 points)?

____

____

____

There are 59 possible points in this worksheet.

• WORKSHEET/ACTIVITY 4

1. Collect pictures of various departments in a medical facility.
2. Glue each picture onto an index card.
3. Write the name of the department on each card.
4. Write what service the department is under (e.g., nursing is therapeutic; medical laboratory is diagnostic).

There are 50 possible points in this worksheet/activity.

• WORKSHEET/ACTIVITY 5

1. Read the labels on five cleaners and identify the difference among a germicidal, a bactericidal, and a bacteriostatic cleaner.
2. List the cleaners in your notebook and explain how they are used.

There are 50 possible points in this worksheet/activity.

• WORKSHEET/ACTIVITY 6

1. Contact three local facilities to see how they handle linen. Do they send out linen that is owned by the facility? Do they have a laundry on site? Do they contract for laundry and linen to be picked up and delivered?
2. Be prepared to discuss the value of each type of linen service.

There are 50 possible points in this worksheet/activity.

Chapter 22 Health Information Technician

• OBJECTIVES

When you have completed this unit, you will be able to do the following:

- Complete all objectives from Part One of this book.
- Match vocabulary words with their correct meanings.
- Explain why customer service is important.
- Differentiate between positive and negative personal appearances.
- Discuss the importance of office appearance.
- Discuss two purposes for writing a letter.
- Explain why a letter is a legal document.
- List nine guidelines when scheduling clients for appointments.
- Describe a tickler file.
- List two kinds of registration forms.
- Discuss the information that is necessary for a medical history form.
- List five filing systems.
- Explain how to reach a "fair dollar amount" for determining fees.
- Define *professional courtesy.*
- Define *insurance assignment.*
- Define *managed care.*
- Differentiate between an HMO, a PPO, and an EPO.
- Define *CPT codes.*
- Define *HCPCS codes.*
- Define *ICD-9 codes.*
- List three types of bookkeeping systems.
- List four items to look for when you receive a check from a client.
- Define *W-4* and *W-2 forms.*
- Match six items that appear on a paycheck.
- Explain how to use a petty cash fund.
- Recognize the difference between medical and administrative supplies.
- Predict what problems might occur if there is no supply ordering procedure.

- Identify the questions to ask regarding business equipment.
- Demonstrate:
  - Looking professional
  - Scheduling appointments
  - Scheduling a new client: first-time visit
  - Scheduling an outpatient diagnostic test
  - Using a pegboard for charges and services
  - Keeping track of petty cash
  - Writing a letter in three styles

• DIRECTIONS

1. Complete vocabulary Worksheet 1.
2. Read this chapter.
3. Complete Worksheets 2 through 4 as directed by your instructor.
4. Ask your instructor for directions to complete Worksheet/Activity 5.
5. Complete Worksheets 6 through 8 and Worksheet/Activity 9 as assigned by your instructor.
6. Practice and demonstrate procedures P22-1 through P22-8 in this chapter.
7. Prepare responses to each item listed in the Chapter Review—Your Link to Success at the end of this chapter.
8. When you are confident that you can meet each objective for this unit, ask your instructor for the unit evaluation.

• EVALUATION METHODS

- Worksheets/Activities
- Class participation
- Written evaluation
- Return demonstrations

• WORKSHEET 1

1. Give an example of when you received good customer service. Explain what made the service good (2 points). ______________________________

____

____

2. Give an example of when you received poor customer service. Explain what made the service poor (2 points). ______________________________

____

____

3. Describe the perception you think others have of you based on how you look (2 points). ______________________________

____

____

4. What will you have to do to your image to give the perception of professionalism (2 points)? ______________________________

____

____

5. Think back to the last time you were in a medical facility. Describe the judgments you made based on what you saw during that visit (2 points).

____

____

____

____

6. Describe observations of a medical environment that give positive feelings (2 points). ______________________________

____

____

7. List five things that you would change in a negative medical environment to make visiting it a positive experience (5 points).

   a. ______________________________

   b. ______________________________

   c. ______________________________

   d. ______________________________

   e. ______________________________

8. Describe why each of the following is a good form of nonverbal body language (3 points).

   a. Maintaining eye contact ______________________________

   ____

   b. Smiling ______________________________

   ____

   c. Maintaining an open stance ______________________________

   ____

9. Name four guidelines to follow when preparing a letter, and explain why each is important (8 points).

   a. ______________________________

   ____

   b. ______________________________

   ____

   c. ______________________________

   ____

   d. ______________________________

   ____

10. Name five items in a block-style letter and where each is located (10 points).

a. ______________________________

b. ______________________________

c. ______________________________

d. ______________________________

e. ______________________________

11. Explain why a letter to a client is considered a legal document (2 points).

____

____

There are 40 possible points in this worksheet.

• WORKSHEET 2

1. List five guidelines to follow when scheduling an appointment, and explain why each is important (10 points).

a. ______________________________

b. ______________________________

c. ______________________________

d. ______________________________

e. ______________________________

2. List the six questions you will ask a new client when scheduling an appointment (6 points).

a. ______________________________

b. ______________________________

c. ______________________________

d. ______________________________

e. ______________________________

f. ______________________________

3. List the information you will give a new client when scheduling an appointment (5 points).

a. ______________________________

b. ______________________________

c. ______________________________

d. ______________________________

e. ______________________________

There are 21 possible points in this worksheet.

• WORKSHEET 3

Select a procedure (e.g., IVP, UGI, BE) that may be scheduled on an outpatient basis. Call a radiology center to get the answers to the following questions.

1. How long does the procedure take? ______
2. What does the client need to do prior to the procedure? ______
3. What time does the client need to arrive at the hospital? ______
4. Where is the x-ray department located? ______
5. What admitting information does the client need to bring? ______
6. When will the procedure report be sent to the provider? ______
7. What information do you need to give the hospital about the client? ______

There are 70 possible points in this worksheet.

• WORKSHEET 4

1. What does the client information form ask for (3 points)?
2. What is the purpose of the medical history form (2 points)?
3. List the information required on the client information form (5 points).
   - a. ______
   - b. ______
   - c. ______
   - d. ______
   - e. ______
4. Call a medical facility or office and ask the following questions (10 points):
   - a. How often is registration information updated? ______
   - b. Why are registration forms routinely updated? ______

There are 20 possible points in this worksheet.

• WORKSHEET/ACTIVITY 5

Match each definition in column B with the correct vocabulary word in column A (8 points).

Column A	*Column B*
____ **1.** Geographic	**a.** Assigning a color.
____ **2.** Numerical	**b.** Order of occurrence.
____ **3.** Alphabetical	**c.** Order by location.
____ **4.** Color coding	**d.** In number order.
____ **5.** Chronological	**e.** Using the alphabet.
____ **6.** Sorting	**f.** Items belonging in a category.
____ **7.** Coding	**g.** Placement according to some system.
____ **8.** Indexing	**h.** Order in which items are filed.

9. Place the numbers in column A in the correct numerical order in column B (10 points).

Column A	**Column B**
236	____________
443	____________
198	____________
245	____________
822	____________
323	____________
543	____________
189	____________
637	____________
935	____________

10. Place the names in column A in correct alphabetical order in column B (10 points).

Column A	**Column B**
Carter	____________
Doors	____________
Dwight	____________
Mitchell	____________
Bradley	____________
Goulle	____________
Christensen	____________
Spencer	____________
Salanger	____________
Lobb	____________

11. Place the names in column A in the correct alphabetical order in column B (12 points).

Column A	**Column B**
Alec Monroe Goldman	________________
Todd C. Sherman	________________
Kellie Bell-White	________________
Timothy Gallagher O'Bannon	________________
Carlos A. DeLeon	________________
Saint Edward	________________
Father Gerald	________________
Queen Erin	________________
Princess Monica	________________
DeeAnn Sherman, M.D.	________________
Kiley Marie Goldman	________________
Steven Edward Gustov	________________

12. Place the numbers in column A in the correct numerical order in column B (10 points).

Column A	**Column B**
0535.60	________________
0935.90	________________
0931.60	________________
0933.80	________________
0932.90	________________
0536.80	________________
0935.60	________________
0937.80	________________
432.80	________________
879.90	________________

13. Using the chronological filing system, place the dates in column A in the correct order in column B (6 points).

Column A	**Column B**
April 8, 1973: Pablo Picasso, one of the greatest artists of the twentieth century, dies.	________________
April 4, 1983: The *Challenger* space shuttle makes its first flight.	________________
January 25, 1971: The U.S. Supreme Court bars discrimination.	________________
August 9, 1974: Richard Nixon resigns as President of the United States.	________________
	________________
	________________

Column A (*cont*)
December 22, 1970: The U.S. Supreme Court rules that 18-year-olds can vote.
December 2, 1982: Barney Clark undergoes the first artificial heart surgery.

There are 56 possible points in this worksheet/activity.

• WORKSHEET 6

1. What is a fee (1 point)? ______________________________

2. Name three resources to check when setting fees at a fair dollar amount (3 points).

   a. ______________________________

   b. ______________________________

   c. ______________________________

Match each definition in column B with the correct vocabulary word in Column A (12 points).

Column A	*Column B*
____ 3. Capitation	a. A discount or no charge extended to a medical professional.
____ 4. Professional courtesy	b. Cost-effective manner of providing medical service.
____ 5. Current procedural terminology	c. Payment to a medical provider per member on a monthly basis.
____ 6. Managed care	d. Plan requires client to see only contracted providers.
____ 7. Accepting assignment	e. Plan pays 90–100 percent.
____ 8. Health maintenance organization	f. Identification of medical services and procedures.
____ 9. International Classification of Disease	g. Alphanumeric code beginning with a letter.
____ 10. Preferred provider organization	h. Identification of diagnosis.
____ 11. Health Common Procedure Coding System	i. Accepting what the insurance allows.
____ 12. Exclusive provider organization	j. Plan requiring client to select a primary care provider.

13. List the questions a billing policy will answer (6 points).

a. ______

b. ______

c. ______

d. ______

e. ______

f. ______

14. Write each term listed below in the space next to the phrase that illustrates it (6 points).

CPT ICD-9-CM HCPCS

a. Describes supplies, material, and services. ______
b. Five-digit alphanumeric. ______
c. Required by Medicare and Medicaid. ______
d. Describes procedures, services, and supplies. ______
e. Three- to five-digit numeric. ______
f. Accepted and required by all insurance carriers. ______

15. Define *delinquent accounts* (1 point). ______

______

16. List the questions to ask regarding a collection policy (4 points).

a. ______

b. ______

c. ______

d. ______

There are 33 possible points in this worksheet.

• WORKSHEET 7

1. Explain what is recorded by a bookkeeping system (2 points).

______

______

______

2. List the material used with the single-entry bookkeeping system (4 points).

a. ______

b. ______

c. ______

d. ______

3. List the information entered on the superbill (4 points).

a. ______________________________

b. ______________________________

c. ______________________________

d. ______________________________

4. List the four items to verify when receiving a check from a client (4 points).

a. ______________________________

b. ______________________________

c. ______________________________

d. ______________________________

There are 14 possible points in this worksheet.

• WORKSHEET 8

Match the definition in column B with the correct vocabulary word in column A (4 points).

Column A	*Column B*
_____ 1. W-4	a. Gross and net pay
_____ 2. Time card	b. Rate of pay and hours worked
_____ 3. Payroll register	c. Actual work time
_____ 4. Employee earnings record	d. Number of exemptions designated by employee

5. List the information on the W-2 form (5 points).

a. ______________________________

b. ______________________________

c. ______________________________

d. ______________________________

e. ______________________________

6. When does an employer need to send a W-2 form to each employee (2 points)?

a. ______________________________

b. ______________________________

7. List the guidelines to follow when setting up a petty cash fund (5 points).

a. ______________________________

b. ______________________________

c. ______________________________

d. ______________________________

e. ______________________________

8. List the steps to follow when replenishing petty cash (4 points).

   a. ______________________________

   b. ______________________________

   c. ______________________________

   d. ______________________________

9. Describe a disbursement form and how it is used (12 points).

   a. ______________________________

   b. ______________________________

   c. ______________________________

   d. ______________________________

   e. ______________________________

   f. ______________________________

10. Place an *M* next to medical supplies and an *A* next to administrative items in the following list (10 points).

_____ **a.** Gloves	_____ **f.** Pens
_____ **b.** Registration forms	_____ **g.** Gowns
_____ **c.** Stationery	_____ **h.** Masks
_____ **d.** Client charts	_____ **i.** Specimen containers
_____ **e.** Exam table sheets	_____ **j.** Gauze

11. List two steps to follow if you unexpectedly run out of gloves (2 points).

   a. ______________________________

   b. ______________________________

12. List four questions to ask regarding a copy machine (4 points).

   a. ______________________________

   b. ______________________________

   c. ______________________________

   d. ______________________________

13. List four questions to ask regarding a fax machine (4 points).

   a. ______________________________

   b. ______________________________

   c. ______________________________

   d. ______________________________

14. List four features a telephone may have (4 points).

   a. ______________________________

   b. ______________________________

   c. ______________________________

   d. ______________________________

There are 56 possible points in this worksheet.

• WORKSHEET/ACTIVITY 9

Your instructor will assign a coding system: CPT, ICD-9-CM, or HCPCS. Write 15 to 25 lines explaining the reason for this coding system and the basics of how it works to a person who knows nothing of it.

There are 25 possible points in this worksheet.

Check-off Sheet:

Looking Professional

Name ______________________________ **Date** ______________

Directions: Practice this procedure, following each step. When you are ready to have your performance evaluated, give this sheet to your instructor. Review the detailed procedure in your textbook.

Procedure	Pass	Redo	Date Competency Met	Instructor Initials
1. Dress according to your facility's dress code.	☐	☐	______	______
2. Jewelry should be kept to a minimum (e.g., watch, stud earrings, and a ring).	☐	☐	______	______
3. Wear your name badge every day, in view of clients.	☐	☐	______	______
4. Wear clean and polished shoes every day.	☐	☐	______	______
5. Keep your hair clean.	☐	☐	______	______
6. Wear your hair up and off your collar.	☐	☐	______	______
7. Use unscented deodorant.	☐	☐	______	______
8. Follow rules for good hygiene:				
a. Brush your teeth at least once a day.	☐	☐	______	______
b. Floss daily.	☐	☐	______	______
c. Use mouthwash or breath mints.	☐	☐	______	______
d. Bathe daily.	☐	☐	______	______
9. Keep your nails short and clean (use light-colored nail polish and repair chips).	☐	☐	______	______
Female				
10. Keep makeup conservative.	☐	☐	______	______
11. Do not use perfume or cologne.	☐	☐	______	______
12. Wear full-length hose without runs.	☐	☐	______	______
Male				
13. Do not use cologne or strong aftershave.	☐	☐	______	______
14. Keep beard or mustache neatly trimmed.	☐	☐	______	______
15. Shave daily. No stubble!	☐	☐	______	______

Chapter 23 Clinical Medical Assistant

• OBJECTIVES

When you have completed this unit, you will be able to do the following:

- Complete all objectives from Part One of this book.
- Match vocabulary words with their correct meanings.
- Measure and record the height and weight of an adult, child, and infant.
- Summarize the importance of measuring the circumference of an infant's head.
- Explain what a drastic change in growth patterns may indicate.
- Explain how to read a visual acuity test and the importance of the results.
- Compare and identify examination positions by name.
- List four basic examination techniques and explain their purposes.
- Compare similarities and differences between a limited and a general physical examination to rule out a condition.
- Identify symptoms of 12 physical conditions and state the appropriate patient education for each.
- Explain two types of pediatric appointment.
- List 13 guidelines to follow when preparing for a surgical procedure.
- Read Chapter 20, Central Supply/Central Processing Worker:
  - Decontamination
  - Preparation area
  - Sterile wraps
  - Sterilization
  - Monitoring effectiveness of sterilization
- Name five public health issues that require an official report with a public agency.
- Match common prescription abbreviations with their meanings.
- Match controlled substances with their assigned schedule level.

- Name four drug reference books.
- Describe methods to ensure safekeeping of medication.
- Write a formula for calculating medication dosage.
- Match metric measures with their equivalent standard measure.
- Name the six "rights" of medication administration.
- Recognize the guidelines for preparing and administering medications.
- Explain why it is important to observe liquid medication and describe what to look for.
- Match the route of administration with its description.
- Explain why injections are given instead of other methods of medication administration.
- Describe body areas where it is not appropriate to give an injection.
- Describe syringe- and needle-handling techniques that prevent accidental needle sticks.
- Recognize different types of parenteral medication containers.
- Name medications commonly administered by the Z-track method.
- Differentiate between intradermal, subcutaneous, intramuscular, and Z-track injections.
- Name and explain the purpose of common immunizations.
- Demonstrate all procedures in this unit.
- Apply all procedural techniques with confidence.

• DIRECTIONS

1. Complete Worksheet 1 before reading this chapter.
2. Read this chapter.
3. Complete Worksheets 3 through 5, 7, 9 through 11, and 13 through 16 as directed by your instructor.
4. Complete Worksheets/Activities 2, 6, 8, and 12 as directed by your instructor.
5. Practice and demonstrate all procedures in this chapter using the skills check-off sheets.
6. Prepare responses to each item listed in the Chapter Review—Your Link to Success at the end of this chapter.
7. When you are confident that you can meet each objective for this unit, ask your instructor for the unit evaluation.

• EVALUATION METHODS

- Worksheets/Activities
- Class participation
- Written evaluation
- Return demonstrations

• WORKSHEET 1

Match each definition in column B with the correct word in column A (38 points).

Column A	*Column B*
1. Circumference	**a.** Clearness or sharpness.
2. Pharmaceutical	**b.** Neck.
3. Administrative	**c.** Not in the digestive system.
4. Acuity	**d.** Distance around.
5. Auscultation	**e.** Pertaining to process, such as handling of paperwork, that assists in client care.
6. Diagnosis	**f.** Having to do with pharmacy.
7. Cervix	**g.** Listening for sounds within the body.
8. Antibiotics	**h.** Opening.
9. Contraceptives	**i.** Identification of a disease or condition.
10. Diuretics	**j.** Substance that provides immunity to a toxin.
11. Parenteral	**k.** Withdrawal of a fluid.
12. Topical	**l.** Weakness or discomfort.
13. Formula	**m.** Liquid added to powder that dissolves the powder.
14. Aspiration	**n.** Adding water to a powdered drug.
15. Reconstituting	**o.** Absence of living organism or inability to produce offspring.
16. Dilutant	**p.** Power or strength to move away or resist.
17. Resistance	**q.** Can be kept from happening.
18. Toxins	**r.** Dead or weakened organisms that stimulate the body to make antibodies.
19. Antibodies	**s.** Poisons.
20. Antigens	**t.** Items that serve to prevent pregnancy.
21. Acquired	**u.** Substances that cause the development of an antibody.
22. Vaccine	**v.** Inflammation of the lungs.
23. Antitoxin	**w.** Substances made by the body that attack foreign bodies or their toxins.
24. Characterized	**x.** Produce the male sex cell.
25. Malaise	**y.** Refers to a condition, disease, or characteristic that began after birth.
26. Paralysis	**z.** Without energy.
27. Epidemic	**aa.** Distinguished by; refers to a trait or quality.
28. Meningitis	**bb.** Inflammation of the joint.
29. Septic	**cc.** Inflammation of the brain.
30. Arthritis	**dd.** Loss of sensation and muscle function.
31. Preventable	
32. Pneumonia	
33. Encephalitis	
34. Gamma globulin	
35. Testicles	

36. Sterility
37. Listless
38. Lumen

ee. Substance that acts as an antibody to increase immunity.
ff. A condition of decay.
gg. Disease that spreads rapidly among people.
hh. Inflammation of the membrane covering the brain.
ii. Surface of the body.
jj. Substances that slow growth of or destroy microorganisms.
kk. Drugs that increase urine output.
ll. Accepted rule.

There are 38 possible points in this worksheet.

• WORKSHEET/ACTIVITY 2

Using a doll, demonstrate to classmates how to measure correctly the weight, length, and head circumference of an infant. Give an explanation of what you are doing and why while you take the measurements.

There are 15 possible points in this worksheet/activity.

• WORKSHEET 3

Place the following information on the growth chart below (12 points).

1. 3 months old, 22″ long, 15 pounds, 38 cm head circumference.
2. 6 months old, 25″ long, 20 pounds, 40 cm head circumference.
3. 12 months old, 30″ long, 28 pounds, 44 cm head circumference.

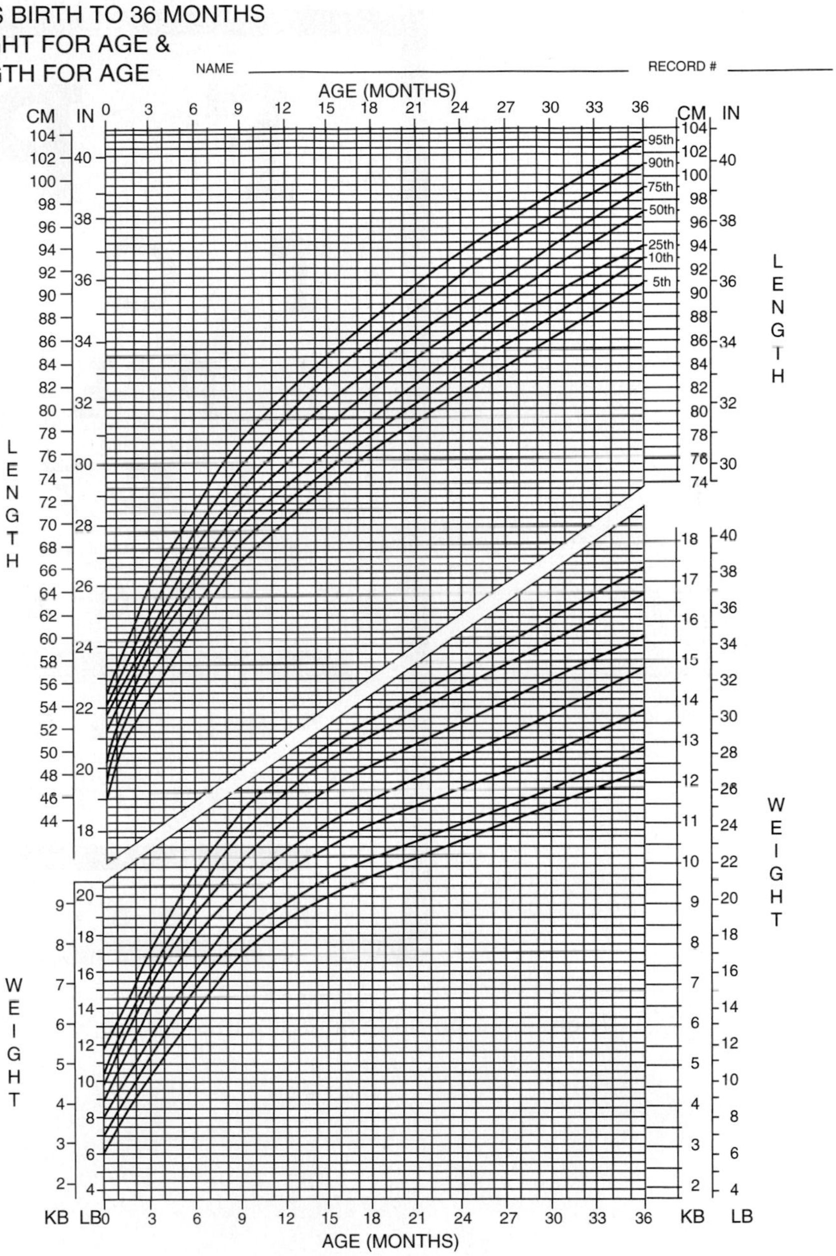

Date	Age in Months	Recumbent Length	Weight	Head Circumference

Department of Health Education, and Welfare, Public Health Service
Health Resources Administration, National Center for Health Statistics, and Center for Disease Control

There are 12 possible points in this worksheet.

• WORKSHEET 4

1. Using the right eye, the patient misses two letters on line 8 and reads all letters in line 7. What is the vision in the right eye (1 point)? ____________

2. Using the left eye, the patient reads all letters in line 5 and misses three letters in line 7 and a letter in line 6. What is the left eye vision (1 point)?

____

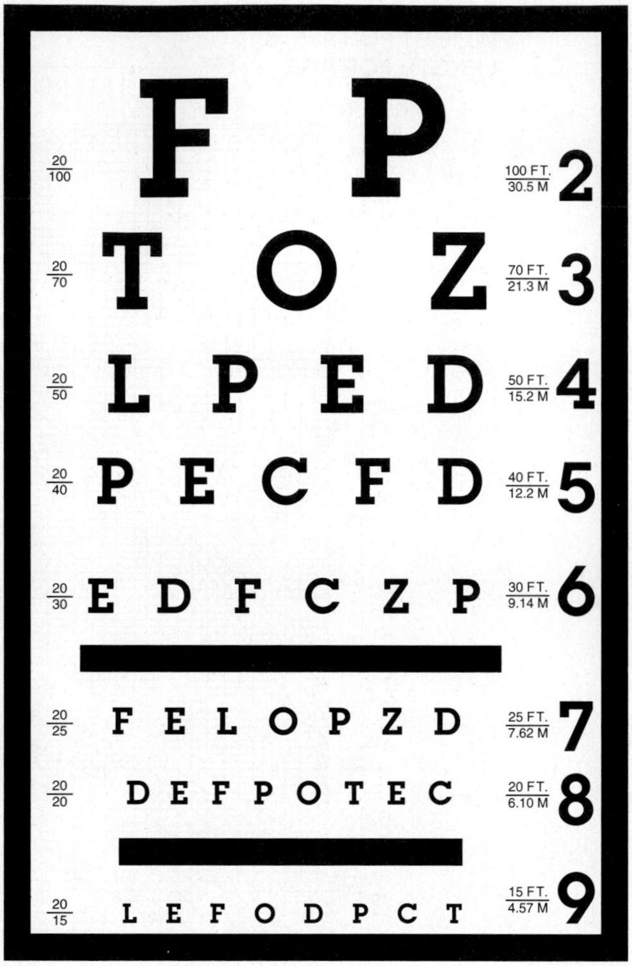

There are 2 possible points in this worksheet.

• WORKSHEET 5

1. Bone size is identified as (3 points):
   a. ______________________________
   b. ______________________________
   c. ______________________________
2. Body weight indicates a person's ____________ status (1 point).
3. A drastic change in the growth pattern can indicate an ____________ (1 point).
4. Vision acuity helps the physician detect ____________ disease (1 point).
5. When a vision acuity test result is 20/50, the top number means that the patient is (a) ____________ (b) ____________ from the chart. The 50 indicates the distance a person with (c) ____________ vision can read that line (3 points).
6. Always follow Standard Precautions to protect yourself when contact with (a) ____________, (b) ____________, nonintact skin, or mucous membrane fluids is possible (2 points).
7. In what risk category are tasks requiring direct contact with blood or other body fluids (1 point)? ____________

There are 12 possible points in this worksheet.

• WORKSHEET/ACTIVITY 6

Find a classmate and role-play filling out a patient questionnaire for the rest of the class. Change roles back and forth between patient and clinical medical assistant. Practice demonstrating a:

- Geriatric client
- Hearing-impaired client
- Mentally disabled client
- Angry client

There are 15 possible points for each participant in this worksheet/activity.

• WORKSHEET 7

Write each word listed below in the space below the picture that illustrates it (6 points).

Dorsal lithotomy	Fowler's	Trendelenburg
Knee-chest	Prone	Left Sim's or left lateral position

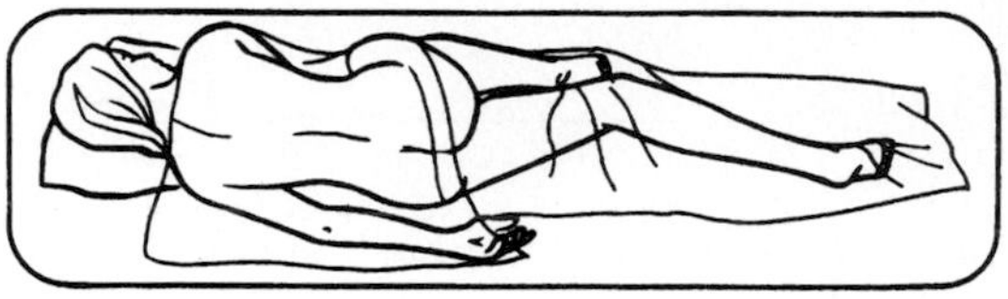

1.______________________________

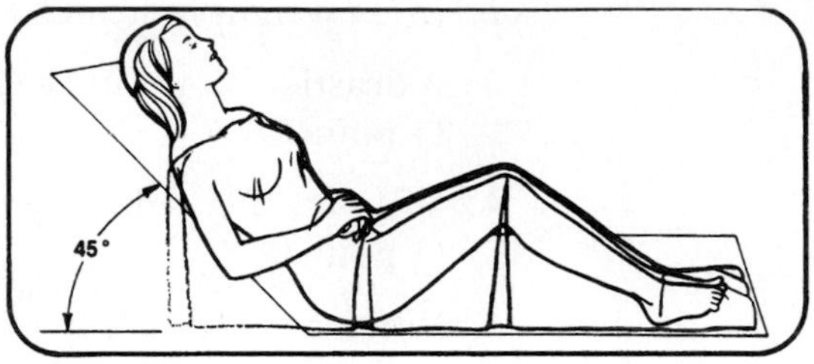

2.______________________________

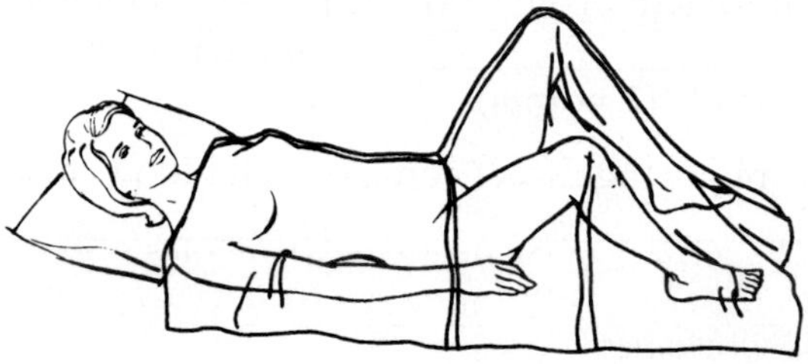

3.______________________________

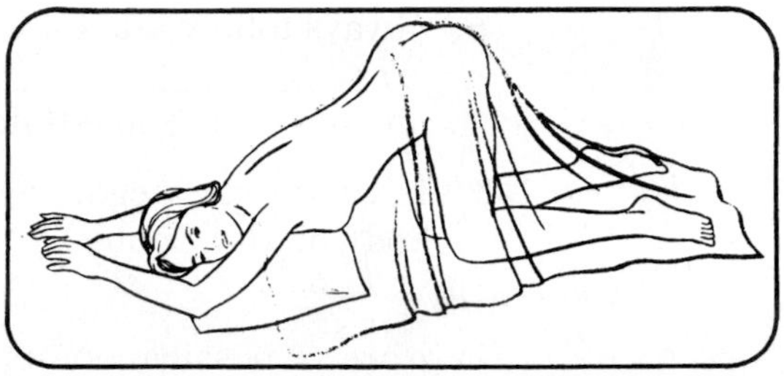

4.______________________________

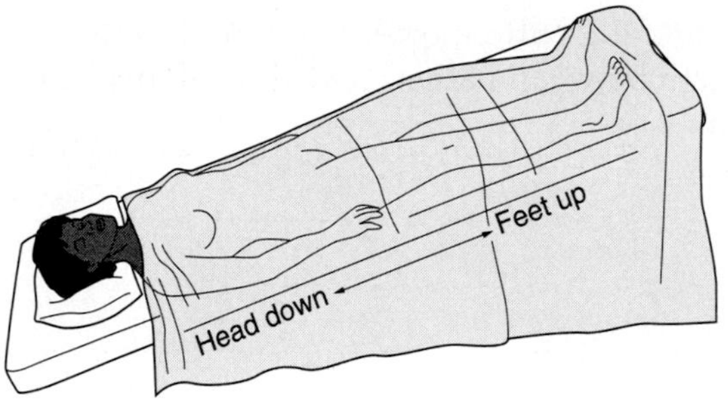

5.______________________________

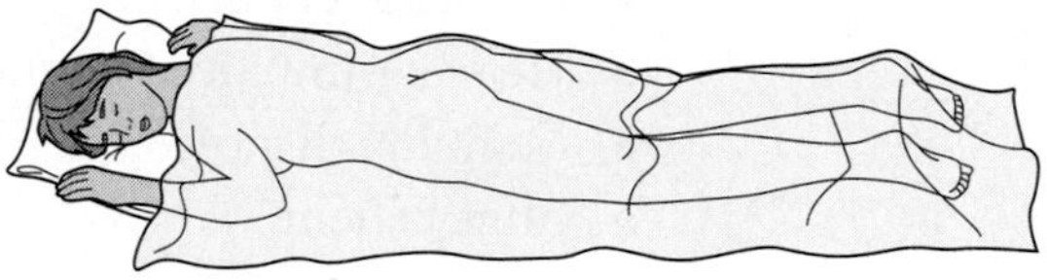

6.______________________________

There are 6 possible points in this worksheet.

• WORKSHEET/ACTIVITY RESOURCES CARD FILE 8

Compile a community resources file on 3-by-5-inch cards with the following information:

Agency name
Address
Telephone number
Services provided

Points are determined by the number of cards filled out.

• WORKSHEET 9

1. Write the examinations, treatments, or surgery the position is used for next to the position names below (9 points).

   a. Horizontal recumbent position ______________________

   b. Fowler's position ______________________

   c. Trendelenburg position ______________________

   d. Dorsal lithotomy position ______________________

   e. Prone position ______________________

   f. Left lateral position ______________________

   g. Sim's position ______________________

   h. Knee-chest position ______________________

   i. Supine position ______________________

2. Explain the following (3 points): ______________________

   a. Rule out (R/O) ______________________

   b. General physical examination ______________________

   c. Client questionnaire ______________________

3. A light eye patch is used to prevent ______________________(1 point).

____

4. Cardiovascular examination focuses on ______________________(1 point).

____

5. Blood tests that tell about the cardiac muscle are (2 points):

a. ____

b. ____

6. A digestive system examination focuses on (2 points): ______________________

____

7. A urinary system examination focuses on (2 points): ______________________

____

8. A male reproductive system examination focuses on (2 points):

____

____

9. A female reproductive system examination focuses on (2 points):

____

____

10. An orthopedic examination focuses on (2 points): ______________________

____

11. Name two types of pediatric appointments (2 points):

a. ____

b. ____

12. Write the 13 guidelines to follow when preparing for a surgical procedure in the office (13 points).

a. ____

b. ____

c. ____

d. ____

e. ____

f. ____

g. ____

h. ____

i. ____

j. ____

k. ____

l. ____

m. ____

13. State the five public health issues that require filing an official report (5 points).

a. ______________________________

b. ______________________________

c. ______________________________

d. ______________________________

e. ______________________________

There are 46 possible points in this worksheet.

• WORKSHEET 10

Match the full term in column B with the abbreviation in column A (29 points).

Column A	*Column B*
_____ **1.** cap(s)	**a.** left eye
_____ **2.** dil	**b.** dextrose in water
_____ **3.** dr	**c.** dram
_____ **4.** D/W	**d.** right eye
_____ **5.** fl or fld	**e.** kilogram
_____ **6.** gal	**f.** tincture
_____ **7.** gt or gtt	**g.** both eyes
_____ **8.** IM	**h.** capsule(s)
_____ **9.** IU	**i.** intramuscular
_____ **10.** IV	**j.** powder
_____ **11.** kg	**k.** gallon
_____ **12.** L	**l.** milliequivalent
_____ **13.** liq	**m.** dilute
_____ **14.** m or min	**n.** fluid
_____ **15.** mcg	**o.** subcutaneous
_____ **16.** mEq	**p.** drop
_____ **17.** mg	**q.** ounce
_____ **18.** ml	**r.** international units
_____ **19.** NS	**s.** liquid
_____ **20.** OD	**t.** ointment
_____ **21.** oint	**u.** liter
_____ **22.** OS	**v.** minim
_____ **23.** OU	**w.** normal saline
_____ **24.** oz	**x.** milligram
_____ **25.** pt	**y.** microgram
_____ **26.** pulv	**z.** intravenous
_____ **27.** sc, subc, subq	**aa.** milliliter
_____ **28.** tinc, tr, tinct	**bb.** pint or patient
_____ **29.** Rx	**cc.** recipe or take

• WORKSHEET 11

Write the letter of the controlled substances schedule listed below next to the appropriate statement. More than one schedule may apply to a statement; include all schedules appropriate for each (20 points).

a. Schedule I **c.** Schedule III **e.** Schedule V

b. Schedule II **d.** Schedule IV

_______________ **1.** Addiction and abuse are limited or not likely.

_______________ **2.** Accepted for medical use in the United States.

_______________ **3.** Marijuana.

_______________ **4.** Low-strength codeine.

_______________ **5.** Limited to approved research.

_______________ **6.** APC with codeine.

_______________ **7.** Drugs are easily addicting and abuse is likely.

_______________ **8.** Chloral hydrate.

_______________ **9.** Butabarbital.

_______________ **10.** Mescaline.

_______________ **11.** Addiction and abuse are possible but less likely.

_______________ **12.** Cocaine.

_______________ **13.** Diazepam.

_______________ **14.** Addiction and abuse are likely.

_______________ **15.** Meperidine.

_______________ **16.** LSD.

_______________ **17.** Methadone.

_______________ **18.** Phenobarbital.

_______________ **19.** Must be witnessed when disposed of.

_______________ **20.** Keep records and inventory that are legally acceptable.

There are 20 possible points in this worksheet.

• WORKSHEET/ACTIVITY 12

Using the PDR reference book, look up three of the following medications and complete the worksheet (27 points).

Zestril	amitriptyline	ibuprofen
Diflunisal	Veetids	Fiorinal with Codeine 3

Medication #1 _______________________

1. Name the resource used _______________________________________

2. Generic name of medication ___________________________________

3. Brand name of medication _____________________________________

4. Color and shape of medication _________________________________

____

5. Dosages ____

6. Frequency of dose ______________________________
7. Side effects ______________________________
8. Indications ______________________________
____
____
9. Contraindications ______________________________
____
____

Medication #2 ____________________

1. Name the resource used ______________________________
2. Generic name of medication ______________________________
3. Brand name of medication ______________________________
4. Color and shape of medication ______________________________
____
5. Dosages ______________________________
6. Frequency of dose ______________________________
7. Side effects ______________________________
8. Indications ______________________________
____
____
9. Contraindications ______________________________
____
____

Medication #3 ____________________

1. Name the resource used ______________________________
2. Generic name of medication ______________________________
3. Brand name of medication ______________________________
4. Color and shape of medication ______________________________
____
5. Dosages ______________________________
6. Frequency of dose ______________________________
7. Side effects ______________________________
8. Indications ______________________________
____
____

9. Contraindications ______________________________

____

____

There are 27 possible points in this worksheet.

• WORKSHEET 13

1. Name the three ways medication and drugs are described (3 points).
   a. ______________________________
   b. ______________________________
   c. ______________________________
2. Name the four most commonly used drug reference books (4 points).
   a. ______________________________
   b. ______________________________
   c. ______________________________
   d. ______________________________
3. State seven ways to ensure the safekeeping of medication (7 points).
   a. ______________________________
   b. ______________________________
   c. ______________________________
   d. ______________________________
   e. ______________________________
   f. ______________________________
   g. ______________________________
4. Write the formula for calculating dosage described in the text (1 point).

   ____
5. Write the six rights of medication administration (6 points).
   a. ______________________________
   b. ______________________________
   c. ______________________________
   d. ______________________________
   e. ______________________________
   f. ______________________________
6. 1 g = ________ gr (1 point).
7. To convert grams to milligrams, move the decimal three places to the ________________ (1 point).

There are 23 possible points in this worksheet.

• WORKSHEET 14

Match the items in column A with column B. Items in column B may be used more than once (20 points).

Column A

1. 1,000 ml
2. 60 mg
3. 4 mL
4. 8 pints
5. 15 mL
6. 240–250 mL
7. 0.5 g
8. 30 g
9. 250 mL
10. buccal
11. inhalation
12. irrigation
13. installation
14. inunction or topical
15. oral
16. parenteral
17. rectal
18. sublingual
19. vaginal
20. 30 mL

Column B

a. 1 fluid ounce.
b. Medication taken by mouth and swallowed.
c. 7 1/2 grains.
d. 8 ounces.
e. Medication applied to skin.
f. 1 grain.
g. Medication applied, inserted, or irrigated into vagina.
h. Medication dropped onto an area.
i. Tablet placed under the tongue to dissolve.
j. 1 L.
k. 8 ounces.
l. 1 gallon.
m. 1/2 ounce.
n. Tablet placed between the gums and cheek.
o. Solution washed through a body cavity or over a membrane.
p. 1 quart.
q. Liquid medications inhaled through nebulizer, respirator, or inhalation device.
r. Medicated solution injected into body tissue and absorbed.
s. Medication solutions or suppositories inserted into the rectum.
t. 1 teaspoon, 1 dram, or 60 drops.
u. 1 ounce.

21. How many times must you read a medication label before giving a medication (1 point)? ______________________

22. When calculating a medication dosage, is it necessary to verify your calculations with a co-worker (1 point)? ______________________

23. What three things are liquid medications observed for (3 points)?

    a. ______________________

    b. ______________________

    c. ______________________

24. When pouring liquid medication, how is the label protected from drips (1 point)? ______________________

25. To achieve an accurate measure of liquid medication, hold the medication cup at ______________ level while pouring (1 point).

26. __________________ the neck of the bottle before recapping (1 point).

27. Never __________________ two or more medications unless ordered (1 point).

28. Never leave medication __________________ (1 point).

29. Watch the patient __________________ the medication (1 point).

30. Never administer medication prepared by __________________ person (1 point).

31. Check with client for __________________ before administering medication (1 point).

32. It is good practice to observe patient for 15 to 20 minutes after administering (4 points):

    a. ______________________________

    b. ______________________________

    c. ______________________________

    d. ______________________________

33. __________________ unused or reused medication (1 point).

There are 38 possible points in this worksheet.

• WORKSHEET 15

1. List five reasons medications are given by injection (5 points).

    a. ______________________________

    b. ______________________________

    c. ______________________________

    d. ______________________________

    e. ______________________________

2. List six places on the body where you should not give injections (6 points).

    a. ______________________________

    b. ______________________________

    c. ______________________________

    d. ______________________________

    e. ______________________________

    f. ______________________________

3. Medication injected just under the skin is an __________________ injection (1 point).

4. Medication injected into the muscle is an __________________ injection (1 point).

5. Medication injected 5/8 to 1 inch into the skin is a __________________ injection (1 point).

6. State five ways to prevent accidental needle sticks (5 points).

a. ______________________________

b. ______________________________

c. ______________________________

d. ______________________________

e. ______________________________

7. Explain the following about ID injections (3 points):

a. Purpose ______________________________

b. Amount ______________________________

c. Common sites ______________________________

8. Explain the following about sub Q injections (3 points):

a. Purpose ______________________________

b. Amount ______________________________

c. Sites ______________________________

9. Explain the following about IM injections (3 points):

a. Purpose ______________________________

b. Amount ______________________________

c. Sites ______________________________

10. Z-track technique is recommended when (3 points):

a. ______________________________

b. ______________________________

c. ______________________________

11. Name the nine medications commonly given with the Z-track method (9 points).

a. ______________________________

b. ______________________________

c. ______________________________

d. ______________________________

e. ______________________________

f. ______________________________

g. ______________________________

h. ______________________________

i. ______________________________

12. Do medical assistants give IV medication (1 point)? ______________

There are 41 possible points in this worksheet.

• WORKSHEET 16

1. List the eight common immunizations (8 points).

a. ______

b. ______

c. ______

d. ______

e. ______

f. ______

g. ______

h. ______

Write the letter of the disease listed below next to the correct statement. Include all diseases appropriate for each. A disease may be used more than once (12 points).

a. pertussis
b. diphtheria
c. tetanus
d. poliomyelitis
e. *Haemophilus influenza B*
f. rubeola
g. mumps
h. rubella

______ **2.** Contagious.

______ **3.** Pregnant women should be notified immediately if exposed to this disease.

______ **4.** Main cause of inflammatory disease in young children.

______ **5.** Produces a false membrane in the throat.

______ **6.** An infection of the central nervous system.

______ **7.** Damaging to the heart and central nervous system.

______ **8.** Cough sounds like a whoop.

______ **9.** Lockjaw.

______ **10.** Pain and paralysis.

______ **11.** Most common in infants and children under four years of age.

______ **12.** German measles.

______ **13.** Preventable by a preparation called gamma globulin.

______ **14.** Glands under the ears swell.

There are 20 possible points in this worksheet.

• MEDICAL INSTRUMENTS

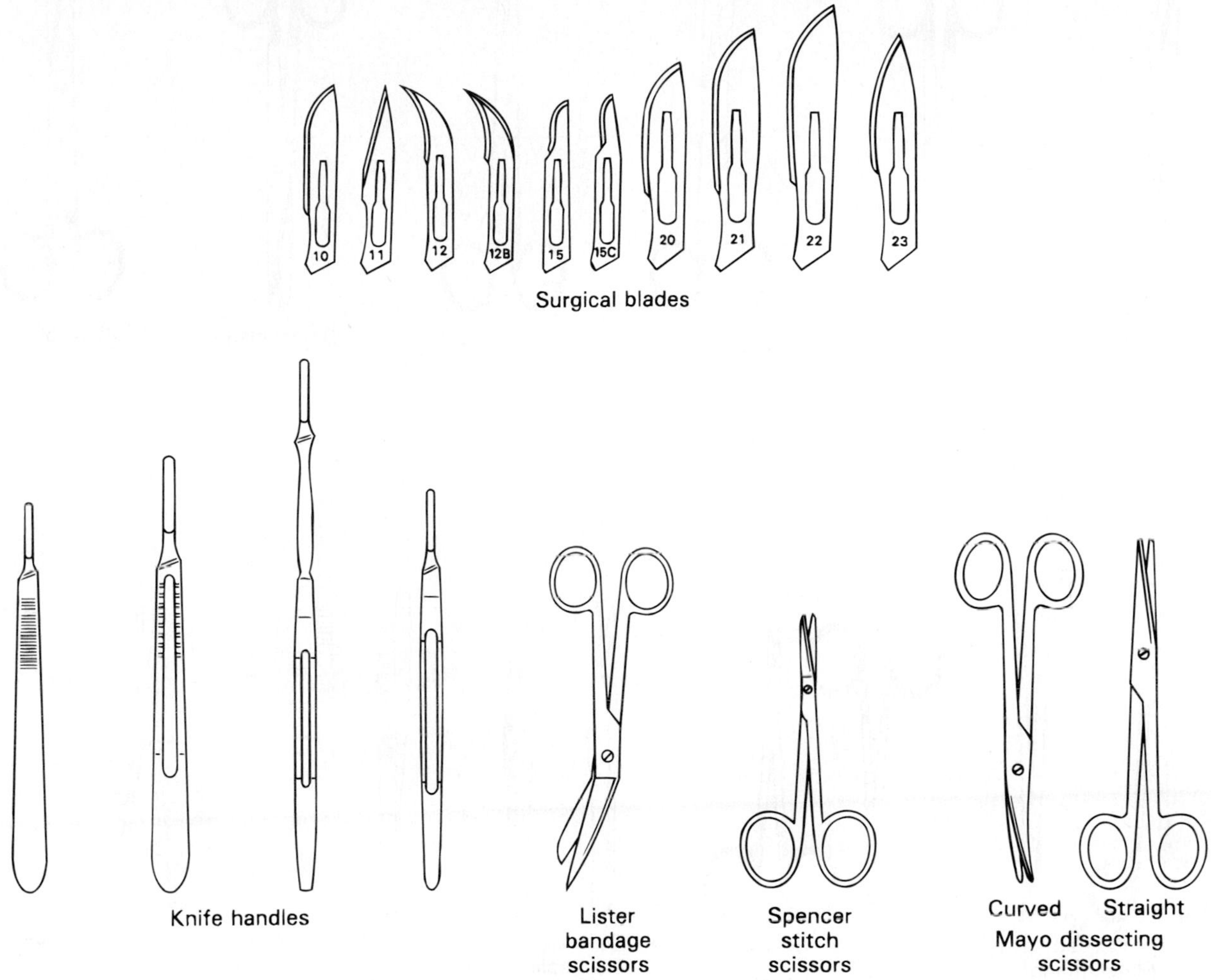

Instruments used for minor surgery. (Courtesy of the Miltex Instrument Co., Lake Success, N.Y.)

• MEDICAL INSTRUMENTS

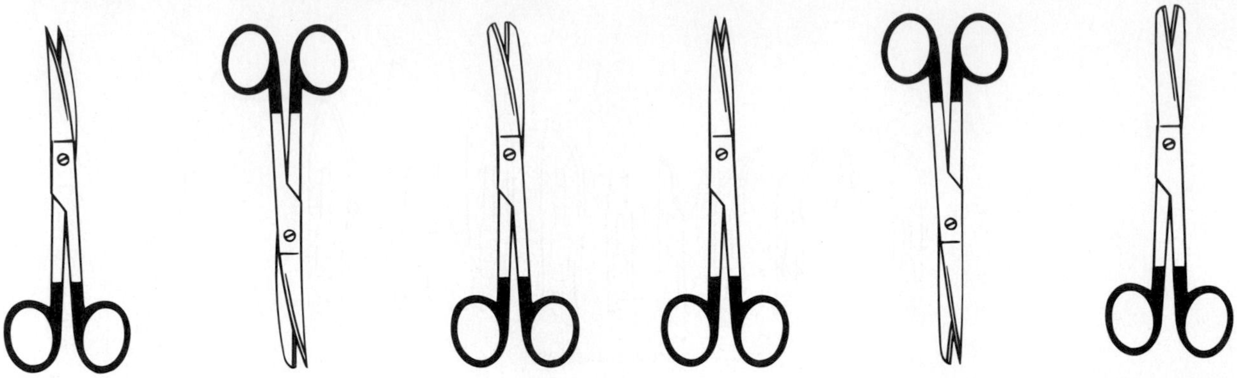

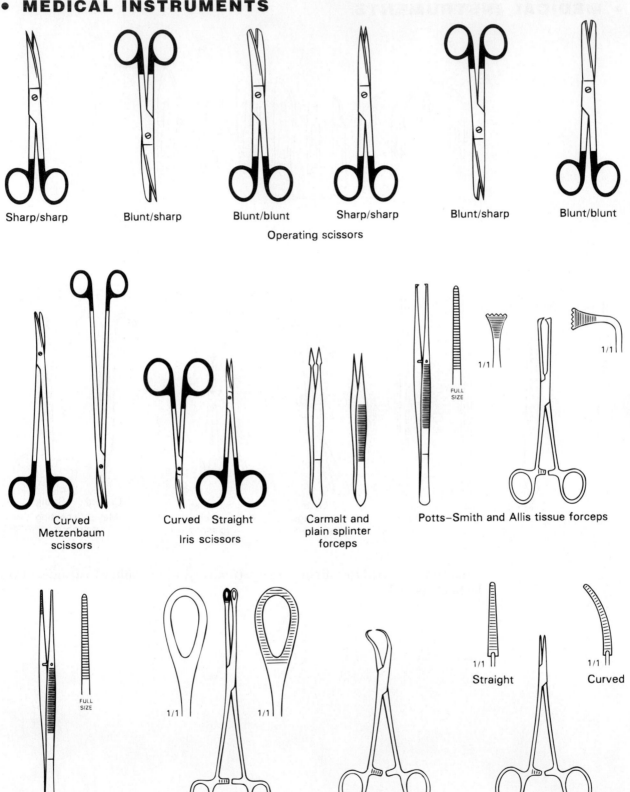

Sharp/sharp | Blunt/sharp | Blunt/blunt | Sharp/sharp | Blunt/sharp | Blunt/blunt

Operating scissors

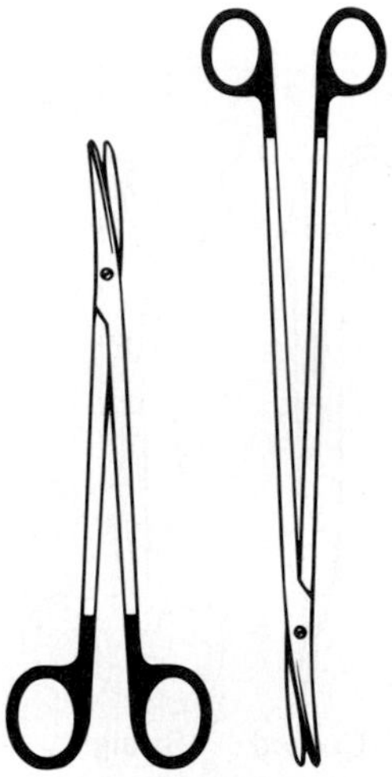

Curved Metzenbaum scissors

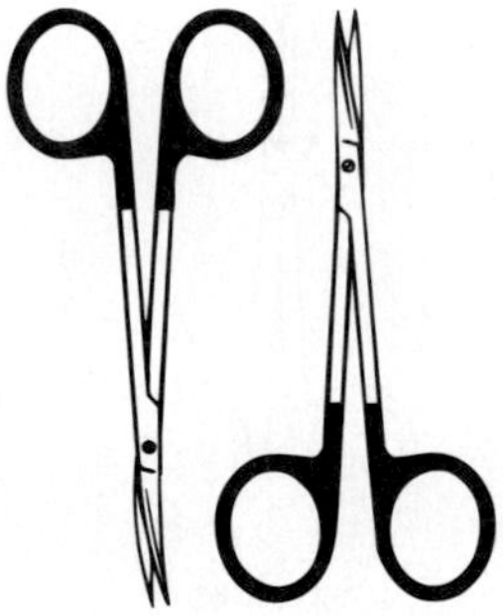

Curved Straight
Iris scissors

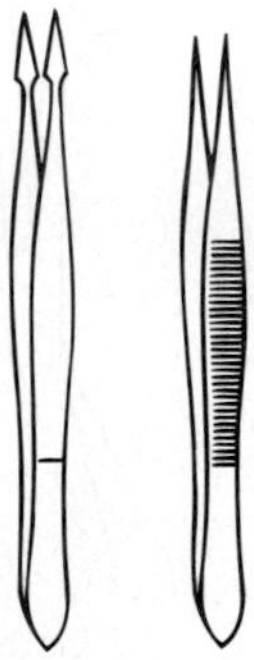

Carmalt and plain splinter forceps

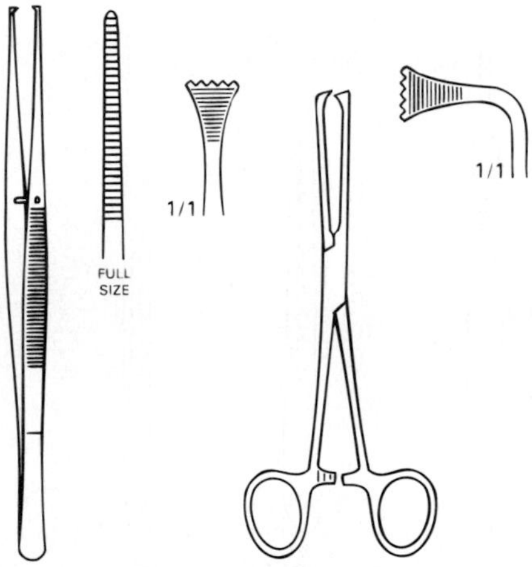

Potts–Smith and Allis tissue forceps

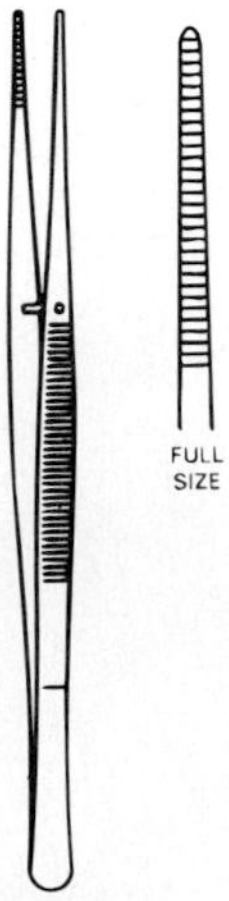

Potts–Smith dressing forceps

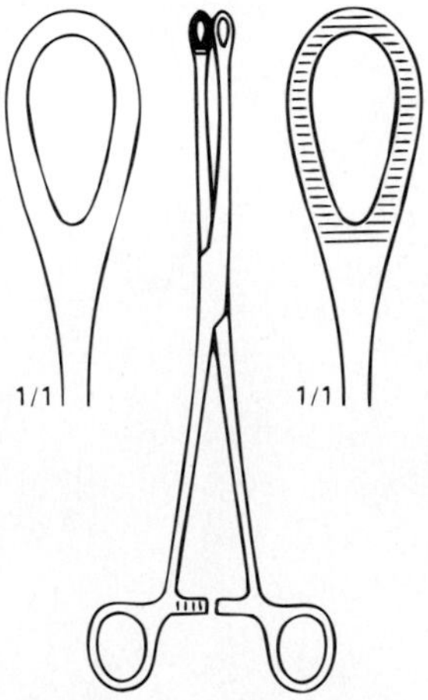

Foerster sponge forceps

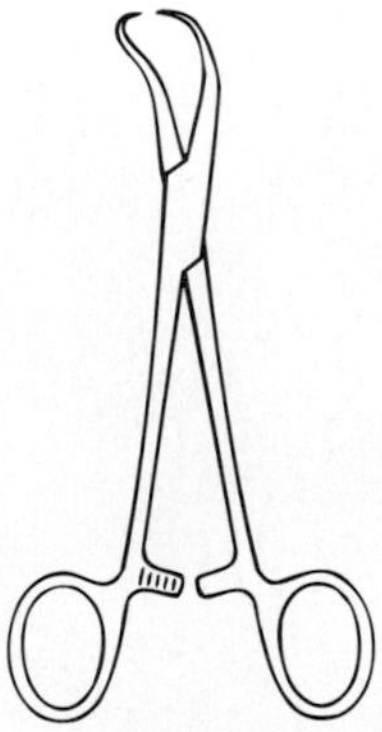

Backhaus towel clamp

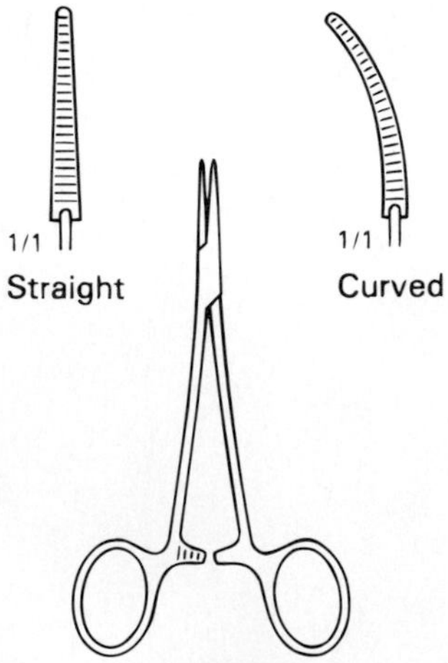

Halsted mosquito forceps

• MEDICAL INSTRUMENTS

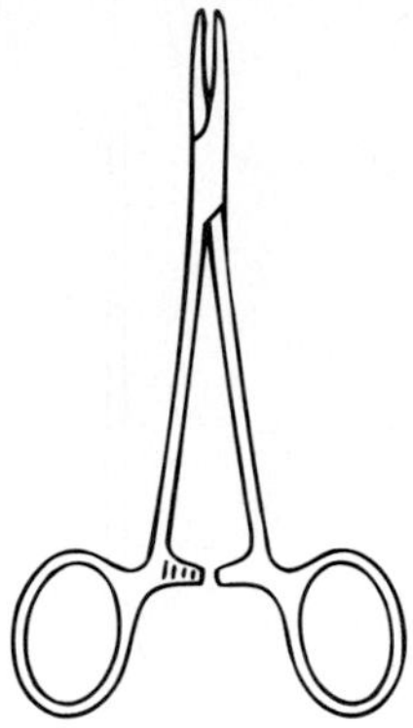

Hemostatic forceps

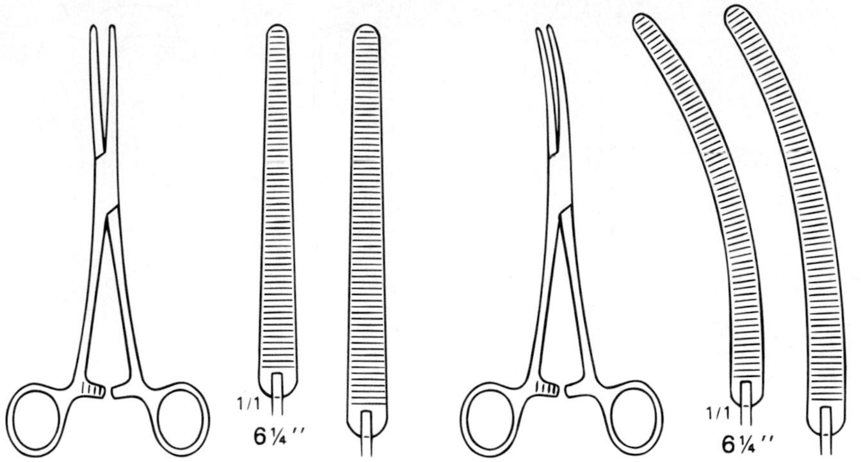

Straight 7¼″ Curved 7¼″

Rochester pean forceps

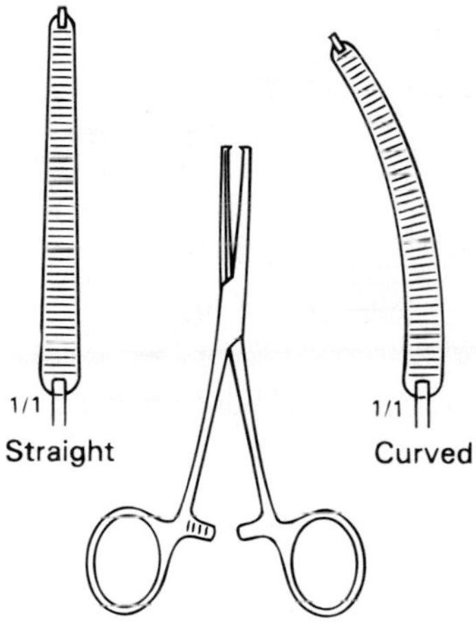

Straight Curved

Kocher forceps

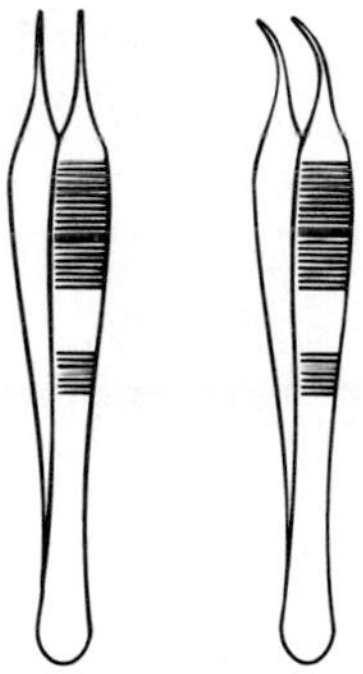

Adson dressing forceps

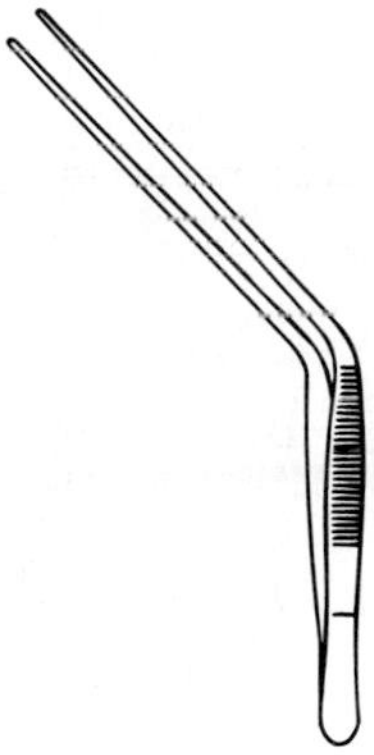

Wilde nasal dressing forceps

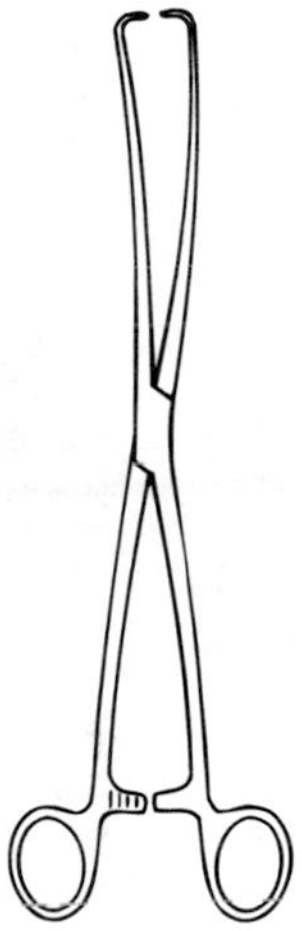

Duplay uterine tenaculum forceps

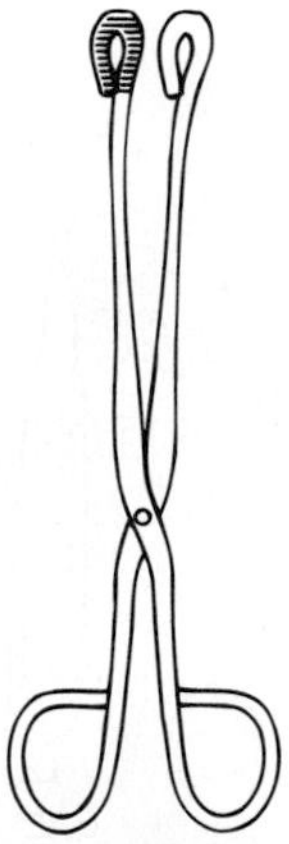

Utility–sterilizer forceps

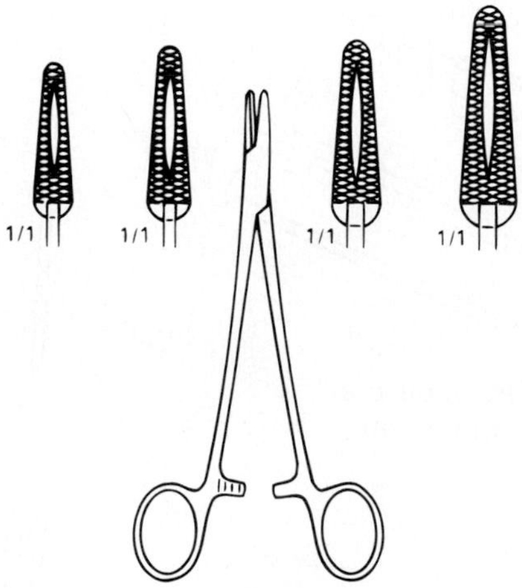

Mayo–Hegar needle holder

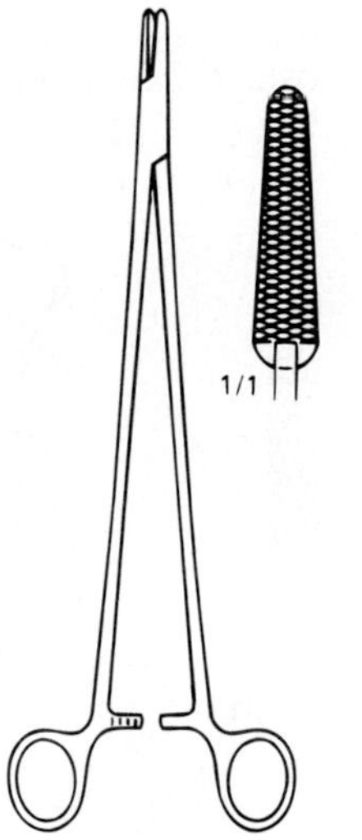

Wangensteen needle holder

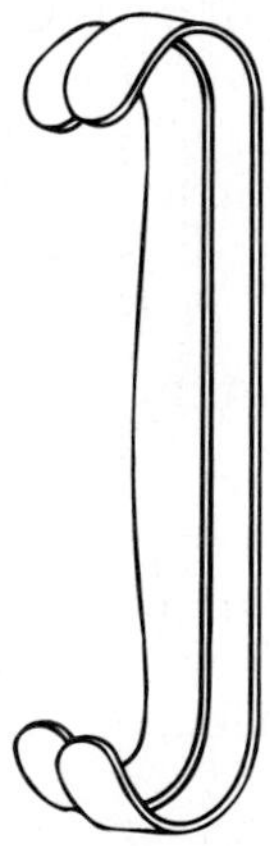

Parker retractors

• MEDICAL INSTRUMENTS

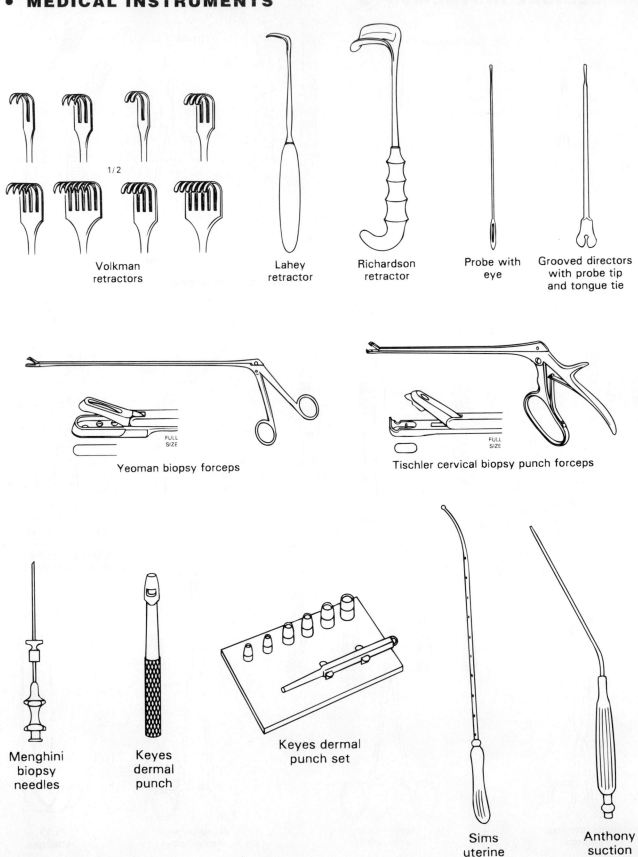

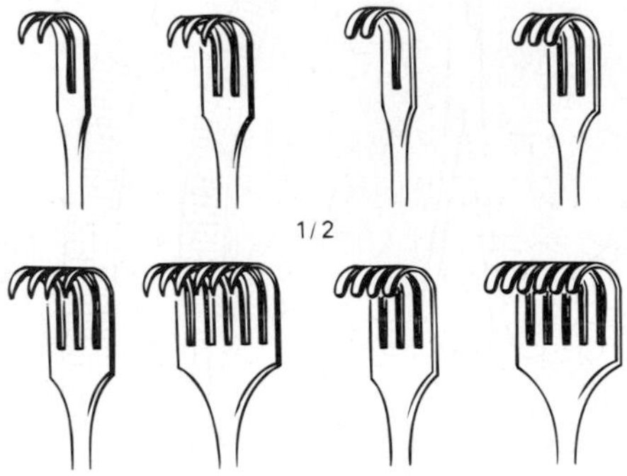

Volkman retractors

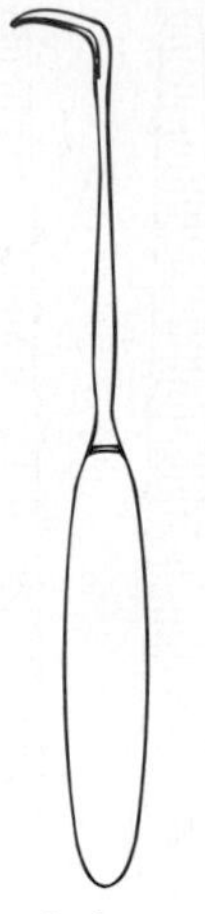

Lahey retractor

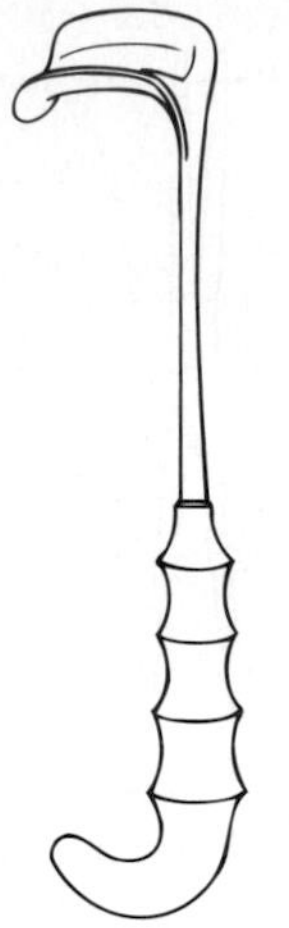

Richardson retractor

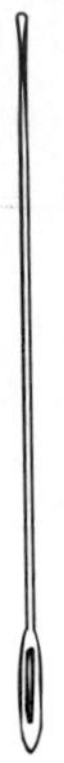

Probe with eye

Grooved directors with probe tip and tongue tie

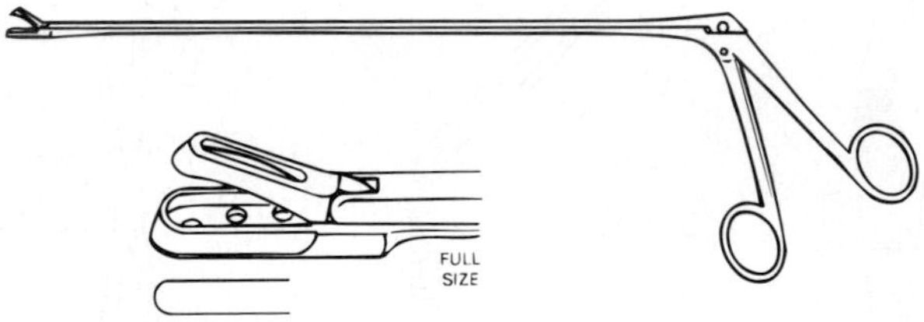

Yeoman biopsy forceps

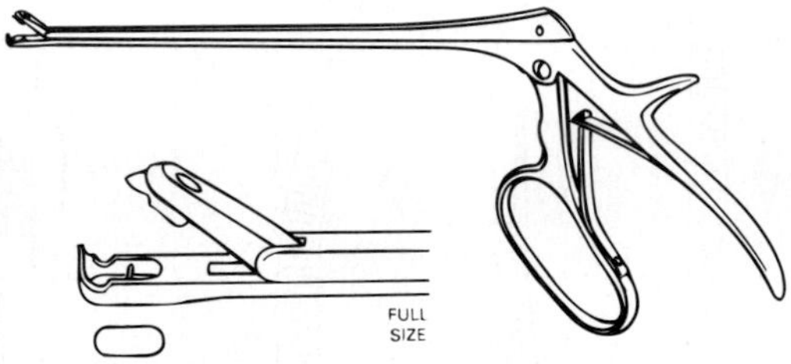

Tischler cervical biopsy punch forceps

Menghini biopsy needles

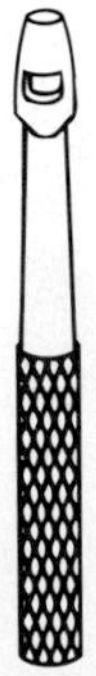

Keyes dermal punch

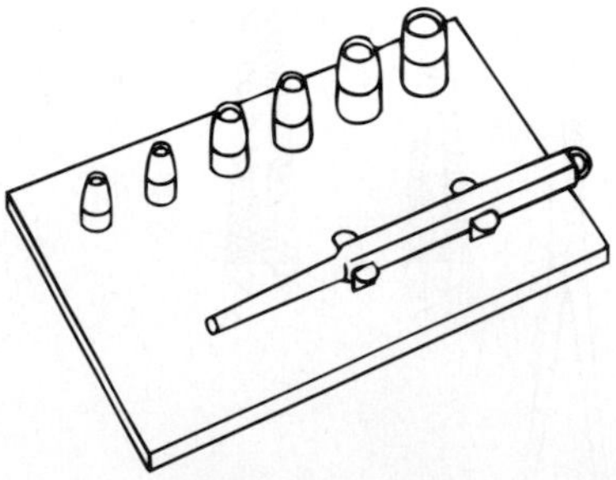

Keyes dermal punch set

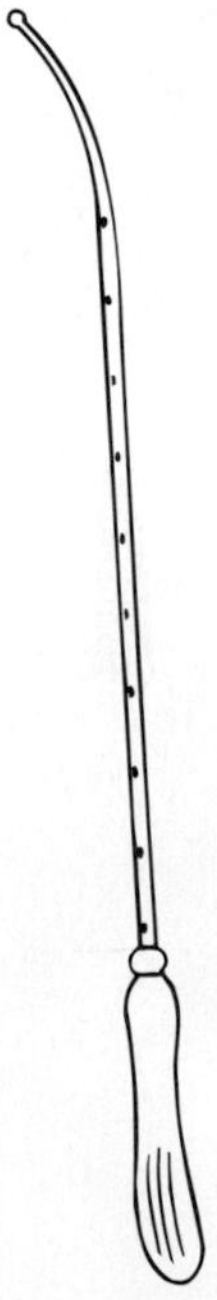

Sims uterine sound

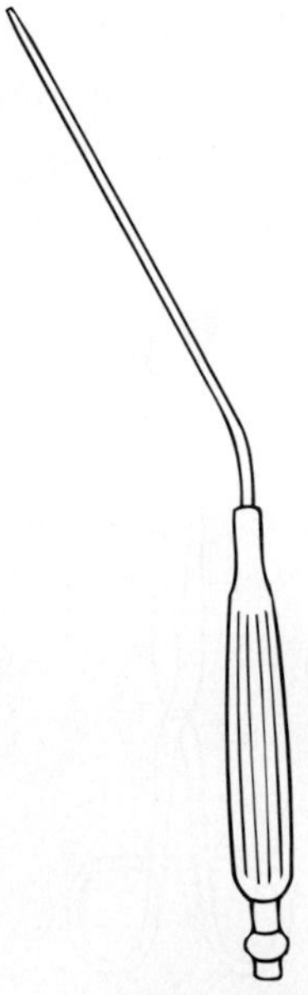

Anthony suction tube

Check-off Sheet:

23-8 Fowler's Position

Name ______________________________ **Date** ______________

Directions: Practice this procedure, following each step. When you are ready to have your performance evaluated, give this sheet to your instructor. Review the detailed procedure in your textbook.

Procedure	Pass	Redo	Date Competency Met	Instructor Initials
Student must use Standard Precautions.	☐	☐	______	______
1. Wash hands.	☐	☐	______	______
2. Explain to patient what you are going to do.	☐	☐	______	______
3. Assist client to a position lying flat on his or her back in good alignment.	☐	☐	______	______
4. Keep patient covered so that he or she is not exposed.	☐	☐	______	______
5. Knees may bend slightly.	☐	☐	______	______
6. Adjust backrest to the correct position according to client's or physician's needs.	☐	☐	______	______
7. Drape cover so that client is not exposed, leaving all edges of drape free.	☐	☐	______	______

Check-off Sheet:

23-12 Left Lateral Position and Left Sims Position

Name ______________________________ **Date** ______________

Directions: Practice this procedure, following each step. When you are ready to have your performance evaluated, give this sheet to your instructor. Review the detailed procedure in your textbook.

Procedure	Pass	Redo	Date Competency Met	Instructor Initials
Student must use Standard Precautions.	☐	☐	______	______
1. Wash hands.	☐	☐	______	______
2. Explain to client what you are going to do.	☐	☐	______	______
3. Assist client to a position lying flat on his or her back.	☐	☐	______	______
4. Cover client so that he or she is not exposed.	☐	☐	______	______
5. Assist client to turn onto left side.	☐	☐	______	______
6. Position client's left arm slightly behind him or her on bed.	☐	☐	______	______
7. Gently bend both knees.	☐	☐	______	______
8. For lateral position, place right leg slightly forward of left leg.	☐	☐	______	______
9. For Sims position, bend right knee toward chest.	☐	☐	______	______

Check-off Sheet:

23-24 Putting on Sterile Gloves and Removing Gloves

Name ______________________________ **Date** ______________

Directions: Practice this procedure, following each step. When you are ready to have your performance evaluated, give this sheet to your instructor. Review the detailed procedure in your textbook.

Procedure	Pass	Redo	Date Competency Met	Instructor Initials
Student must use Standard Precautions.	☐	☐	______	______
1. Wash hands.	☐	☐	______	______
2. Pick up wrapped gloves.	☐	☐	______	______
3. Check to be certain that they are sterile:				
a. Package intact	☐	☐	______	______
b. Seal of sterility	☐	☐	______	______
4. Place on clean, flat surface.	☐	☐	______	______
5. Open wrapper by handling only the outside.	☐	☐	______	______
6. Use your left hand to pick up the right-handed glove.	☐	☐	______	______
7. Put glove on right hand.	☐	☐	______	______
8. Use gloved right hand to pick up left-handed glove.	☐	☐	______	______
9. Place finger of gloved right hand under cuff of left-handed glove.	☐	☐	______	______
10. Lift glove up and away from wrapper to pull onto left hand.	☐	☐	______	______
11. Continue pulling left glove under wrist.	☐	☐	______	______
12. With gloved left hand, place fingers under cuff of right gloves and pull cuff up over right wrist.	☐	☐	______	______
13. Adjust fingers of gloves as necessary.	☐	☐	______	______
If either glove tears, remove and discard. Begin with new gloves!				
14. Turn gloves inside out as you remove them, and put them with hazardous materials.	☐	☐	______	______

Check-off Sheet:

23-11 Prone Position

Name ______________________________ Date ______________

Directions: Practice this procedure, following each step. When you are ready to have your performance evaluated, give this sheet to your instructor. Review the detailed procedure in your textbook.

Procedure	Pass	Redo	Date Competency Met	Instructor Initials
Student must use Standard Precautions.	☐	☐	______	______
1. Wash hands.	☐	☐	______	______
2. Explain to client what you are going to do.	☐	☐	______	______
3. Assist client to a position lying flat on his or her back.	☐	☐	______	______
4. Cover client so that he or she is not exposed.	☐	☐	______	______
5. Assist client to turn onto stomach, keeping him or her covered.	☐	☐	______	______

Chapter 24 Dental Assistant

• OBJECTIVES

When you have completed this unit, you will be able to do the following:

- Complete all objectives from Part One of this book.
- Match vocabulary words with their correct meanings.
- Describe the responsibilities of a dental assistant.
- List eight recognized dental specialties.
- Label parts of the oral cavity on a diagram.
- Differentiate between posterior and anterior teeth and their functions.
- Identify deciduous and permanent teeth by name on a diagram.
- Label teeth on a diagram using the universal method.
- Label anatomical structures of a tooth on a diagram.
- Identify surfaces of a tooth.
- Identify charting symbols and abbreviations.
- Apply charting symbols and abbreviations to indicate conditions of teeth on a dental chart.
- Identify dental office equipment by name.
- Identify specific OSHA infection control guidelines for the dental office.
- Describe steps to clean the treatment room following procedures and between patients.
- Identify common dental instruments.
- Identify basic dental tray setups.
- Describe admitting and seating a patient/client for a dental procedure.
- Explain how to position a patient/client for a dental procedure.
- Describe the dental assistant's position in relation to the patient/client and the dentist during a procedure.
- Demonstrate basic instrument transfer techniques.

- Demonstrate preparation and transfer of an anesthetic syringe.
- Explain the importance of observing patients/clients before, during, and after procedures.
- Describe oral evacuation, rinsing, and drying techniques.
- Demonstrate the procedure for completion of treatment and dismissing a patient/client.
- Prepare impression materials.
- Demonstrate how to make a study model.
- Demonstrate assisting techniques during basic restorative procedures.
- Teach the following:
  - How to use disclosing tablets or solution
  - The Bass tooth brushing technique
  - Dental flossing techniques
- Mount a full-mouth and bite-wing x-ray series.
- Apply all procedural techniques with confidence.

• DIRECTIONS

1. Complete Worksheet 1 before beginning text.
2. Read this chapter.
3. Complete Worksheets 2 through 6, and 9 through 10 as assigned.
4. Complete Worksheets/Activities 7, 8, and 11 as assigned.
5. Prepare responses to each item listed in the Chapter Review—Your Link to Success at the end of this chapter.
6. When you are confident that you can meet each objective listed, ask your instructor for the unit evaluation.

• EVALUATION METHODS

- Worksheets/Activities
- Class participation
- Written evaluation
- Return demonstrations

• WORKSHEET 1

Match each definition in column B with the correct vocabulary word in column A (23 points).

Column A	*Column B*
____ 1. Apex	a. American Dental Association.
____ 2. Ala	b. Intended to help.
____ 3. ADA	c. Destined to fall out.
____ 4. Deciduous	d. Natural teeth in the dental arch.
____ 5. Posterior	e. The outer side of the nostril.
____ 6. Visible	f. Within the oral cavity.
____ 7. Seating	g. Stress to tooth caused by its normal function.
____ 8. Caries	h. An opening in the apex.
____ 9. Proximal	i. To the back.
____ 10. Saturating	j. Nearest or next to.
____ 11. Rheostat	k. A record that can be used in a lawsuit.
____ 12. Aspirate	l. Decay.
____ 13. Exposure	m. Contact with radiation.
____ 14. Alginate	n. Able to be seen.
____ 15. Palpation	o. Soaking.
____ 16. Accessory	p. Material for making impressions.
____ 17. Dentition	q. Hand used for writing, eating, and so on.
____ 18. Intraoral	r. Hand not used for writing, eating, and so on.
____ 19. Apical foramen	s. Putting firmly in place to prevent moving.
____ 20. Functional stress	t. Examination by feeling for unusual or abnormal conditions
____ 21. Legal record	u. Control for flow of electric current.
____ 22. Dominant hand	v. Remove substances.
____ 23. Nondominant hand	w. Area at the end of the tooth root.

There are 23 possible points in this worksheet.

• WORKSHEET 2

Fill in the crossword puzzle using the vocabulary words from Chapter 24 and the clues on the next page (25 points).

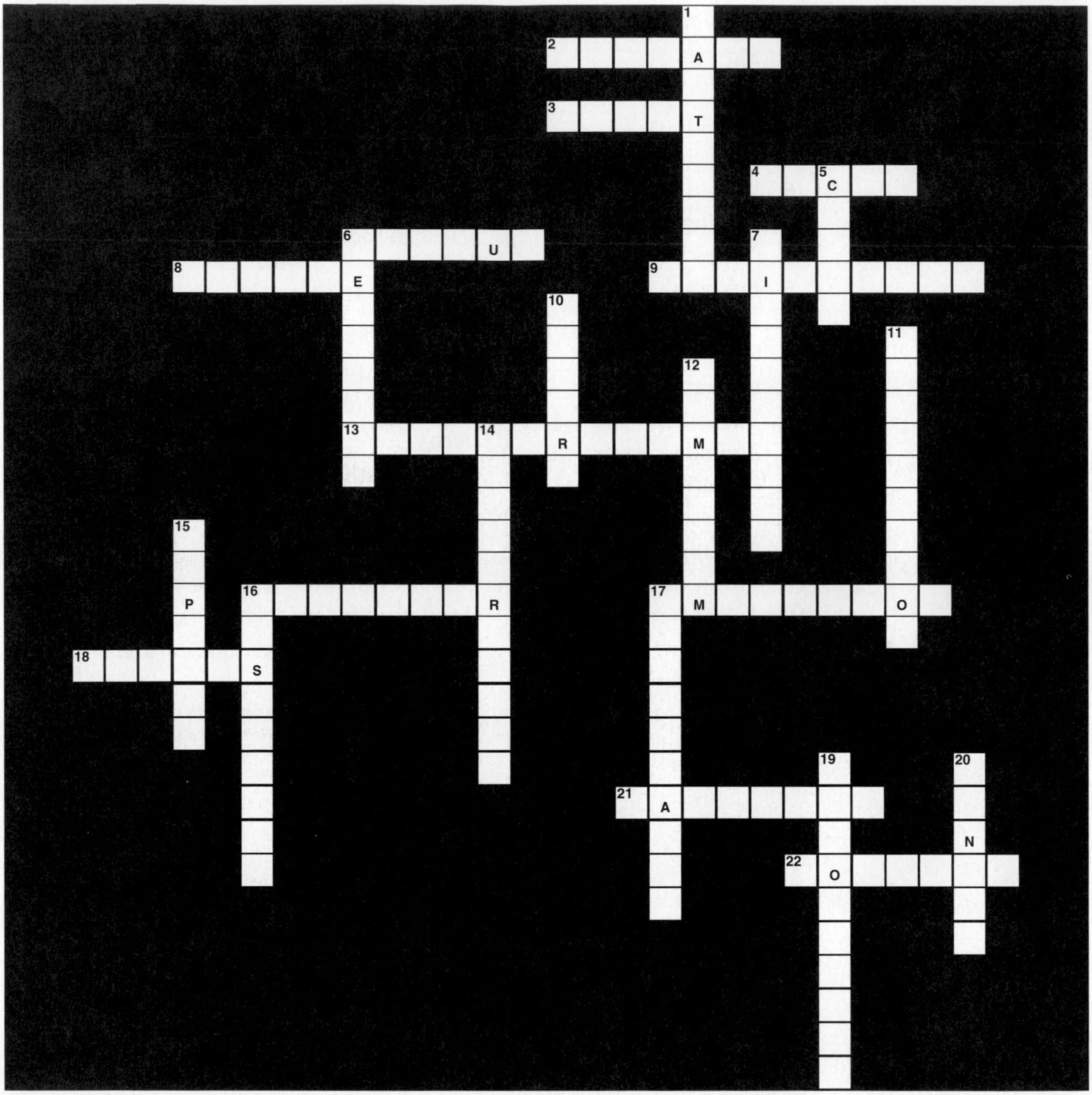

Clues

Across

2. First.
3. Push through.
4. Breaking down, rot.
6. Soft deposit of bacteria and bacteria products on teeth.
8. Calm.
9. Tissue around the apex of the tooth.
13. Sides between teeth.
16. Toward the front.
17. Any tooth that does not erupt when it normally should.
18. Depression, groove, area where gingival tip meets tooth enamel.
21. Same direction and at a distance so two points do not touch.
22. Indented.

Down

1. Chew.
5. Pointed or rounded, raised areas on the surface of the tooth.
6. At regular times, with time in between.
7. Ability to clearly see structures in the mouth.
10. Moving in a circular motion.
11. Removal.
12. Hard, thin covering or shell that covers the root.
14. Returning to as close to normal as possible.
15. Applied to surface.
16. Pockets of pus in a limited area.
17. Type of medication given by needle.
19. Loss of substance or bone.
20. Raised.

There are 25 possible points in this worksheet.

• WORKSHEET 3

1. Write the three ways teeth are identified (3 points).
   a. ______________________________
   b. ______________________________
   c. ______________________________
2. Name two arches in the mouth (2 points).
   a. ______________________________
   b. ______________________________
3. Name the anterior teeth, and explain their function (4 points).
   a. ______________________________
   b. ______________________________
4. Name the posterior teeth, and explain their function (4 points).
   a. ______________________________
   b. ______________________________
5. There are ______________ teeth in the deciduous dentition (1 point).
6. There are ______________ teeth in the permanent dentition (1 point).

There are 15 possible points in this worksheet.

• WORKSHEET 4

Identify the teeth listed below as deciduous, permanent, or both by placing the appropriate letter next to each tooth name (9 points).

a. deciduous **b.** permanent **c.** both deciduous and permanent

_______________ **1.** Central incisors
_______________ **2.** Lateral incisors
_______________ **3.** Cuspids
_______________ **4.** Bicuspids
_______________ **5.** 1st premolar
_______________ **6.** 2nd premolar
_______________ **7.** 1st molar
_______________ **8.** 2nd molars
_______________ **9.** 3rd molars

Label the following teeth by the universal method (52 points).

Deciduous Teeth

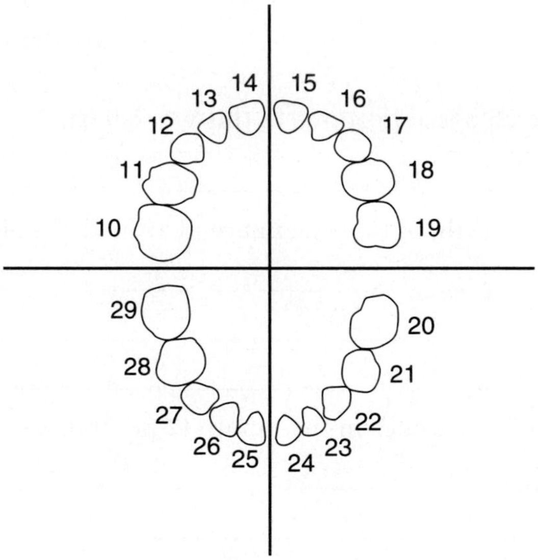

10. _______________ **20.** _______________
11. _______________ **21.** _______________
12. _______________ **22.** _______________
13. _______________ **23.** _______________
14. _______________ **24.** _______________
15. _______________ **25.** _______________
16. _______________ **26.** _______________
17. _______________ **27.** _______________
18. _______________ **28.** _______________
19. _______________ **29.** _______________

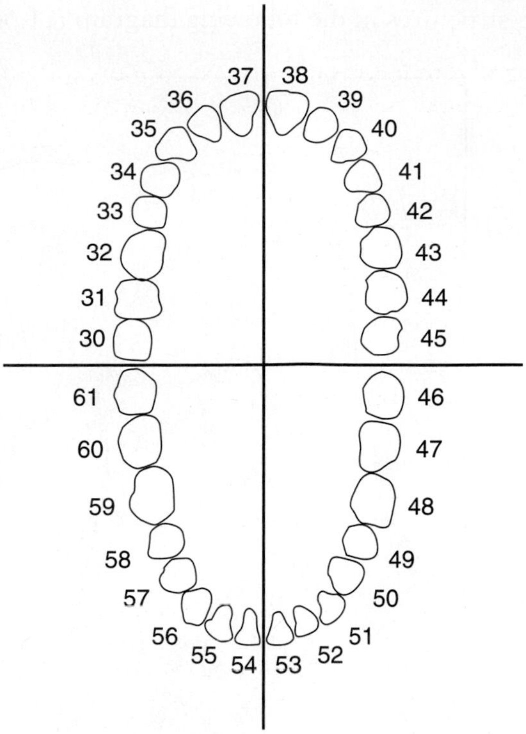

30. ____________	41. ____________	52. ____________
31. ____________	42. ____________	53. ____________
32. ____________	43. ____________	54. ____________
33. ____________	44. ____________	55. ____________
34. ____________	45. ____________	56. ____________
35. ____________	46. ____________	57. ____________
36. ____________	47. ____________	58. ____________
37. ____________	48. ____________	59. ____________
38. ____________	49. ____________	60. ____________
39. ____________	50. ____________	61. ____________
40. ____________	51. ____________	

There are 61 possible points in this worksheet.

• WORKSHEET 5

Part 1

Label the three main sections of a tooth on the following diagram (3 points).

1. ________________

2. ________________

3. ________________

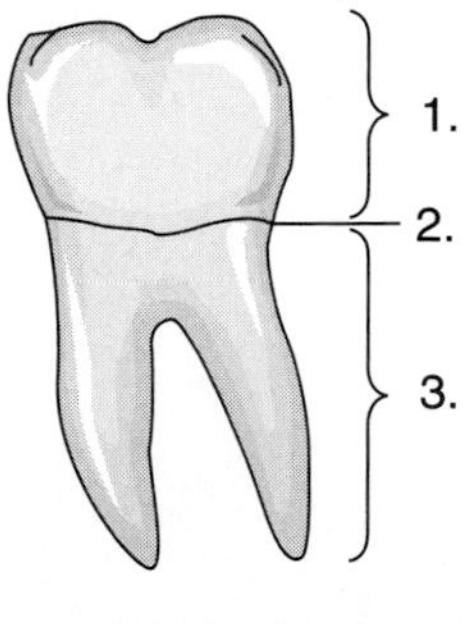

Label the structures in the following diagram (11 points).

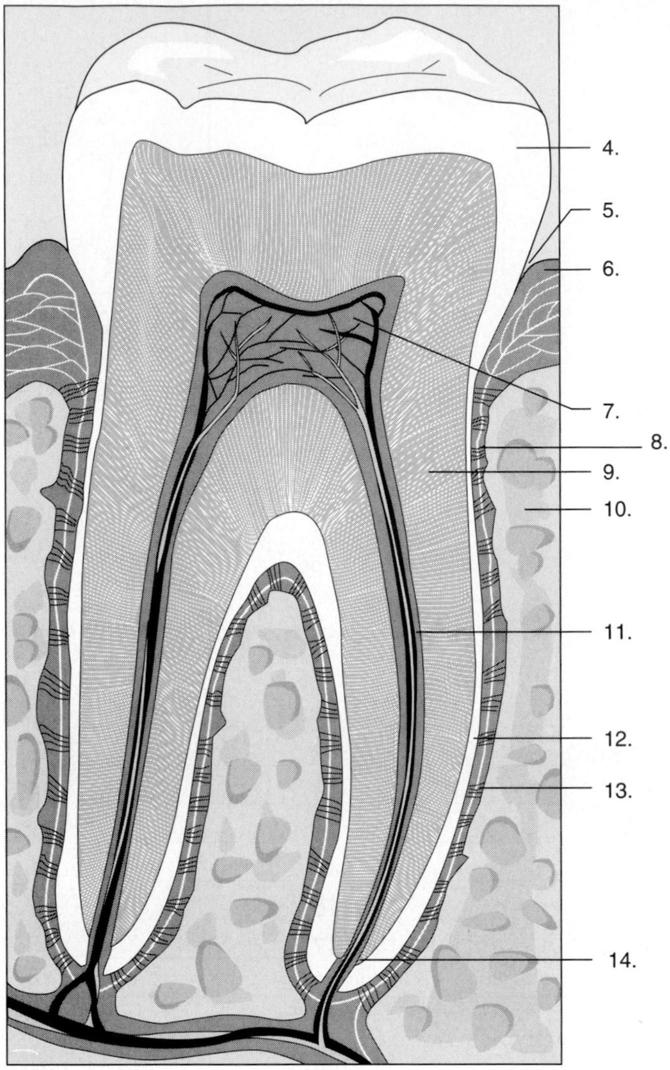

4. ____________________
5. ____________________
6. ____________________
7. ____________________
8. ____________________
9. ____________________
10. ____________________
11. ____________________
12. ____________________
13. ____________________
14. ____________________

Part 2

The surfaces of anterior crowns are indicated below. Photocopy the diagram, cut diagram out, and fold into the shape of a tooth (5 points). See diagram 24-10.

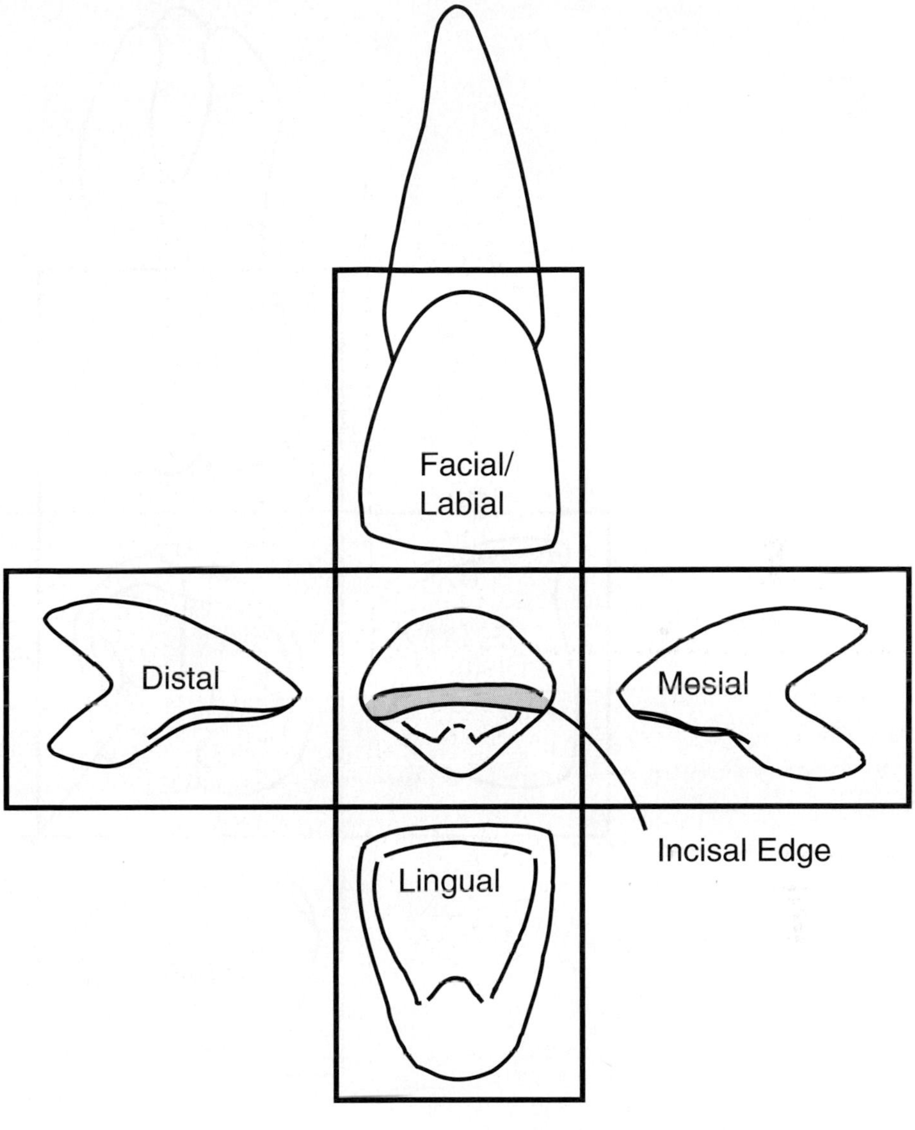

Part 3

The five surfaces of the posterior crown are indicated below. Photocopy the diagram, cut diagram out, and fold into the shape of a tooth (5 points). See diagram 24-10.

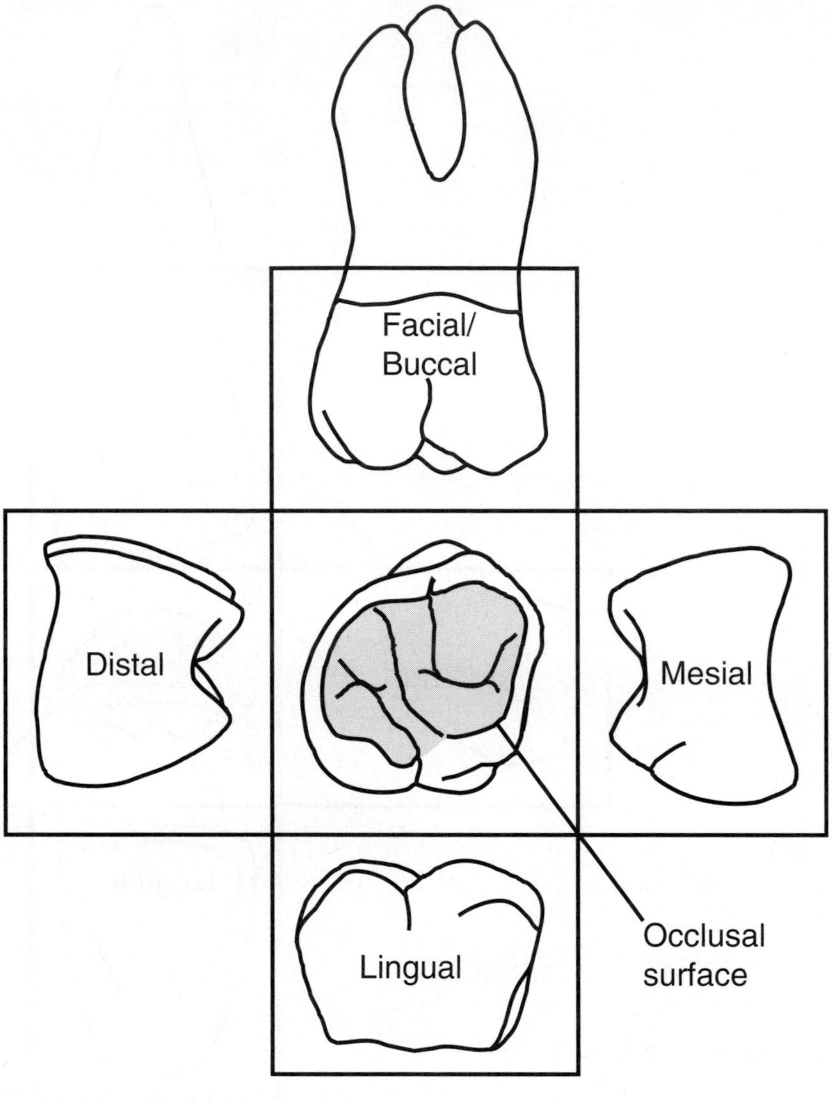

There are 24 possible points in this worksheet.

• WORKSHEET 6

Write the correct abbreviation next to each word (24 points).

____________ 1. Denture
____________ 2. Anesthetic
____________ 3. Oral surgery
____________ 4. Preparation
____________ 5. Temporary
____________ 6. Abscess
____________ 7. Sedative treatment
____________ 8. Corrective appliance
____________ 9. Gold inlay
____________ 10. Fixed bridge
____________ 11. Impression
____________ 12. Removable
____________ 13. Root canal therapy
____________ 14. Full mouth
____________ 15. Gingiva/gums treatment
____________ 16. Porcelain fused to metal
____________ 17. Examination
____________ 18. Crown and bridge
____________ 19. Adjustment
____________ 20. Estimate
____________ 21. Prophylaxis
____________ 22. Xylocaine
____________ 23. Full gold crown
____________ 24. Partial lower

There are 24 possible points in this worksheet.

• WORKSHEET/ACTIVITY 7

Find a partner and ask your instructor if you may organize a class spelling bee when you are close to finishing the dental assisting chapter. Get a list of dental terms:

- Read out a term.
- Have your partner select a class volunteer to spell the term and write it on the board.
- Select another volunteer to define the term.
- Keep a list on the board of the people who correctly spelled or defined terms.

There are 10 possible points for each organizer of the worksheet/activity. Volunteers get 1 point for each correct spelling or definition.

• WORKSHEET/ACTIVITY 8

Cut out and paste each symbol on a 3-by-5-inch index card to use as a flash card. Write the meaning of each symbol on the opposite side of the card and indicate if it is an anatomical or geometrical diagram.

ANATOMICAL DIAGRAMS	GEOMETRICAL DIAGRAMS	ANATOMICAL DIAGRAMS	GEOMETRICAL DIAGRAMS
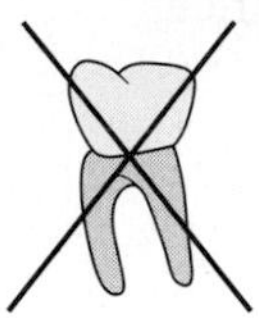	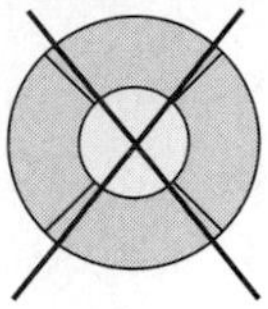	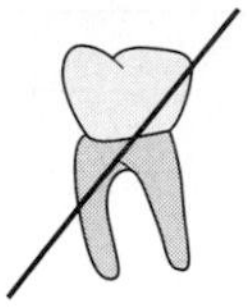	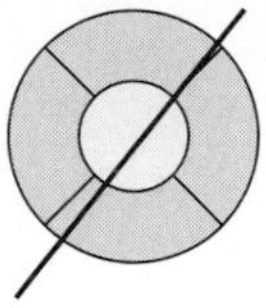
Missing Tooth	Missing Tooth	To Be Extracted	To Be Extracted
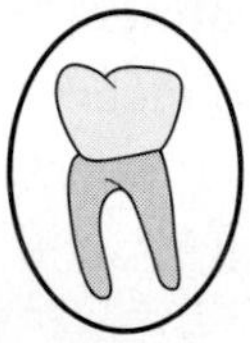	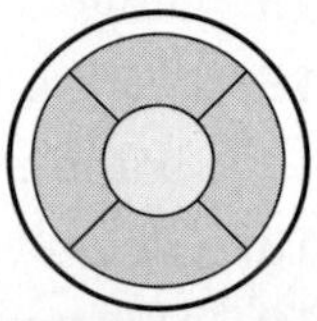	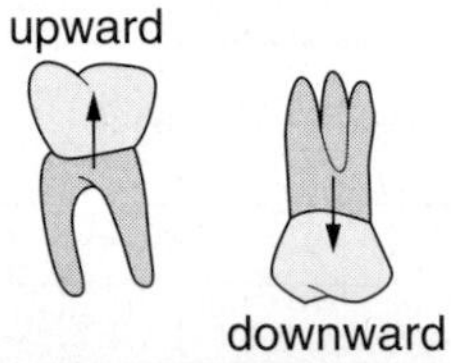	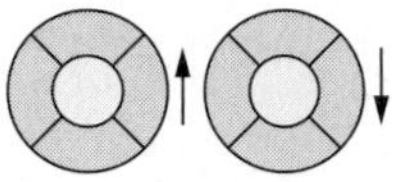
Unerupted or Impacted	Unerupted or Impacted	Upward/Downward Drifting	Upward/Downward Drifting
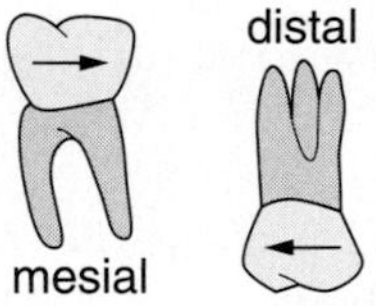	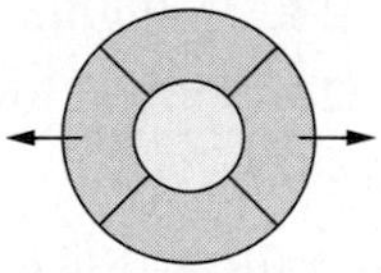	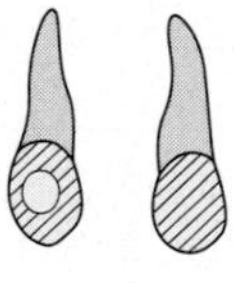	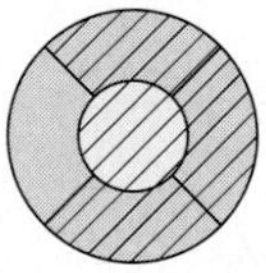
Mesial Distal Drifting Tooth	Mesial Distal Drifting Tooth	Buccal Lingual 3/4 Crown	Buccal Lingual 3/4 Crown

• WORKSHEET/ACTIVITY 8 (CONTINUED)

ANATOMICAL DIAGRAMS	GEOMETRICAL DIAGRAMS	ANATOMICAL DIAGRAMS	GEOMETRICAL DIAGRAMS
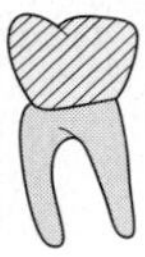	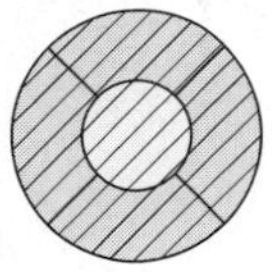	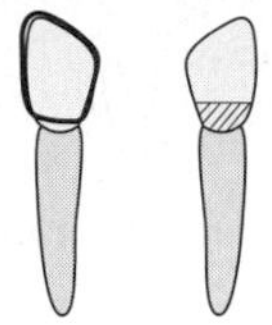	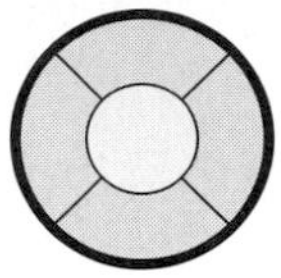
Full Crown	Full Crown	Porcelain Crown Fused to Metal	Porcelain Crown Fused to Metal
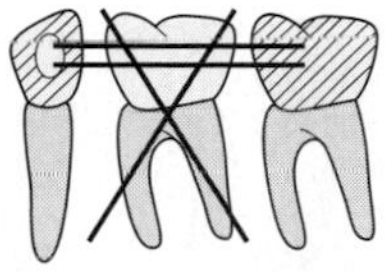	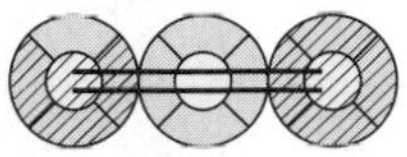	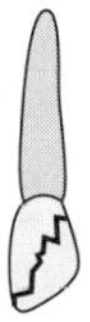	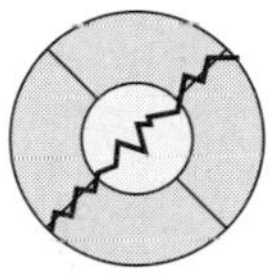
3/4 Crown Full Crown Fixed Bridge	Unerupted or Impacted	Fracture	Fracture
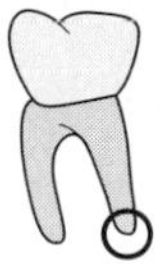	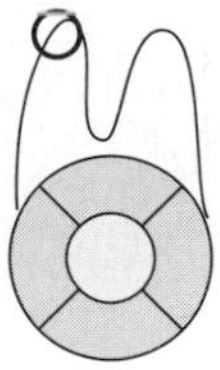	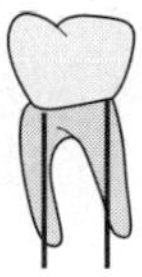	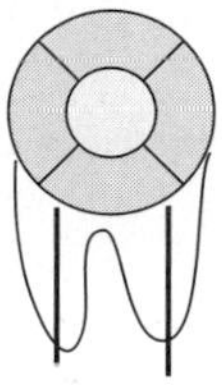
Abscess	Abscess	Root Canal	Root Canal

• WORKSHEET/ACTIVITY 8 (CONTINUED)

ANATOMICAL DIAGRAMS	GEOMETRICAL DIAGRAMS	ANATOMICAL DIAGRAMS	GEOMETRICAL DIAGRAMS
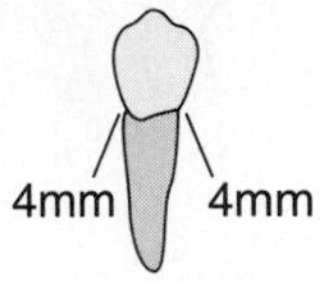	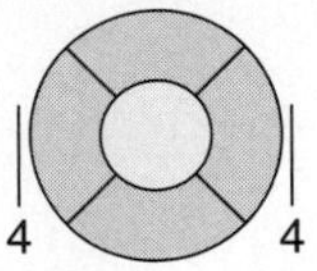	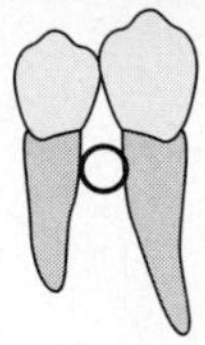	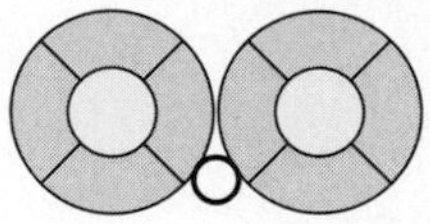
Periodontal Pocket	Periodontal Pocket	Periodontal Abscess	Periodontal Abscess
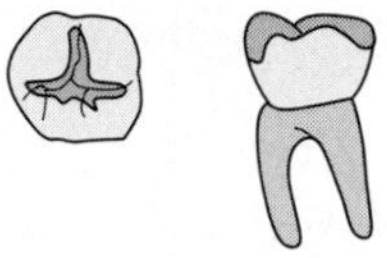	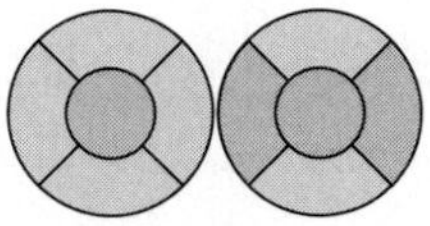	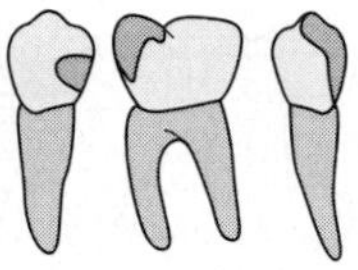	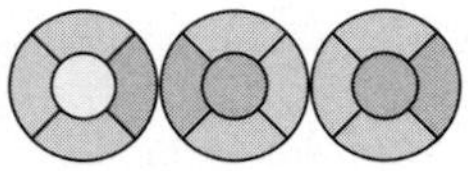
Occ MOD Amalgam Restoration	Occ MOD Amalgam Restoration	D(III) MO(II) MI(IV) Composite Restoration	D(III) MO(II) MI(IV) Composite Restoration
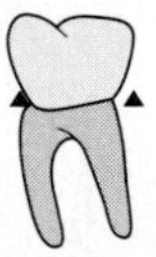	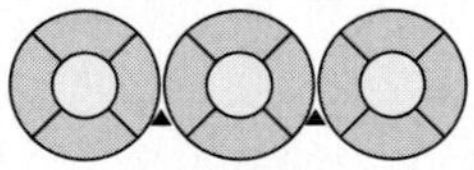		
Overhanging margin	Overhanging Margin		

• WORKSHEET 9

Identify what each chart symbol means. Then place an *A* for anatomical diagram or *G* for a geometrical diagram in the space provided (32 points).

1. Symbol ____________________
   Diagram ________

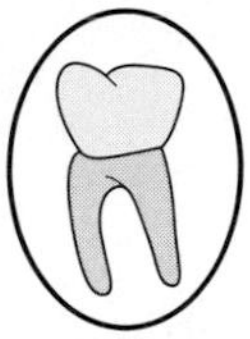

2. Symbol ____________________
   Diagram ________

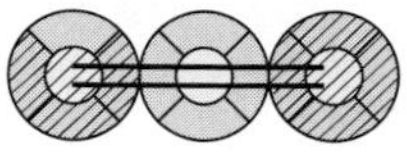

3. Symbol ____________________
   Diagram ________

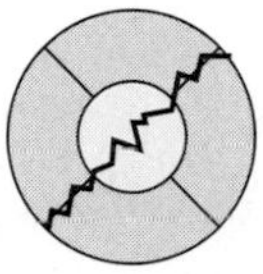

4. Symbol ____________________
   Diagram ________

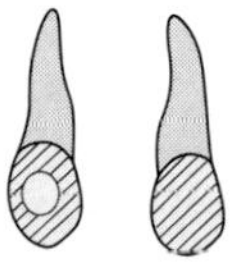

5. Symbol ____________________
   Diagram ________

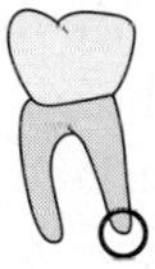

6. Symbol ____________________
   Diagram ________

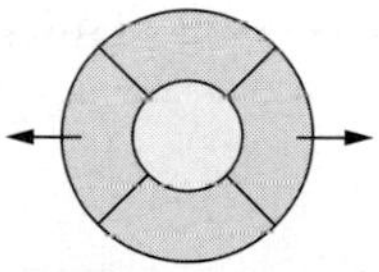

7. Symbol ____________________
   Diagram ________

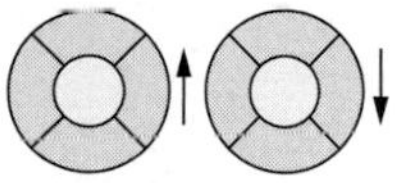

8. Symbol ____________________
   Diagram ________

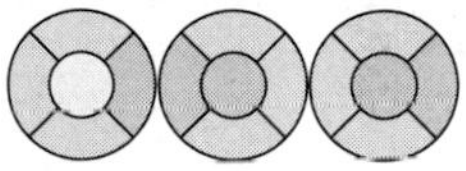

9. Symbol ____________________
   Diagram ________

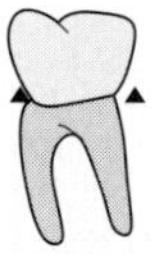

10. Symbol ____________________
    Diagram ________

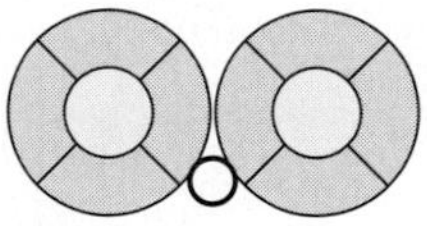

11. Symbol ____________________
    Diagram ________

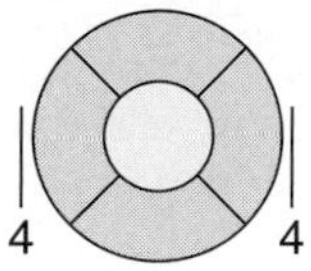

12. Symbol ____________________
    Diagram ________

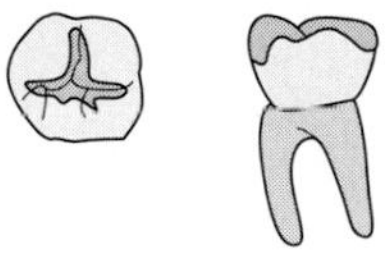

13. Symbol ____________________
Diagram ________

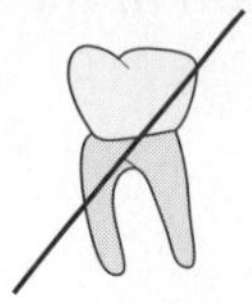

14. Symbol ____________________
Diagram ________

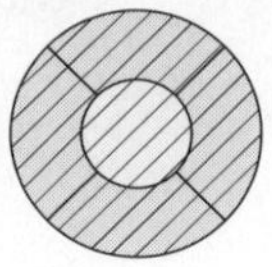

15. Symbol ____________________
Diagram ________

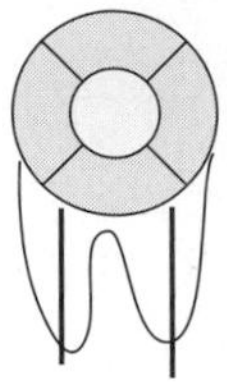

16. Symbol ____________________
Diagram ________

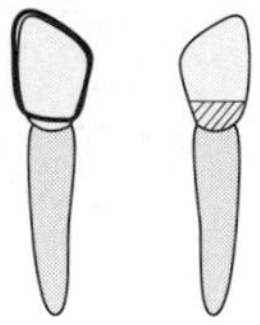

Write the correct abbreviation listed below next to the definition that best illustrates it (6 points).

(L/Li/Lin) lingual	(La/F) labial	(i) incisal
(D) distal	(M) mesial	(O/Occ) occlusal

_______________ **17.** Surface that touches the lips.
_______________ **18.** Surface toward the midline.
_______________ **19.** Large chewing surface.
_______________ **20.** Edge of the tooth used to bite with.
_______________ **21.** Surface toward the tongue.
_______________ **22.** Surface away from the midline.

23. Name the three parts of a dental chart (3 points).

a. ____

b. ____

c. ____

24. Charting in red on a dental diagram indicates (1 point) ________________

____.

25. Charting in blue on a dental diagram indicates (1 point) ________________

____.

There are 43 possible points in this worksheet.

• WORKSHEET 10

1. What do OSHA standards provide (1 point)? ____________________
2. Name four items used to protect yourself when Standard Precautions are followed (4 points).
   a. ____________________
   b. ____________________
   c. ____________________
   d. ____________________
3. Name the instruments or supplies used to do the following (7 points):
   a. To feel teeth for decay: ____________________
   b. To keep mouth dry and structures visible: ____________________
   c. To reflect light to see oral surfaces: ____________________
   d. To pick up gauze or cotton to dry areas of mouth and teeth: __________
   e. To check and measure the sulcus area: ____________________
   f. To dry and hold slippery tissues: ____________________
   g. To check contacts between teeth: ____________________
4. How far away is the light positioned from the mouth (1 point)? __________
5. Compared to a clock, what is the position of the (3 points):
   a. Patient's/client's head during treatment or examination? __________
   b. Dentist during treatment or examination? __________
   c. Dental assistant during treatment or examination? __________
6. Name two types of local anesthetic (2 points).
   a. ____________________
   b. ____________________
7. A maxillary infiltration requires how many injections for each tooth (1 point)? ____________________
8. How long is the needle for a maxillary infiltration (1 point)? __________
9. How does a mandibular block prevent pain (1 point)? __________
   ____
10. How long is the needle for a mandibular block (1 point)? __________
    ____
11. When passing a syringe to the dentist, always pass it __________ (1 point).____________________
12. Explain four things for which to inspect the carpule during preparation (4 points).
    a. ____________________
    b. ____________________

c. ______________________

d. ______________________

There are 27 possible points in this worksheet.

• WORKSHEET/ACTIVITY 11

Part 1

Student's name: ______________________

Peer evaluation of instruction. Use the procedure in your text to rate your partner on the scale below. Check the appropriate performance level. In the space provided, write hints to help improve the instruction technique or indicate what made the instruction especially good. All ratings must have a comment.

TASK Bass Toothbrushing Instruction	LOW 1	2	3	4	HIGH 5
1. Wash hands. ______________________					
2. Assemble equipment and PPE. ______________________					
3. Explain importance of toothbrushing. ______________________					
4. Demonstrate, using model. ______________________					
5. Answer patient questions correctly. ______________________					
6. Remove and clean equipment. ______________________					
7. Remove and dispose of protective wear. ______________________					
8. Wash hands. ______________________					
9. Chart, using abbreviations. ______________________					
10. Ask patient to demonstrate brushing teeth following your instructions. ______________________					

Part 2

Student's name: ______________________________

Peer evaluation of instruction. Rate your partner on the scale below by checking the appropriate level. In the space provided, write hints to help improve the instruction technique or indicate what made the instruction especially good. All ratings must have a comment.

TASK Disclosing Tablet/Solution Procedure	LOW 1	2	3	4	HIGH 5
1. Wash hands. ______________________					
2. Assemble equipment and PPE. ______________________					
3. Explain importance of disclosing tablets. ______________________					
4. After patient/client brushes teeth, ask him or her to use a disclosing tablet or solution. ______________________					
5. Instruct patient/client to rinse mouth. ______________________					
6. Using a mirror, show patient/client the red areas left on the teeth. ______________________					
7. Explain plaque residue, and reinforce toothbrushing technique. ______________________					

Student's name: ______________________________

Peer evaluation of instruction. Rate your partner on the scale below by checking the appropriate level. In the space provided, write hints to help improve the instruction technique or indicate what made the instruction especially good. All ratings must have a comment.

TASK Flossing Instruction	LOW 1	2	3	4	HIGH 5
1. Wash hands. ______________________________					
2. Assemble equipment and PPE. ______________________________					
3. Explain importance of flossing. ______________________________					
4. Demonstrate, using model. ______________________________					
5. Explain that bleeding may occur. ______________________________					
6. Ask if patient/client has questions. ______________________________					
7. Remove and dispose of protective wear. ______________________________					
8. Wash hands. ______________________________					
9. Chart, using abbreviations. ______________________________					